MACROELEMENTS, WATER, *and* ELECTROLYTES
in Sports Nutrition

NUTRITION in EXERCISE and SPORT

Edited by Ira Wolinsky and James F. Hickson, Jr.

Published Titles

Nutrients as Ergogenic Aids for Sports and Exercise,
Luke Bucci

Nutrition in Exercise and Sport, Second Edition,
Ira Wolinsky and James F. Hickson, Jr.

Exercise and Disease,
Ronald R. Watson and Marianne Eisinger

Nutrition Applied to Injury Rehabilitation and Sports Medicine,
Luke Bucci

Nutrition for the Recreational Athlete,
Catherine G.R. Jackson

NUTRITION in EXERCISE and SPORT

Edited by Ira Wolinsky

Published Titles

Nutrition, Physical Activity, and Health in Early Life:
Studies in Preschool Children,
Jana Parizkova

Exercise and Immune Function,
Laurie Hoffman-Goetz

Sports Nutrition: Minerals and Electrolytes,
Constance V. Kies and Judy A. Driskell

Nutrition and the Female Athlete,
Jaime S. Ruud

Body Fluid Balance: Exercise and Sport,
E.R. Buskirk and S. Puhl

Sports Nutrition: Vitamins and Trace Elements,
Ira Wolinsky and Judy A. Driskell

Amino Acids and Proteins for the Athlete—The Anabolic Edge,
Mauro G. DiPasquale

Nutrition in Exercise and Sport, Third Edition,
Ira Wolinsky

Gender Differences in Metabolism: Practical and Nutritional Implications,
Mark Tarnopolsky

NUTRITION in EXERCISE and SPORT

Edited by Ira Wolinsky

Forthcoming Titles

High Performance Nutrition: Diets and Supplements for the Competitive Athlete,
Mauro DiPasquale

Sports Nutrition,
Judy A. Driskell

Energy-Yielding Macronutrients and Energy Metabolism in Sports Nutrition,
Judy A. Driskell and Ira Wolinsky

Nutrients as Ergogenic Aids for Sports and Exercise, Second Edition,
Luke Bucci

MACROELEMENTS, WATER, *and* ELECTROLYTES
in Sports Nutrition

edited by

JUDY A. DRISKELL
IRA WOLINSKY

CRC Press
Boca Raton London New York Washington, D.C.

Library of Congress Cataloging-in-Publication Data

Catalog information may be obtained from the Library of Congress

DEDICATION

This book is dedicated to all the athletes and others who, by their questions, have encouraged researchers to expand knowledge of the relationships between nutrition and exercise. Those who have approached the co-editors, including our students, have helped us to realize the need for a book that relates macroelement, water, and electrolyte nutrition to athletic performance. We thank them for their encouragement. We also thank the authors for contributing the excellent chapters found in this book.

SERIES PREFACE

The CRC series, Nutrition in Exercise and Sport, provides a setting for in-depth exploration of the many and varied aspects of nutrition and exercise, including sports. The topic of exercise and sports nutrition has been a focus of research among scientists since the 1960s, and the healthful benefits of good nutrition and exercise have been appreciated. As our knowledge expands, it will be necessary to remember that there must be a range of diets and exercise regimes that will support excellent physical condition and performance. There is not a single diet–exercise treatment that can be the common denominator, or the single formula for health, or panacea for performance.

This series is dedicated to providing a stage upon which to explore these issues. Each volume provides a detailed and scholarly examination of some aspect of the topic.

Contributors from any bona fide area of nutrition and physical activity, including sports and the controversial, are welcome.

Ira Wolinsky, Ph.D.
Series Editor

PREFACE

This book addresses the relationships between macroelements, water, and electrolyte needs and interactions in sports and exercise. Actually, electrolytes are macroelements but most frequently are considered in terms of fluid replacement. A body of research indicates that work capacity, oxygen consumption, muscular strength, and other measures of physical performance of individuals including athletes are affected by deficiency or borderline deficiency of specific essential macroelements. Athletes as well as the public in general often have low dietary intakes of many of the essential macroelements. Athletes and nonathletes frequently consume too little water or fluids, thus affecting exercise performance as well as overall health. Physiological effects are observed when the water content of the body falls by 1 to 2%. The findings of some researchers indicate that large doses of certain essential macroelements given to individuals who had adequate status of those macroelements improved various measures of physical performance. Other researchers have reported conflicting findings. A critical review of these reports is included in this book.

This volume includes a collection of chapters written by scientists from various academic disciplines, each an expert in an area of macroelement and water nutrition as it relates to sports and exercise. The book reviews the convincing evidence that exercise and sport activities do affect the macroelement, including electrolyte, and water status of individuals and vice versa. Following an introduction are reviews of exercise and sport as they relate to calcium, phosphorus, magnesium, water, sodium, potassium, chloride, fluid and electrolyte replacement, and magnesium, phosphate, and calcium supplementation. The usage of sports beverages is discussed, followed by a summary chapter. Researchers, practitioners, students, the educated layperson, and athletes, both professional and recreational, will benefit from reading the book.

Judy A. Driskell, Ph.D., R.D.
Ira Wolinsky, Ph.D.

THE EDITORS

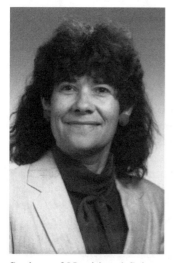

Judy Anne Driskell, Ph.D., R.D., is Professor of Nutritional Science and Dietetics at the University of Nebraska. She received her B.S. degree in biology from the University of Southern Mississippi in Hattiesburg and her M.S. and Ph.D. degrees from Purdue University. She has served in research and teaching positions at Auburn University, Florida State University, Virginia Polytechnic Institute and State University, and the University of Nebraska. She has also served as the Nutrition Scientist for the U.S. Department of Agriculture/Cooperative State Research Service and as a Professor of Nutrition and Food Science at Gadjah Mada and Bogor Universities in Indonesia.

Dr. Driskell is a member of numerous professional organizations including the American Society of Nutritional Sciences, the Institute of Food Technologists, the American College of Sports Medicine, and the American Dietetic Association. In 1993 she received the Professional Scientist Award of the Food Science and Human Nutrition Section of the Southern Association of Agricultural Scientists. In addition, she was the 1987 recipient of the Borden Award for Research in Applied Fundamental Knowledge of Human Nutrition. She is listed as an expert in B-complex vitamins by the Vitamin Nutrition Information Service.

Dr. Driskell recently co-edited *Sports Nutrition: Minerals and Electrolytes* with Constance V. Kies (deceased) and *Sports Nutrition: Vitamins and Trace Elements* with Ira Wolinsky. She has published about 100 refereed research articles and 10 book chapters as well as several publications intended for lay audiences and has given numerous professional and lay presentations. Her current research interests center around vitamin metabolism and requirements, including the interrelationships between exercise and water-soluble vitamin requirements.

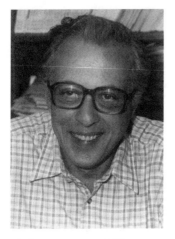

Ira Wolinsky, Ph.D., is Professor of Nutrition at the University of Houston. He received his B.S. degree in chemistry from the City College of New York and his M.S. and Ph.D. degrees in biochemistry from the University of Kansas. He has served in research and teaching positions at the Hebrew University (Medical School and Faculty of Agriculture), the University of Missouri, and Pennsylvania State University and has conducted basic research in NASA life sciences facilities.

Dr. Wolinsky is a member of the American Society of Nutritional Sciences, among other honorary and scientific organizations. He has contributed numerous nutrition research papers in the open literature. His current major research interests relate to the nutrition of bone and calcium and to sports nutrition. He has been the recipient of research grants from both public and private sources and several international research fellowships, including a Fulbright Senior Scholar Fellowship.

Dr. Wolinsky has co-authored a book on the history of the science of nutrition, *Nutrition and Nutritional Diseases.* He edited the third edition of *Nutrition in Exercise and Sport* and co-edited *Sports Nutrition: Vitamins and Trace Elements* with Judy A. Driskell and *Nutritional Concerns of Women* with Dorothy Klimis-Tavantzis. He is also the editor of the CRC Series on Nutrition in Exercise and Sport, the CRC Series on Modern Nutrition, and the CRC Series on Exercise Physiology.

CONTRIBUTORS

John J.B. Anderson, Ph.D.
Department of Nutrition
School of Public Health and Medicine
University of North Carolina
Chapel Hill, North Carolina

Jacqueline R. Berning, Ph.D., R.D.
Department of Biology
University of Colorado,
　Colorado Springs
Colorado Springs, Colorado

L. Mallory Boylan, Ph.D., R.D., L.D.
Department of Education, Nutrition,
　Restaurant/Hotel Management
Texas Tech University
Lubbock, Texas

Lorraine R. Brilla, Ph.D.
Department of Physical Education,
　Health and Recreation
Western Washington University
Bellingham, Washington

Felix Bronner, Ph.D., Dr.(h.c.)
Department of Biostructure and Function
School of Dental Medicine
University of Connecticut Health
　Center
Farmington, Connecticut

Julie H. Burns, M.S., R.D.
SportFuel, Inc.
Western Springs, Illinois and
Department of Nutrition
Rush University at Rush-Presbyterian-
　St. Luke's Medical Center
Chicago, Illinois

Elsworth R. Buskirk, Ph.D.
Noll Physiological Research Center
Pennsylvania State University
University Park, Pennsylvania

Judy A. Driskell, Ph.D., R.D.
Department of Nutritional Science
　and Dietetics
University of Nebraska
Lincoln, Nebraska

William B. Farquhar, M.S.
Noll Physiological Research Center
Pennsylvania State University
University Park, Pennsylvania

John R. Halliwill, Ph.D.
Department of Anesthesia Research
Mayo Clinic and Foundation
Rochester, Minnesota

Dorothea J. Klimis, Ph.D.
Department of Food Science and
　Human Nutrition
University of Maine
Orono, Maine

Richard B. Kreider, Ph.D.
Exercise & Sport Nutrition Laboratory
Department of Human Movement
　Sciences and Education
University of Memphis
Memphis, Tennessee

V. Patteson Lombardi, Ph.D.
Department of Biology
University of Oregon
Eugene, Oregon

Henry C. Lukaski, Ph.D.
U.S. Department of Agriculture
Agricultural Research Service
Grand Forks Human Nutrition
   Research Center
Grand Forks, North Dakota

Christopher T. Minson, Ph.D.
Department of Anesthesia Research
Mayo Clinic and Foundation
Rochester, Minnesota

Leo C. Senay, Jr., Ph.D.
Department of Pharmacological and
   Physiological Sciences, Emeritus
St. Louis University School of Medicine
St. Louis, Missouri

**Carmen R. Roman-Shriver, Ph.D.,
R.D., L.D.**
Department of Education, Nutrition,
   Restaurant/Hotel Management
Texas Tech University
Lubbock, Texas

Paul N. Taylor, Ph.D.
Department of Nutrition
Simmons College
Boston, Massachusetts

Ira Wolinsky, Ph.D.
Department of Human Development
University of Houston
Houston, Texas

CONTENTS

Introduction

Macroelements

Water and Electrolytes

Supplements Containing Macroelements

INTRODUCTION

Chapter **1**

INTRODUCTION TO MACROELEMENTS, WATER, AND ELECTROLYTES IN SPORTS NUTRITION

John J.B. Anderson

CONTENTS

0-8493-8196-7/99/$0.00+$.50
© 1999 by CRC Press LLC

I. INTRODUCTION

Athletes need an array of nutrients to meet the needs of their finely tuned organ systems. Although recommended allowances for nutrients and energy have been developed for each gender at most age-specific periods of life, these allowances are based on moderate activity only, as opposed to the high levels of activity required for performance in competitive athletics.[1] Typically, recommendations for athletes are increased to meet their requirements for energy, and, hopefully, protein and the essential micronutrients (i.e., vitamins and minerals) will be ingested in the amounts needed to support body structures and functions. Unfortunately, this scenario does not hold when examining the dietary intakes of U.S. athletes in practically all sports. In general, athletes tend to consume several micronutrients from foods in amounts considerably lower than the recommended levels. For many athletes who take a supplement every day, micronutrient intakes should meet tissue requirements.

The science of nutrition clearly has not been incorporated into the teachings or training methods of athletic coaches and trainers in the U.S., nor has it progressed very far in the realm of sports medicine. The sport that probably utilizes nutritional guidelines for micronutrient consumption the most is wrestling, but common knowledge confirms that wrestlers typically deny themselves adequate intakes of energy and fluids. The education of sports personnel in the field of nutrition needs to be greatly improved if injuries and other physical problems of athletes are to be prevented.

This introductory section outlines a few important concepts.

A. CONCEPT OF LINKING NUTRIENT INTAKES TO ENERGY CONSUMPTION

Athletes, as opposed to nonathletes, need to consume energy (kilocalories) in amounts that meet their utilization of energy in their sports activities, both training sessions and competitive events. If energy intake matches energy expenditure, athletes should theoretically obtain enough of all the micronutrients on a daily basis. This linkage, however, seldom occurs because many of the foods selected to provide energy are energy-dense and not nutrient-dense, at least in the U.S., as shown for male and female triathletes.[2] Many of the highly processed foods available on the market today have low amounts of essential vitamins, macrominerals, and trace elements because of the processing of these foods. If fortification of these foods occurs, typically only a few of the nutrients lost in processing are added back. An example is wheat flour, extracted at 72% of the original; many nutrients are removed at this level (the highest used in breads and related cereal products), and only iron, thiamin, riboflavin, and niacin are put back as fortificants. A few breads do add calcium, and in the future most breads will include folic acid as a fortificant. Many breakfast cereals and fruit drinks fortify with numerous vitamins and minerals, but few other foods are fortified.

Because several micronutrients are inadequately consumed by a large majority of the population, including athletes, they are appropriately called problem nutrients (see Section IV). These are the nutrients that need to be increased in the diets of athletes in order to optimize their performance. In many cases, multinutrient supplements are recommended in an effort to remedy the insufficiencies, but caution must be exercised here to avoid potential adverse interactions and to avoid missing a nutrient or two in a specific formulation of a supplement (see Section III.C).

In summary, diets that provide sufficient energy to meet the Recommended Dietary Allowances should also supply adequate amounts of protein and the micronutrients, both minerals and vitamins. This correlation does not generally exist for several micronutrients in the intakes of adolescents and adults in the U.S. Data to support this statement are provided later in this chapter for selected macrominerals that are problem nutrients.

B. CURRENT RECOMMENDED DIETARY ALLOWANCES OR NEW DIETARY REFERENCE INTAKES FOR NUTRIENTS

The Recommended Dietary Allowances (RDAs),[1] last published in 1989, for micronutrients are currently undergoing revision, and the new recommended Dietary Reference Intakes for most micronutrients are expected to be fully published in 1999.[3] The limited new information on nutrients has been published in one document that deals only with bone-related micronutrients (i.e., calcium, phosphorus, vitamin D, magnesium, and fluoride).[3] Instead of using RDAs for all of these nutrients, as in previous publications, the Food and Nutrition Board has assigned Adequate Intakes (AIs) to the recommendations for calcium, vitamin D, and fluoride. (RDAs continue to be used for phosphorus and magnesium.) AIs were used for these nutrients because compelling data on the actual requirements were not available so that RDAs could be estimated to exceed the mean requirements by a factor of ±2 SD. The recommended values for consumption of these five nutrients are listed in Table 1. As new documents on other nutrients and energy are published, close attention should be paid to the distinction made between RDA and AI for each nutrient.

C. POTENTIAL ADVERSE INTERACTIONS FROM EXCESSIVE INTAKES OF SUPPLEMENTS

An issue of major importance in nutrition is the potential for one nutrient, when taken in large amounts (i.e., greater than 100% of the RDA or AI), to

TABLE 1   Recommended Values[a] for Consumption of Five Bone-Related Nutrients (Food and Nutrition Board, 1998)

Age (years)	Calcium (mg/day) AI	Phosphorus (mg/day) RDA	Magnesium (mg/day) RDA		Vitamin D (μg/day) AI	Fluoride (mg/day) AI	
1–3	500	460	80		5	0.7	
4–8	800	500	130		5	1.1	
			M	F		M	F
9–13	1300	1250	240	240	5	2.0	2.0
14–18	1300	1250	410	360	5	3.2	2.9
19–30	1000	700	400	310	5	3.8	3.1
31–50	1000	700	420	320	5	3.8	3.1
51–70	1200	700	420	320	10	3.8	3.1
>70	1200	700	420	320	15	3.8	3.1

[a] AI = Adequate Intake, RDA = Recommended Dietary Allowance.

adversely affect the absorption or utilization of another nutrient. This issue applies in particular to the minerals, because many individuals take calcium supplements in amounts that meet or exceed the AI. The concern is that calcium, in the form of divalent cations, may interfere with the absorption of several different divalent minerals, such as iron, zinc, or magnesium. Scant published data on these interactions exist, but data typically point to potentially reduced amounts of absorbed iron, zinc, and magnesium caused by the high calcium consumption. Much more experimental work is needed to better appreciate the significance of these potential interactions.

II. OVERVIEW OF FACTORS THAT AFFECT THE NEEDS OF ESSENTIAL NUTRIENTS

Nutrient requirements of humans have been difficult to establish because of the stringent requirements for doing so. For example, requirements can be determined in rodent models by controlling the environment of the animals, feeding them different levels of a specific nutrient, and housing them in a way that keeps them happy and permits adequate exercise. These conditions cannot be maintained for human subjects for longer than approximately 4 weeks in special metabolic units. Therefore, much of the human data on mineral requirements is based on the quantitation of biomarkers of function or other surrogate measures as opposed to balance data which measure input and output of a nutrient over time. Additionally, much of the human research on requirements has focused on young healthy adults, although much new information is being published on the nutrient needs of adults and the elderly.

A. MEASUREMENT ESTIMATES OF NUTRIENT BALANCES

The difficulties in conducting balance studies of nutrients are well known. For example, measuring macrominerals in fecal collections, not urinary collections, gives great individual variability in estimating requirements. Another complicating factor is the uncertainty of the endogenous fecal (EF) secretion of macromineral elements. EF secretion encompasses those minerals secreted by various gastrointestinal (GI) glands, including the liver or gallbladder and pancreas. In addition, the sloughing of epithelial cells at senescence can be traced in the EF route of excretion. These categories do not include any "leakage" of a mineral because of a break in the epithelial barrier of the gut mucosa. For example, distance runners are thought to be frequently iron-insufficient because of the loss of blood through the GI epithelium as a result of the pounding or stress on gut tissue caused by running on hard surfaces. If an iron balance study were performed on distance runners while in heavy training, more precise estimates of iron requirements might be made if a good estimate of GI losses could be measured. Losses of calcium and other macrominerals may also occur in distance runners, who undergo much road "pounding" on their internal organs, because of breaks in the gut barrier.

Mineral balance studies are difficult to perform because of errors associated with fecal excretion and sweat losses, and the validity of requirement estimates remains unclear for most minerals. Additionally, very few studies using rigid scientific protocols have been undertaken using athletes in prime condition.

B. MAINTAINING NUTRIENT BALANCES IN ATHLETES

Nutrient balances must, by definition, be achieved by taking in an amount of a nutrient that meets or exceeds an individual's requirement. The best way to estimate the requirement is to do repeat studies on the same individuals, varying only the dose or the amount of the nutrient ingested over a minimum of 2 weeks. Few such studies have been performed on athletes. Therefore, using the current RDAs or AIs as the starting guidelines for intakes, these recommendations should be increased by a factor (or percentage) that is proportional to the greater amount of energy consumed by an athlete during typical training periods. For example, if the energy RDA for a 21-year-old male distance runner is 2900 kcal/day, but dietary record analysis indicates that he actually consumes 4300 kcal/day, then the mineral and vitamin intakes should be increased by approximately 50% over the current RDA or AI. If the mineral in question were calcium, the young man should consume almost 1800 mg of calcium a day to meet his needs. In practice, he may not need quite as much as 1800 mg because calcium is considered a nutrient with a threshold,[4] beyond which additional intake has little or no benefit, but his requirements would almost certainly be increased compared to more sedentary males of his age because of increased losses through sweat and other excretions.

C. SUMMARY

The issue of achieving nutrient balances, while clearly important for the athlete, is difficult to measure because of the many factors that must be controlled to achieve a carefully monitored study. In the vast majority of cases, it would be satisfactory if usual intakes of a specific nutrient approximately equaled its RDA or AI values. In reality, few athletes consume enough of many of the nutrients to meet their recommended amounts (RDAs or AIs). Exceptions to this statement apply to protein, phosphorus or phosphates, and sodium, for which excessive intakes are the rule for most individuals. Ideal intakes of nutrients would almost always be proportionate to the energy intake. This scenario, however, is very difficult to achieve. The best goal is to try to get athletes to improve their intakes of nutrients to at least the recommended levels (RDAs or AIs) for their age, even slightly exceeding these limits. For protein and a few minerals (see below), it is difficult for most Americans not to consume excessive amounts of these nutrients.

III. FOOD ISSUES THAT MAY IMPACT ATHLETES

Many reports on the dietary intakes of athletes have revealed poor diet quality, especially with respect to the consumption of micronutrients, such as calcium and magnesium. Many athletes, especially females, have insufficient intakes of the minerals and vitamins mentioned above. Improvements in nutrition education are necessary to achieve the desired level of performance of athletes and to maintain generally good health status. Much more attention must be paid to achieving the recommended numbers of servings of the Food Guide Pyramid[5] and to taking nutrient supplements, if recommended by a health professional. In at least one study of female athletes, nutrient supplements were shown to improve the intakes of nutrients that were below 100% of the RDAs from foods alone.[6]

A. FOOD GUIDE PYRAMID RECOMMENDATIONS

The Food Guide Pyramid is a good nutrition tool for educating people to recognize the basic food groups and the numbers of servings that should be consumed daily from each group. Because many athletes, particularly female athletes, consume a form of a vegetarian diet, more guidance concerning the proper selection of vegetarian foods is necessary. For example, a female vegan who consumes no meat, poultry, fish, or dairy products must get all of her micronutrients from fruits, vegetables, grains, and legumes, unless she is taking a multinutrient supplement. These plant foods tend to be much lower in calcium and a few other micronutrients.

The Vegetarian Food Guide Pyramid[7] can help these athletes recognize other good sources of minerals and vitamins when the more traditional Food Guide Pyramid is not as useful. Figure 1 shows where many of the major minerals and

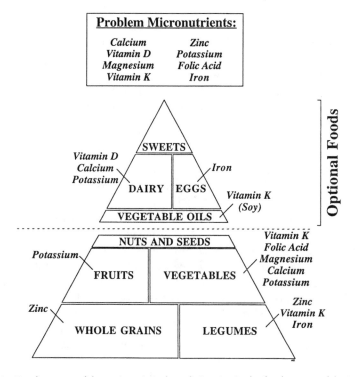

FIGURE 1 Food sources of the major minerals and vitamins in the food groups of the Vegetarian Food Guide Pyramid.[7] If milk, other dairy products, and eggs are consumed, then more choices are available for obtaining adequate amounts of the essential minerals and vitamins. Caution: A reliable source of vitamin B_{12} should be included if no dairy products or eggs are consumed.

most vitamins are found in the Vegetarian Food Guide Pyramid. Despite somewhat lower energy intakes than recommended, distance runners and endurance athletes may have better diets with respect to micronutrients than most other types of athletes,[8,9] in part because of their selection of foods that approaches vegetarian patterns of food selection, but not all studies support this conclusion.[10]

B. FAST FOODS AND SNACK FOODS

Fast foods tend to be high in energy, especially from fats, and protein, but low with respect to micronutrients. Again, wise food choices need to be made to obtain adequate amounts of all the minerals and vitamins, and it is unlikely that athletes make the effort to achieve balanced intakes.

Often, nonnutritious snack foods replace healthy snacks, such as an apple, orange, or carrots, that could have provided fairly good amounts of micronutrients. In general, snack foods provide sufficient amounts of calories from macronutrients but proportionately much less of the micronutrients. Not only are they often high in fat and sodium, but they tend to be poor in almost all other minerals. The exception is some snack foods that are fortified with iron, thiamin, riboflavin, and niacin and, in the future, folic acid. In a prospective study of female varsity athletes at the University of North Carolina,[11] snacks consisted of primarily energy-dense foods that were low in micronutrients. Problem micronutrients, such as magnesium and potassium (see Section IV), are low in practically all of the snack foods.

C. NUTRIENT SUPPLEMENTS

Multinutrient supplements that contain minerals and vitamins at approximately 100% of the current RDAs may be recommended to athletes to assure they get adequate intakes of these essential dietary components. (Calcium in these supplements exists in amounts that are much lower than the old RDAs or the new AIs for calcium, because the amount of calcium would make the pill too large to swallow.) These nutrient supplements apparently have no ergogenic effects.[12] In a prospective study of female varsity athletes at the University of North Carolina, low percentages of both athletes and control subjects reported that they took supplements.[11] Excessive amounts (i.e., greater than the RDAs) are not recommended for general use. Only a physician's prescription for higher intake of one or more minerals would, of course, override this recommendation. The concern about excessive intakes is the potential interaction between two nutrients that results in an insufficient intake of one of the micronutrients. This concern applies in particular to the minerals that exist as divalent ions in body fluids.

D. SUMMARY

Athletes do not, in general, have good intakes of specific minerals, especially calcium, magnesium, and potassium, because of unwise food selections that contribute to poor or less than adequate nutritional status of these minerals. Many athletes rely heavily on fast foods and snack foods without proper attention to obtaining balanced intakes of nutrients, especially minerals, in particular the plant foods. Female athletes may be at greater risk than male athletes, but neither gender is faring well with respect to dietary intakes. Better nutrition education with the use of food guides, including the Vegetarian Food Guide Pyramid, is needed by athletes across the U.S. Sports personnel need to help athletes meet nutritional needs by getting them to consume healthier diets. Attention to these efforts could improve performance levels of athletes and reduce the risk of injuries. A diet good for bone health should also be good for cardiovascular function and skeletal muscle action. Supplements may be recommended to assure a balanced intake of micronutrients when food consumption does not adequately provide these required nutrients.

IV. PROBLEM NUTRIENTS FOR ATHLETES, ESPECIALLY FEMALE ATHLETES

Problem nutrients for athletes exist because of poor consumption patterns. These patterns, however, are similar to those of the U.S. population as a whole. Energy is commonly inadequately consumed by runners and athletes in most other sports, except swimming, crew, cycling, and football. For example, calcium is a classic underconsumed micronutrient and has been identified as such for almost 50 years. The situation may be getting even worse for calcium. The reason for the underconsumption and insufficiency of calcium is simple: food behaviors are such that dairy products, the richest sources of calcium in the U.S. diet, are being consumed less by each succeeding generation. It is now estimated that a majority of adolescent girls and a large percentage (~25%) of adolescent boys are consuming less than 67% of the RDAs (the old RDA was 1200 mg/day and the new AI is 1300 for adolescents).[13] These low intakes are of great concern to nutritionists because peak bone development (i.e., the maximal accumulation of bone mass) cannot be optimized at such low levels. If the same low intakes for other micronutrients exist, and some evidence suggests this is so for magnesium and potassium, then our youth are not consuming sufficient amounts of several essential nutrients. These moderate insufficiencies, rather than severe (frank) deficiencies, probably also affect competitive athletes, both adolescents and young adults. The greater concern lies with female athletes, who typically are much more conscious of their body weight and fat composition and therefore frequently skip meals and/ or consume too little food energy. Disordered eating behaviors of females clearly can affect athletic performance as well as menstrual cycles and bone health.[14]

This section provides brief reviews of several macrominerals that have been found to be either insufficiently or excessively consumed by athletes. Other nutrients, not considered here, may also be problem macrominerals, but more research is needed to establish the basis of insufficient intakes.

A. CALCIUM: INSUFFICIENT INTAKES

Calcium intakes are typically low in adolescents after age 11 and in adults living in the U.S.[13] Only dairy products provide rich sources of calcium, but a few others foods, especially fortified foods, contain significant amounts of calcium. Increasingly, adolescents, in particular those becoming partial vegetarians, are not consuming dairy foods in sufficient amounts to reach their age-specific RDAs. Young athletes, especially females, need calcium to optimize their skeletal development. At the low intakes of calcium currently being consumed, optimal bone health could be sacrificed. In a prospective study of female intercollegiate athletes at the University of North Carolina, mean calcium intakes approximated 70% of the RDA over 2 years, a value similar to that of nonathletes.[11] Those who have low calcium intakes typically have diets that are inadequate in several other micronutrients.[15] For many low consumers of calcium, multinutrient supplements will be needed to reach the 1200-mg/day recommendation, as well as to provide other essential micronutrients. This supplemental approach appears to be reasonable for female athletes.[14]

B. MAGNESIUM: INSUFFICIENT INTAKES

Magnesium is widely distributed in the food supply, but it is consumed at levels well below the RDAs by both males and females. Vegetarians obtain more magnesium than nonvegetarians, because dark green, leafy vegetables provide rich sources of this mineral. Magnesium is found in plant foods because this macromineral is required in the photosynthetic process.

C. POTASSIUM: INSUFFICIENT INTAKES

Because potassium is found in very good amounts in plant foods, particularly fruits and vegetables, this electrolyte tends to be low in the diets of those who are predominantly meat-eaters. Vegetarians have no trouble getting adequate amounts of potassium, because this electrolyte exists primarily in the intracellular space of foods. High salt consumption may, however, increase the requirement for potassium because of renal conservation of sodium at the expense of potassium (and also calcium). Athletes need adequate intakes of potassium to replace the amounts of this electrolyte lost in sweat, urine, and fecal secretions.

D. SODIUM: EXCESSIVE INTAKES

Sodium intakes of athletes may be excessive, but because of excessive sweating in sports activities and other regulatory mechanisms operating in well-tuned bodies, sodium is typically not a problem nutrient for athletes. Heavy users (those who use the salt shaker excessively) may have a problem that could eventually lead to hypertension. Excessive sodium use should be avoided because of potential health consequences later in life.

E. PHOSPHATES: EXCESSIVE INTAKES

Phosphates are increasingly being used in highly processed foods in the marketplace today. Concern about excessive consumption of phosphates (listed as phosphorus on food labels) relates to the calcium-to-phosphorus (Ca:P) ratio in the diet. When the ratio goes much below 0.5 to 1, parathyroid hormone is increasingly secreted by the parathyroid glands, and the elevation of this hormone typically contributes to increased losses of bone mineral. This complex interaction between the nutrients and bone has not been studied in athletes, but it has been studied in young adult women who have adverse hormonal responses to a low Ca:P ratio in the diet.[16]

TABLE 2   Major Food Sources That Provide the Problem
Nutrients Commonly Deficient in the Diets of
Athletes

	Food Sources	
Nutrient	Animal	Plant
Calcium	Milk, cheese, yogurt	Fortified orange juice
Magnesium	Meats	Dark green, leafy vegetables
Potassium	Meats	Fruits, vegetables

F. OTHER MICRONUTRIENTS

A few other micronutrients, such as iron, zinc, folic acid, vitamin D, and
vitamin K, may also be insufficient in the diets of athletes (see Figure 1).

G. SUMMARY

Table 2 summarizes the major food sources that provide insufficient amounts
of the specific problem nutrients, as well as the excessive problem nutrients, and
emphasizes the importance of consuming a balanced diet that contains many different foods, especially plant foods, in amounts that meet human requirements.
Plant foods contain numerous nutrients that are not adequately ingested by individuals who either avoid or eat fruits and vegetables sparingly. Other plant sources,
such as nuts and seeds, also tend to be high in some micronutrients that benefit
body health and athletic performance.

V. CONCLUDING REMARKS

Athletes in the U.S. fall short in intake of several mineral and vitamin nutrients because of poor dietary choices. Nutrition education of athletes is deficient.
Athletes need to learn more about the benefits of diverse foods and the importance
of obtaining balanced intakes on a daily basis. Use of the Food Guide Pyramid or
Vegetarian Food Guide Pyramid to help athletes make the most of their meal
selections could help optimize athletic performance. In addition to foods, athletes
may need to take a daily nutrient supplement that contains approximately 100%
of the recommended intakes of the essential micronutrients. One of the important
benefits of consuming foods as opposed to supplements is that plant foods also
contain many nonnutrient molecules, such as dietary fibers and diverse
phytomolecules. Together with the essential nutrients they contain, these
nonnutrients in plants may contribute to health and most likely contribute to performance, but additional research on the potential benefits of nonnutrients to athletes is needed.

ACKNOWLEDGMENTS

Appreciation is expressed to several individuals who helped in the development and fine-tuning of this manuscript, namely, Lauren Grimes, Lee Thrash, Carolyn Barrett, and Bryan Smith, M.D. Sanford Garner, Ph.D., prepared the figures.

REFERENCES

1. Food and Nutrition Board, National Research Council, *Recommended Dietary Allowances*, 10th ed., National Academy Press, Washington, D.C., 1989.
2. Green, D.R., Gibbons, C., O'Toole, M., and Hiller, W.B.O., An evaluation of dietary intakes of triathletes: are RDAs being met? *J. Am. Diet. Assoc.*, 89, 1653, 1989.
3. Food and Nutrition Board, Institute of Medicine, *Dietary Reference Intakes*, National Academy Press, Washington, D.C., in press.
4. Matkovic, V. and Heaney, R.P., Calcium balance during human growth: evidence for threshold behavior, *Am. J. Clin. Nutr.*, 55, 992, 1992.
5. Cronin, F., Shaw, A., Krebs-Smith, S., Marsland, P., and Light, L., Developing a food guidance system to implement the dietary guidelines, *J. Nutr. Educ.*, 19, 281, 1987.
6. Nowak, R.K., Knudsen, K.S., and Schulz, L.O., Body composition and nutrient intakes of college men and women basketball players, *J. Am. Diet. Assoc.*, 88, 575, 1988.
7. Whitten, C., Haddad, E., and Sabate, J., Developing a vegetarian food guide pyramid: a conceptual framework, *Vegetarian Nutr.*, 1, 25, 1997.
8. van Erp-Baart, A.M.J., Saris, W.M.H., Binkhorst, A., Vos, J.A., and Elvers, J.W.H., Nationwide survey on nutritional habits in elite athletes. II. Mineral and vitamin intake, *Int. J. Sports Med.*, 10 (Suppl.), S11, 1989.
9. Nieman, D.C., Butler, J.V., Pollett, L.M., Dietrich, S.J., and Lutz, R.D., Nutrient intake of marathon runners, *J. Am. Diet. Assoc.*, 89, 1273, 1989.
10. Keith, R.E., O'Keeffe, K.A., Alt, L.A., and Young, K.L., Dietary status of trained female cyclists, *J. Am. Diet. Assoc.*, 89, 1620, 1989.
11. Anderson, J.J.B., Stender, M.W., Smith, B.W., Grimes, L., and Wang, E.X., Nutrient intakes and bone measurements of female intercollegiate athletes: a prospective study, *FASEB J.*, 11(3), A572, 1997 (Abstr. #3310).
12. Beltz, S.D. and Doering, P.L., Efficacy of nutritional supplements used by athletes, *Clin. Pharmacol.*, 12, 900, 1993.
13. U.S. Department of Agriculture, *Continuing Survey of Food Intake by Individuals (CSFII): Diet and Health Knowledge Survey 1991*, National Technical Information Service, Springfield, VA, 1994.
14. Anderson, J.J.B., Stender, M., Rondano, P., Bishop, L., and Duckett, A.B., Nutrition and bone in physical activity and sport, in *Nutrition in Exercise and Sport*, 3rd ed., Wolinsky, I., Ed., CRC Press, Boca Raton, FL, 1998, 219.
15. Barger-Lux, M.J., Heaney, R.P., Packard, P.T., Lappe, J.M., and Recker, R.R., Nutritional correlates of low calcium intake, *Clin. Appl. Nutr.*, 2, 39, 1992.
16. Calvo, M.S. and Park, Y.K., Changing phosphorus content of the U.S. diet: potential for adverse effects on bone, *J. Nutr.*, 126, 1168, 1996.

MACROELEMENTS

Chapter 2

CALCIUM IN EXERCISE AND SPORT

Felix Bronner

CONTENTS

I. INTRODUCTION

Calcium is the fifth most abundant element on the globe. It is found in a variety of rocks and throughout most waters. The concentration of calcium in sea water varies from 1 to 10 mM and averages almost 1 mol/kg in the earth's crust. More than 80% of the calcium found in the crust is in the form of limestone ($CaCO_3$) deposits.

As cells evolved, they learned to get rid of excess calcium, adapting calcium extrusion to a variety of cellular processes: protein secretion, intracellular signaling, and the many calcium-dependent processes that have come to light in recent years. Thus the conquest of the ocean by living systems, uni- and multicellular, was paralleled by their ability to deal with the calcium in their surroundings. When organisms began to leave the ocean to conquer the land, they required mechanisms of support and developed external and ultimately internal skeletons. These calcium deposits also served as storage depots (i.e., for the accumulation and release of calcium).

II. CALCIUM NUTRITION AND METABOLISM

The adult human body contains about 1 kg of calcium, over 99% of which is found in the skeleton in solid form. Calcium in the tissues is either bound to a variety of organic or inorganic molecules or is free (i.e., as ion in solution).

Calcium in blood is found almost entirely in the plasma, where about half is bound to proteins such as albumin, with most of the remainder in ionic form and a small fraction (<7%) as citrate, phosphate, or other complexes.[1] Calcium traffic in the body therefore changes in state from solid to fluid and back. Moreover, because calcium concentrations vary from nanomolar in the cell cytoplasm to millimolar in the fluids and in cell organelles and components, calcium traffic also involves multiple steps in changes of gradients of concentration. These changes occur in the face of the body making a major effort to maintain the plasma calcium concentration constant, at 2.5 mM. This is termed extracellular calcium homeostasis. The calcium concentration of the cell sap (i.e., the free intracellular calcium concentration) is maintained at ~100 nM. Extracellular calcium homeostasis is accomplished with the help of the skeleton, the major storage place of body calcium. Intracellular calcium homeostasis depends on cellular structures binding and holding calcium. For example, a typical muscle cell may contain 3 mmol calcium per kilogram wet weight, yet the free intracellular calcium content approximates 100 nmol/l, a gradient of 30,000. The gradient between body fluid calcium and free intracellular calcium is about 10,000.

Figure 1 summarizes in schematic form the pathways followed by calcium as it is ingested, absorbed, transported to and from the skeleton, and excreted from the body.

Calcium-rich foods include milk, cheese and cheese-containing foods, ice cream, broccoli, kale, and cream of wheat. In the U.S. diet, dairy products contribute about 55% of total dietary calcium[2] and may reach 70% for those who eat diets that contain foods enriched with milk powder, as is true of certain baked goods. Women in the U.S. on the average consume only two-thirds of the Recommended Dietary Allowance (RDA) of 800 mg of calcium per day. If the RDA is raised to 1200 mg/day, as is likely, mean calcium consumption by U.S. females will be closer to 50% of the RDA. Men and boys tend to consume amounts of calcium that come closer to their RDA. Low intake of dairy foods by women often is due to their avoidance of fat, even though dairy foods with reduced fat content are now widely available.

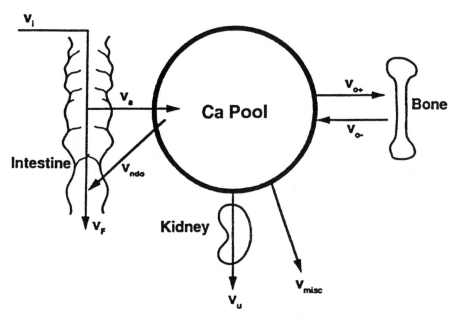

FIGURE 1 Schematic diagram of the flow of calcium through the body. The Ca pool includes calcium in solution in blood plasma, in the extracellular fluid, and in, or associated with, bone, described in units of mass (e.g., mmol). v_i = Ca ingested in food; v_a = Ca absorbed from food; v_{ndo} = endogenous Ca lost in stool; v_u = Ca excreted in urine; v_F = Ca excreted in stool; v_{misc} = Ca lost from the body via sweat, semen, menstrual fluid, and milk; v_{o+} = Ca deposited in bone; and v_{o-} = Ca resorbed from bone, described in units of mass per unit time (e.g., mmol/day). v_T = rate at which Ca enters or leaves the pool (i.e., = $v_a + v_{o-}$ = $v_u + v_{ndo} + v_{o+} + v_{misc}$). In a nonlactating organism, v_{misc} is generally negligibly small. (From Bronner, F., in *Handbook of Nutritionally Essential Mineral Elements,* O'Dell, G.B. and Sunde, R. A., Eds., Marcel Dekker, New York, 1997, 13. With permission.)

Another reason relates to lactose intolerance, yet appropriately treated dairy foods that will not produce the symptoms of lactose intolerance are also available.

A. CALCIUM ABSORPTION[3]

Calcium that enters the small intestine is absorbed via two independent routes, transcellular and paracellular. The transcellular route is localized to the proximal duodenum and is absent in the distal jejunum and ileum. Calcium moves via the paracellular route throughout the length of the small intestine, with essentially all calcium that is absorbed in the jejunum and ileum traveling paracellularly. The transcellular pathway is the regulated route, inasmuch as it is upregulated when calcium intake is low and downregulated when calcium intake is high. Upregulation occurs via a cytosolic protein, calbindin D_{9K} ($\approx$9 kDa), which functions as a calcium carrier. Biosynthesis of calbindin D_{9K} is totally vitamin D dependent. Consequently, the transcellular absorption mechanism is essentially nonfunctional in total vitamin D deficiency, with transcellular absorption directly proportional to the cellular content of calbindin D_{9K}.

The transcellular route involves three sequential steps: (1) calcium entry, (2) intracellular diffusion, and (3) calcium extrusion. Calcium entry is down a chemical gradient, inasmuch as the free intracellular calcium concentration is at least four orders of magnitude below the lowest luminal calcium concentration. Calcium entry is via calcium channels. Once inside the cell, the calcium ion must diffuse through the cytoplasm to the serosal pole of the intestinal cell. There it is extruded by a calcium pump, the Ca–ATPase. Calcium extrusion is against an electrochemical gradient and therefore requires metabolic energy. Energy, derived from phosphorylation, brings about a conformational change and permits calcium to be extruded through the transmembrane elements of the Ca–ATPase, which act like a calcium channel.

Intracellular diffusion of the calcium ion is the limiting rate, and in the absence of calbindin D_{9K}, self-diffusion of the calcium ion is too slow to permit transcellular absorption to proceed at the experimentally observed rate. Calbindin D_{9K} acts in a bucket-brigade fashion. As the calbindin D_{9K} concentration increases, more calcium gets bound to it, the intracellular concentration of total and free calcium is raised, and the calcium gradient between the luminal and serosal poles of the intestinal cell is raised so that the extrusion pump can act at maximum efficiency.

The bulk of calcium absorption in the small intestine is via the paracellular route; the amount absorbed is a function of the chemical gradient between intestinal lumen and the calcium concentration in the body fluids, approximately 1.1 mmol/l. The amount absorbed is also a function of the time spent by the chyme in a given intestinal location.[4] When calcium intake is moderately high, the paracellular route accounts for at least two-thirds of the total calcium absorbed. The amount of calcium absorbed in the large intestine is not well established, but probably does not amount to more than 10% of total calcium absorption.

In people eating the usual U.S. diets that contain between 600 and 1000 mg calcium per day, calcium absorption is some 20 to 25% of the amount digested. It is higher in children, especially when actively growing. It is depressed in the elderly, especially during winter, when exposure to ultraviolet light is minimal. Calcium absorption by athletes tends to be similar to that of nonathletes. However, amenorrheic women athletes have significantly lower calcium absorption than women athletes with normal menses.

B. CALCIUM IN BLOOD AND BONE[5,6]

The plasma calcium is very closely regulated, typically at 2.5 mmol/l (10 mg calcium per 100 ml). Deviations of even ±20% are cause for major concern and, if they persist, are indications of disease (e.g., hypo- or hyperparathyroidism).

The plasma calcium is in extremely rapid, dynamic equilibrium with calcium in the extracellular fluid. Plasma constitutes about 17% of the extracellular fluid volume. If a calcium load is injected intravenously, half of the load would be disposed of in 27 circulations, almost all of it taken up by the bone mineral. The circulation time in adults is approximately 40 sec, so that an intravenous calcium load would be reduced to half in about 18 min.

Under normal conditions (i.e., with no calcium load), the amount of calcium taken up by bone mineral from the blood is identical to the amount released, thereby maintaining the plasma calcium constant. The fact that calcium uptake and release occur can be deduced from isotope experiments which showed that half of the isotope inflow is taken up by bone, yet total plasma calcium does not change.

Three hormones are directly involved in the regulation of plasma calcium: parathyroid hormone (PTH), calcitonin (CT), and 1,25-dihydroxyvitamin D_3 (1,25-$(OH)_2D_3$), the most bioactive metabolite of vitamin D. PTH action on bone leads to increased release of calcium from bone mineral. CT action on bone causes diminished calcium release from bone mineral. 1,25-$(OH)_2D_3$ causes increased calcium release from bone. Receptors for PTH are found exclusively on osteoblasts, the cells responsible for bone formation. Receptors for CT are found exclusively on osteoclasts, the cells responsible for bone mineral lysis. Receptors for 1,25-$(OH)_2D_3$ are found not only on osteoblasts but also on parathyroid cells, so that 1,25-$(OH)_2D_3$ acts directly on bone cells and indirectly via action on the parathyroid gland.

To explain the action of the hormones and the rapid response (within an hour) to PTH and CT (the action of 1,25-$(OH)_2D_3$ is slower), it has been proposed[7] that shape changes by bone cells free up more mineral surface for rapid calcium release or uptake by bone mineral sites. These sites are postulated to differ in their calcium affinity. Thus osteoblasts are thought to be associated with low-affinity calcium-binding sites, whereas osteoclasts are thought to be associated with high-affinity calcium-binding sites. PTH causes osteoblasts to round up, thereby permitting osteoclasts to spread out. As a result, more low-affinity binding sites are exposed. This causes the apparent half-concentration (K_m, which describes the equilibrium of bone calcium-binding sites) to go up and plasma calcium goes up. When, as a result of the action of CT, osteoclasts contract, osteoblasts can then expand. Thus less low-affinity and more high-affinity binding sites become available. The K_m of the bone calcium-binding sites goes down and plasma calcium drops.

Contraction by either osteoblasts or osteoclasts causes reduction or cessation of metabolic activity; expansion leads to greater metabolic activity. Shape changes are only the first step in a metabolic cascade. Osteoblasts, when stimulated and expanded, synthesize more collagen, which, when extruded, assembles into fibrils that undergo calcification. Osteoclasts, when stimulated, expand and their podosomes seal off a region into which the cells extrude lysosomes and protons. This in turn solubilizes the bone mineral, with the bone matrix then undergoing destruction.

Although PTH and CT have opposing actions, plasma calcium regulation does not involve a push–pull situation. Rather, PTH is the major hormone regulating plasma calcium homeostasis acutely. CT is released in response to calcium overloads, but does not appear to play a significant role acutely.

Calcium, along with phosphate, constitutes the principal structural mineral of the skeleton that gives vertebrates their internal support and allows people to be erect. The skeleton makes up about 16% of an adult's body weight; 47% of the skeletal weight is dry, fat-free bone, 25% of which is calcium. The principal forms or phases in which calcium occurs in bone are, in decreasing order of solubility, brushite, octacalcium phosphate, amorphous calcium phosphate, whitlockite, and hydroxyapatite. The latter is an apatitic type of calcium phosphate that also contains calcium carbonate on the surface.

Calcium exists in bone in two forms: in solution, as part of the fluid that surrounds and exists in bone, and in a solid state, as the phases of calcium phosphate described above. The bone calcium pool contains five to six times more calcium than is found in the extracellular fluid, but constitutes only a small fraction of the total body calcium.

The bone calcium pool serves two functions: as the source of calcium that becomes deposited as bone salt and as the source of exchangeable calcium (i.e., the calcium that leaves and reenters blood), with the concentration of blood plasma calcium determined by the average calcium-binding capacity of the bone salt.

The fraction of calcium that enters the bone calcium pool undergoes a phase transformation to become bone salt. This fraction diminishes with age more than the total flow of calcium into the bone calcium pool does.

Bone calcium resorption (i.e., the phase transformation of solid to solution and the return of that calcium into the circulation) also decreases with age, but somewhat less rapidly than the bone calcium deposition rate. As a result, the individual goes into negative bone calcium balance (i.e., the bone mass decreases).

Modeling and remodeling of bone also involve structural changes (i.e., osteoclast-mediated dissolution of calcium and partial or total degradation of the extracellular matrix from which the bone salt has been removed). These structural changes proceed necessarily more slowly than the initial steps which involve calcium binding and release by the bone salt.

Thus bone formation and bone resorption each refer to a cascade of events, with calcium constituting the principal cation of bone salt, the major product of the osteoblasts.

C. CALCIUM EXCRETION
1. Urine[8]
Of the calcium circulating in the blood, less than 0.1% is typically excreted in the urine. Thus, in a 70-kg adult man, the plasma volume is about 2.5 l and contains about 6 mmol calcium. Of the 20 to 25% of cardiac output presented to the kidney, half of that amount is filtered at the glomerulus. Thus the nephron handles approximately 1.5 mmol of calcium per minute or some 2100 mmol of calcium per day. The urinary calcium output of the typical 70-kg man might be 7 mmol/day or 0.3% of the filtered load. Actual calcium excretion in the urine is a complicated function of an individual's prior calcium intake, vitamin D and

nutritional status, sex, and reproductive status (if female), as well as age and therefore skeletal maturity.

Most of the calcium in the kidney is reabsorbed by a passive, paracellular mechanism. Active calcium reabsorption occurs principally in the distal convoluted tubule and is mediated by calbindin D_{28K}. This calbindin is a different gene product than the intestinal calbindin. The renal calbindin, whose biosynthesis is also totally vitamin D dependent, is a larger molecule (28 kDa) and has four calcium-binding sites.

A major regulator of calcium reabsorption in the kidney is parathyroid hormone with action in the distal tubule.

2. Stool[6]

Calcium in the stool originates from two sources: food calcium that has escaped intestinal absorption and endogenous calcium that also has escaped absorption. The term endogenous calcium refers to calcium that has entered the intestinal tract as a constituent of cellular debris or various body fluids such as bile, pancreatic juices, *succus entericus,* etc. In people, the quantity of endogenous calcium lost daily with the feces is approximately equal to the daily output of calcium in the urine and constitutes only a small fraction of the total fecal calcium if calcium intake is adequate.

Under conditions of hypogravity, the amount of calcium that is excreted increases. Urinary calcium increases because plasma calcium tends to rise and active calcium reabsorption in the distal tubule is diminished. Fecal calcium also increases, because active calcium absorption in the intestine has been downregulated. Endogenous fecal calcium may increase because of a rise in body fluid calcium, but that is modest at best. In general, it is best to characterize the endogenous fecal calcium as a nonregulated route.

III. RELATIONSHIP BETWEEN MUSCLE AND BONE

Muscles and weight-bearing bones exist in an intimate relationship to one another. As muscles increase in mass due to stress exercise, so does bone mass. Tennis arms of professional tennis players are always larger in circumference than the opposite arm, because of heavier musculature and stouter bones. Conversely, individuals subjected to long periods of microgravity lose muscle mass and bone. Indeed, readaptation to the gravity conditions prevailing on earth is a major challenge to astronauts returning to earth after prolonged space sojourns.

Research in recent years has shown that the relationship between muscle and bone prevails not only under extreme conditions, as in stress exercise or microgravity, but in all situations. For example, in a cross-sectional study of 18-year-old healthy females,[9] bone mineral density was shown to be positively and significantly associated with body weight and muscle strength. Indeed, body size, an expression of body weight, has the strongest correlation with bone mineral density.[10]

The effects of exercise tend to be specific to the muscles and bones specifically involved in the exercise. Thus, bone mineral density was higher in the legs of endurance runners than of matched controls, but this was not true for other bones, such as lumbar spine or the forearm.[11] Prolonged bed rest, on the other hand, has long been known to weaken muscles and bones. Bloomfield[12] reviewed the effects of prolonged bed rest on muscle structure and function and concluded that the muscle mass undergoes dramatic change with 4 to 6 weeks of bed rest, accompanied by significant decreases in bone mineral density of the lumbar spine, femoral neck, and calcaneus, bones that are subject to load stress in the erect individual.

One of the complicating factors in the muscle–bone relationship is the effect of gonadal hormones. Do women athletes who become amenorrheic have bones with lower density than eumenorrheic women athletes? Postmenopausal osteoporosis has, since the path-breaking studies of Albright et al.,[13] been associated with diminished gonadal function. A number of studies have indeed shown that amenorrheic women runners have lower bone mineral density than eumenorrheic athletes.[14,15] Okano et al.,[16] however, matched their amenorrheic athletes with women of the same age range and body weight and found little difference in the bone mineral density of the two types. Nevertheless, bone turnover of the amenorrheic athletes was lower than that of the eumenorrheic controls. Okano et al.[16] therefore expect a long-term bone mass deficit in the amenorrheic as compared to the eumenorrheic subjects. Caballero et al.[17] showed that 5 months of moderate physical exercise in postmenopausal women led to increased muscle strength and flexibility, as well as a modest but statistically significant decrease in the plasma levels of the sex-hormone-binding globulin. High levels of the latter in postmenopausal women are thought to be related to increased bone loss. Because osteoporosis frequently is a complication of heart transplants, although without direct involvement of the gonadal hormones, Braith and colleagues[18] placed heart transplant patients on a resistance exercise program for 6 months. The exercise regimen consisted of a lumbar extension exercise done 1 day/week and variable resistance exercises, done with the Nautilus machine 2 days/week. Whereas bone mineral density of the total body, the femur neck, and lumbar vertebrae decreased significantly within 2 months in all patients, it was restored to nearly pretransplantation levels in the exercised group. Prince et al.[19] reported that calcium supplementation of women who were more than 10 years postmenopausal resulted in cessation of bone loss at both the trochanteric and intertrochanteric hip sites. Exercise plus calcium supplementation had a more positive effect than calcium supplementation alone. There was no significant loss of bone at the spine site in any group. Calcium supplementation in the absence of hormonal replacement therapy seems more effective in reducing cortical bone loss than trabecular bone loss. Women who are 10 years beyond their menopause are likely to have lost whatever trabecular bone they are going to lose.[20] Because the spine contains more trabecular bone than the other sites, it is not surprising that the spine was unaffected by calcium supplementation or added exercise.

The relationship between muscle mass and strength, on the one hand, and bone mass and strength, on the other, seems well established, at least for weight-bearing bones. What is less well known, however, are the mechanisms by which muscle can act on bone and by which bone tissue adapts to mechanical demands. How bone tissue senses mechanical stimuli and translates them into remodeling is as yet not known. It is known that the cytoskeleton of cells generally can undergo structural deformation. This in turn acts on ion channels[21] which cause signals like ionic calcium to enter the cell or be released from cellular stores and to travel to intracellular receptors. The receptors initiate a further cascade of changes, beginning with a kinase complex. It has been reported[22] that osteoblasts specifically respond to mechanical stimulation via cyclic AMP and cyclic GMP. More recently, it has been suggested that osteocytes (bone cells deep inside bone) are the principal mechanosensory cells in bone.[23] However, muscles insert on the surface of bones, and it is these surface cells — osteoblasts and osteoblast-derived cells — that are likely to initiate the response to mechanical stimuli. Vibrational forces have been shown to induce rapid upregulation of mRNA expression of two growth-related protooncogenes.[24] Future work is therefore likely to uncover the molecular pathways that lead from muscular contraction to changes in bone metabolism.

IV. ROLE OF MICROGRAVITY

From the preceding discussion, the loss of bone associated with prolonged bed rest with immobilization, as in patients with scoliosis treated with whole body casts, or with weightlessness, as in space flight, is well established. It may however be useful to describe the effects of weightlessness in somewhat greater detail, because space flight is and will be the major exploration activity by humankind.

From a review by Bikle et al.,[25] it is evident that loss in the calcaneus, a weight-bearing heel bone, amounts to about 8% of mineral density of the bone over a period of 100 days of space flight (Skylab). Changes in nonweight-bearing bones, as in the lumbar spine, appear to be minimal. Changes in the calcium metabolism of the astronauts included a negative calcium balance, largely the result of increased urinary losses, although fecal losses also increased. Increased urinary losses can be attributed to an increase in plasma calcium and to diminished calcium reabsorption. Increased fecal calcium output can be attributed to diminished absorption. Because plasma PTH levels diminished as a result of the increase in plasma calcium, as did plasma $1,25\text{-}(OH)_2D_3$ levels, the decrease in intestinal calcium absorption and renal calcium reabsorption must have resulted from a diminution in the biosynthesis of the intestinal calbindin D_{9K} and renal calbindin D_{28K}. In their review, Bikle et al.[25] conclude that the principal effect of weightlessness is a greater reduction in bone formation than resorption. Interestingly, this is also true in osteoporosis and the age-dependent decrease in bone mass.[20]

An as yet unanswered question is how easily and quickly the muscle and bone sequelae of prolonged space flight are overcome once the astronaut returns to earth. Current indications are that the return to preflight bone mineral density is relatively slow and, over the median term, may be incomplete. In current space flights that last weeks or months, as on Mir, astronauts do resistance exercises for about 1 hr/

day and therefore minimize loss, but it is not clear whether they continue exercise once on earth to rebuild the lost muscle and bone. If one considers that the absolute rates of bone calcium formation and resorption peak at about menarche in girls[26] and that bone mass peaks in the third decade of life in both men and women,[20] it is not surprising that return to earth, exercise, and appropriate calcium intake do not result in rapid remineralization to preflight status.

V. CALCIUM NUTRITION IN SPORTS

The calcium intake of American women, on the average, is substantially below the RDA.[6] Teenage girls in particular and young women fail to take in sufficient calcium to achieve their genetically programmed bone mass and density. This is also the age range of the majority of women who are actively engaged in competitive sports. Moreover, because active sportspersons are likely to have a higher rate of bone turnover, at least of weight-bearing bones, it is important that coaches encourage their charges to eat adequate amounts of calcium. The easiest and least expensive food source of calcium is milk and dairy products. Concern about fat intake can be alleviated by recommending skim milk or milk with reduced fat content. Lactose intolerance can be overcome by the use of lactose-treated milk or dairy products made from it. The advantage of the use of milk is that it also provides a high-quality protein.

The recommended daily calcium intake is between 1.0 and 1.5 g for most adults and somewhat less for growing children. Athletes should be encouraged to consume enough calcium near the upper limit of the RDAs. Males generally consume quantities of calcium that come closer to the RDA. If calcium is taken as a supplement, it is desirable to have the calcium in a relatively soluble form (e.g., as citrate). The most common form of calcium in tablet form is calcium carbonate. When taken with food, absorption may be adequate, but a more soluble calcium salt can be taken at any time and is preferable, especially in the elderly.

The recommended daily intake of vitamin D is 400 international units (1 μg). This is the quantity added to 1 quart (0.94 l) of milk in the U.S. and is considered adequate to meet the RDA of most individuals. Persons who are confined indoors during long dark winters and do not drink fortified milk need to supplement their intakes with vitamin D and calcium. This situation may not apply to most people engaged in active sports but is a possibility that trainers and coaches should keep in mind. There are no indications that active sportspeople need larger quantities of vitamin D.

VI. CONCLUSIONS

Calcium intakes between 1.0 and 1.5 g are considered adequate to ensure appropriate bone health if there are no other health problems, such as gonadal deficiency. At those calcium intake levels, active transcellular calcium absorption in the duodenum is likely to be downregulated. Nevertheless, enough calcium is absorbed by the passive, paracellular pathway to assure adequate calcium absorption. Amenorrheic women athletes need to be treated by adequate nutrition counseling, hormone replacement therapy, and a reduction in exercise.[27] Individuals who have been subjected to prolonged periods of bed rest, immobilization, or hypogravity need to replace gradually the calcium they lost while engaging in an appropriate exercise program that would strengthen weakened muscles and, with time, thinned bones.

REFERENCES

1. Walser, M., Ion association. VI. Interaction between calcium, magnesium, inorganic phosphate, citrate and protein in normal human plasma, *J. Clin. Invest.*, 40, 723, 1961.
2. Block, G., Dresser, C.M., Hartman, A.M., and Carroll, M.D., Nutrient sources in the American diet: quantitative data from the NHANES II survey. I. Vitamins and minerals, *Am. J. Epidemiol.*, 122, 13, 1985.
3. Bronner, F., Intestinal calcium absorption: mechanisms and applications, *J. Nutr.*, 117, 1347, 1987.
4. Pansu, D., Duflos, C., Bellaton, C., and Bronner, F., Solubility and intestinal transit time limit calcium absorption in rats, *J. Nutr.*, 123, 1396, 1993.
5. Bronner, F., Bone and calcium homeostasis, *NeuroToxicology*, 13, 775, 1992.
6. Bronner, F., Calcium, in *Handbook of Nutritionally Essential Mineral Elements*, O'Dell, G.B. and Sunde, R.A., Eds., Marcel Dekker, New York, 1997, 13.
7. Bronner, F. and Stein, W.D., Calcium homeostasis — an old problem revisited, *J. Nutr.*, 125, 1987S, 1995.
8. Bronner, F., Renal calcium transport: mechanisms and regulation — an overview, *Am. J. Physiol.*, 257 (*Renal Fluid Electrolyte Physiol.* 26), F707, 1989.
9. Henderson, N.K., Price, R.I., Gutteridge, J.H., and Bagat, C.I., Bone density in young women is associated with body weight and muscle strength but not dietary intakes, *J. Bone Miner. Res.*, 10, 384, 1995.
10. Glastre, C., Braillon, P., David, L., Cochat, P., Meunier, P.J., and Delmas, P.D., Measurement of bone mineral content of the lumbar spine by dual energy X-ray absorptiometry in normal children: correlation with growth parameters, *J. Clin. Endocrinol. Metab.*, 70, 1330, 1990.
11. Brahm, H., Strom, H., Piel-Aulin, K., Mallwin, H., and Ljunghall, S., Bone metabolism in endurance-trained athletes: a comparison to population-based controls based on DXA, SXA, quantitative ultrasound, and biochemical markers, *Calcif. Tissue Int.*, 61, 448, 1997.
12. Bloomfield, S.A., Changes in musculoskeletal structure and function with prolonged bedrest, *Med. Sci. Sports Exercise*, 29, 197, 1997.
13. Albright, F., Bloomberg, F., and Smith, P.H., Postmenopausal osteoporosis, *Trans. Assoc. Am. Physicians*, 55, 298, 1940.
14. Drinkwater, B.L., Nilson, K., Chesnut, C.H., III, Brenner, W.J., Shainholz, S., and Southworth, M.B., Bone mineral content of amenorrheic and eumenorrheic athletes, *N. Engl. J. Med.*, 311, 277, 1984.
15. Marcus, R., Cann, C., Madvig, P., Minkoff, J., Goddard, M., Bayer, M., Martin, M., Gandiani, L., Haskell, W., and Genant, H., Menstrual function and bone mass in elite women distance runners, *Ann. Intern. Med.*, 102, 158, 1985.
16. Okano, H., Mizunuma, H., Soda, M., Matsui, H., Aoki, I., Honjo, S., and Ibuki, Y., Effects of exercise and amenorrhea on bone mineral density in runners, *Endocr. J.*, 42, 271, 1995.

17. Caballero, M.J., Mahedero, G., Hernandez, R., Alvarez, J.L., Rodriguez, J., Rodriguez, I., and Maynar, M., Effects of physical exercise on some parameters of bone metabolism in postmenopausal women, *Endocr. Res.*, 22, 131, 1996.

18. Braith, R.W., Mitlo, R.M., Welsch, M.A., Keller, J.W., and Pollock, M.L., Resistance exercise training restores bone mineral density in heart transplant recipients, *J. Am. Coll. Cardiol.*, 28, 1471, 1996.

19. Prince, R., Devine, A., Dick, I., Criddle, A., Kerr, D., Kent, N., Price, R., and Randell, A., The effects of calcium supplementation (milk powder or tablets) and exercise on bone density in postmenopausal women, *J. Bone Miner. Res.*, 10, 1068, 1995.

20. Bronner, F., Calcium and osteoporosis, *Am. J. Clin. Nutr.*, 60, 831, 1994.

21. Sachs, F., Ion channels as mechanical transducers, in *Cell Shape. Determinants, Regulation and Regulatory Role,* Stein, W.D. and Bronner, F., Eds., Academic Press, San Diego, 1989, 63.

22. Rodan, G.A., Bourret, L.A., Harvey, A., and Mensi, T., 3′,5′ Cyclic AMP and 3′,5′ cyclic GMP: mediators of the mechanical effects on bone remodeling, *Science,* 189, 467, 1975.

23. Burger, E.H., Klein-Nulend, J., van der Plas, A., and Nijweide, P.J., Function of osteocytes in bone — their role in mechanotransduction, *J. Nutr.*, 125, 2020S, 1995.

24. Tjandrawinata, R.R., Vincent, V.L., and Hughes-Fulford, M., Vibrational force alters mRNA expression in osteoblasts, *FASEB J.*, 11, 493, 1997.

25. Bikle, D.D., Halloran, B.P., and Morey-Holton, E., Space flight and the skeleton: lessons for the earthbound, *Gravit. Space Biol. Bull.*, 10, 119, 1997.

26. Bronner, F. and Abrams, S.A., Development and regulation of calcium metabolism in healthy girls, *J. Nutr.*, 128, 1474, 1998.

27. Anderson, J.J.B., Stender, M., Rondano, P., Bishop, L., and Duckett, A.G., Nutrition and bone in physical activity and sport, in *Nutrition in Exercise and Sport,* 3rd ed., Wolinsky, I., Ed., CRC Press, Boca Raton, FL, 1998, 219.

Chapter 3

PHOSPHORUS IN EXERCISE AND SPORT

Richard B. Kreider

CONTENTS

I. INTRODUCTION

Over the past 20 years, a significant amount of research has been devoted to identifying medically safe nutritional ergogenic aids. One of the most promising nutritional ergogenic substances appears to be phosphorus.[1] Phosphorus is intimately involved in numerous metabolic pathways. Consequently, researchers have been interested in the potential ergogenic value of phosphorus since the early 1920s. Most of this research has evaluated the role of phosphorus in energy metabolism as well as the effects of either sodium or calcium phosphate supplementation on exercise capacity. Sodium and/or calcium phosphate loading prior to exercise (4 to 10 g/day for 3 to 6 days) has been reported to affect exercise capacity in a number of ways (see Table 1). Although not all studies have reported ergogenic benefit (particularly with calcium phosphate), most studies indicate that sodium phosphate supplementation is an effective ergogenic aid during certain exercise conditions. The purpose of this chapter is to discuss the theoretical rationale of phosphate supplementation and to provide an overview of the literature relative to the effect of phosphate loading on human performance.

II. NUTRITIONAL ROLE OF PHOSPHORUS

A. DIETARY SOURCES

Phosphorus is a nonmetallic element found in a variety of foods. Animal meats, dairy products, and eggs provide approximately 60% of the daily intake of phosphorus in industrialized societies because they contain high levels of phospholipids such as phosphatidylcholine (lecithin), which are excellent sources of phosphorus. Grains also contain substantial amounts of phosphorus, but are not considered as good a source as animal products because part of the phosphorus exists as inositol hexaphosphate (phytate), which is not as highly absorbable. Phosphates are commonly added to food in processing. For example, lecithin is a major emulsify-

TABLE 1   Proposed Theoretical Ergogenic Value of Phosphate Supplementation

- Elevates extracellular and intracellular phosphate concentrations
- Stimulates glycolysis and energy metabolism
- Increases the availability of phosphate for oxidative phosphorylation and creatine phosphate synthesis
- Increases 2,3-diphosphoglycerate synthesis and peripheral extraction of oxygen
- Enhances myocardial and cardiovascular responses to exercise
- Serves as a metabolic buffer
- Increases anaerobic threshold and maximal oxygen uptake
- Improves endurance exercise performance and/or efficiency
- May enhance psychological responses to exercise

ing agent, and carbonated drinks also contain phosphoric acid. Consequently, phosphorus obtained from food additives typically constitutes about 30% of the daily dietary intake.[2]

The Joint Nutrition Monitoring Evaluation Committee has reported that phosphorus intake in the U.S. is generally adequate and requires less monitoring than other nutrients.[3] The Recommended Dietary Allowance for adults in the U.S. is 800 mg/day, while the mean daily intake of phosphorus is 1536 and 966 mg/day in males and females, respectively.[4,5] Generally, about 60 to 70% of dietary phosphorus is absorbed. However, absorption of phosphorus may increase to 90% when blood serum levels are low. Phosphorus toxicity is rare but may occur in individuals who ingest more than 12 g/day.

B. REGULATION OF PHOSPHORUS

Because phosphorus acts as a threshold substance, serum levels of phosphorus are regulated in part by an overflow mechanism.[2,6] The normal serum concentration of phosphorus ranges from 0.75 to 1.35 mmol/l with a mean of 1.1 mmol/l. When serum levels are low, additional phosphorus is absorbed from the intestines and/or the proximal tubules of the nephron.[2,6] When serum levels of phosphorus are high, extra phosphorus is typically excreted by the kidney.[6] Normal urinary excretion of phosphorus is approximately 175 to 300 mmol/day.[2,6] Hormonal regulation also affects serum phosphorus levels. For example, the interaction of parathyroid hormone and 1,25-dihydroxyvitamin D_3, which is intimately involved in maintaining calcium levels, influences serum phosphate levels. Moreover, cortisol and estrogen are also involved in phosphorus regulation.[2,6]

Approximately 50% of serum phosphorus exists as free phosphate, while the remaining phosphorus is bound with sodium, calcium, magnesium, and protein. Serum phosphorus levels normally fluctuate by 0.3 to 0.6 mmol/l. The fluctuation generally reflects shifts between intracellular and extracellular concentrations. Because phosphorus is found in a wide variety of foods and serum phosphorus levels are generally well regulated, hypophosphatemia is rare. However, hypophosphatemia may be observed in alcoholism and with excessive consumption of non-absorbable antacids.[2] Hypophosphatemia may lead to serious medical consequences, such as hemolytic anemia, congestive heart failure, myopathy, kidney malfunction, respiratory distress, and central nervous system abnormalities.[2] In the absence of chronic renal disease, hyperphosphatemia is rare[2,4–6] and exhibits no specific signs or symptoms.[2,6]

III. THEORETICAL ERGOGENIC VALUE OF PHOSPHATE SUPPLEMENTATION

The average adult contains approximately 11 to 14 g of phosphorus per kilogram fat-free body weight. About 85% is stored in the skeletal system, mostly as inorganic orthophosphate complexed with calcium into a crystalline salt, hydroxyapatite. The remaining amount of phosphorus is contained in soft tissues, mainly as organic compounds in conjunction with proteins and amines as well as inorganic phosphate. Although maintenance of bone integrity is important in certain athletic populations susceptible to premature bone mass loss, the theoretical ergogenic value of phosphate supplementation primarily resides in the metabolic role of phosphorus in soft tissues. In this regard, it has been theorized that altering extracellular and intracellular availability of organic phosphorus compounds and/ or inorganic phosphate may enhance exercise metabolism, leading to improved performance.[1]

In support of this contention, serum phosphate levels have been reported to increase in response to intense anaerobic and aerobic exercise.[7-10] The increase in serum phosphate is related in part to phosphate efflux from the intracellular stores in the muscle to the blood.[2,10] Furthermore, endurance athletes have been reported to have elevated resting serum phosphate levels or to be hyperphosphatemic (i.e., >1.35 mmol/l).[8,10-13] The cause of the elevated serum phosphate levels in trained endurance athletes has not been determined. However, Dale and associates[10] have suggested that it may represent a metabolic training effect and/or an inborn metabolic advantage. The following discussion examines the major hypotheses by which phosphate loading has been suggested to affect exercise performance.

A. ENHANCED METABOLIC REGULATION

Phosphate is the major anion of the intracellular fluids,[6] and the proportion of intracellular phosphate available for energy metabolism depends upon the extracellular concentration.[14] Phospholipids, which are the major component of cell membranes,[15] may also serve as donors of phosphate radicals when they are needed for different chemical reactions in the tissues.[1,5] Phosphate binds reversibly with a number of coenzyme systems and other compounds involved in metabolism.[5] For example, protein phosphorylation (phosphoprotein) is believed to be a precursor to cellular changes induced by some extracellular signals, particularly as an allosteric regulator of many enzymes.[3,15] Several vitamins involved in the metabolic regulation of intracellular carbohydrate metabolism are also phosphate dependent, particularly thiamin pyrophosphate (vitamin B_1) during glycolysis and pyridoxal phosphate, a derivative of pyridoxine (vitamin B_6), during glycogenolysis. Additionally, several of the second messengers in the cell are phosphate dependent, such as cyclic adenosine monophosphate and inositol-1,4,5-triphosphate, both of which can initiate a cascade of metabolic events in the cell by modifying intracellular calcium metabolism.[15,16]

Intracellular phosphate is also involved in the regulation of energy metabolism in a variety of ways.[5,17-19] For example, phosphate is an important component of phosphocreatine (PCr), which is intimately involved in the phosphagen energy system employed during intense exercise as well as oxidative phosphorylation employed during aerobic exercise.[18] Moreover, glucose is phosphorylated upon entry into the muscle cell, while pyridoxal phosphate is needed for glycogenolysis. Enhanced glycogenolysis, glycolysis, and oxidative phosphorylation may increase the rate of adenosine triphosphate (ATP) production and possibly improve cellular metabolism during exercise. There is evidence that phosphate supplementation may stimulate the activity of a variety of enzymes in the erythrocyte, such as phospho-fructokinase (PFK) and glyceraldehyde 3-phosphate (G-3-P), involved in glycogen metabolism,[20-22] any may also increase hemoglobin levels.[8] Collectively, increasing the availability of extracellular and intracellular phosphate through phosphate supplementation could theoretically provide an ergogenic effect during intense and endurance exercise by enhancing energy metabolism and/or efficiency.

B. ENHANCED ATP AND PCR SYNTHESIS

Phosphate is integrally involved in the formation of purines and pyrimidines and thereby DNA and RNA synthesis.[16] In this regard, phosphate contributes to the development of adenine, a component of adenosine, and also provides high energy bonds in ATP and PCr. The phosphorylation potential, given as the ratio of [ATP] to [ADP + P_i], is an index for the energy status of the cell and is dependent upon the concentration of P_i. The phosphorylation potential is directly related to the free energy available from ATP.[16] Theoretically, phosphate supplementation may increase the cellular concentrations of ATP and/or PCr as well as provide additional inorganic phosphate for replenishment of ATP and PCr during exercise. Because ATP and PCr are depleted rapidly during high-intensity sprint exercise,[23-25] rapid restoration of ATP and PCr during and following intense exercise may enhance performance capacity. Additionally, increased availability of phosphate in the electron transport system may promote oxidative phosphorylation.[18] Collectively, phosphate loading may theoretically provide ergogenic benefit during anaerobic and aerobic exercise.

C. ENHANCED 2,3-DIPHOSPHOGLYCERATE SYNTHESIS

2,3-Diphosphoglycerate (2,3-DPG) is a highly anionic organic phosphate which binds to hemoglobin in the erythrocyte. 2,3-DPG serves to lower the oxygen affinity of oxygen by a factor of 26, thereby facilitating the release of oxygen to the tissues.[16] Several studies have shown increased 2,3-DPG levels in the adaptation to hypoxia at altitude.[19,26] One of the most espoused hypotheses regarding the ergogenic value of phosphate loading suggests that phosphate supplementation may increase erythrocyte 2,3-DPG content, thereby facilitating oxygen delivery to the muscle during exercise.[27-31] Although most studies have reported increased 2,3-DPG levels following phosphate supplementation,[27-31] others have reported no effects on 2,3-DPG levels.[7,8]

D. ENHANCED CARDIOVASCULAR RESPONSES TO EXERCISE

Phosphate supplementation has also been suggested to affect myocardial function at rest and during exercise. In this regard, hypophosphatemia is associated with depressed myocardial contractility and cardiac output.[34] Reversal of hypophosphatemic states has been reported to markedly improved myocardial responses in the canine.[35,36] In addition, several reports indicate that sodium or calcium phosphate supplementation enhances peripheral extraction of oxygen,[28] reduces submaximal cardiac output[29,37,38] and/or stroke volume,[7] and increases myocardial contractility and ejection fraction[39] during intense endurance exercise. Improving cardiovascular efficiency and/or performance would theoretically provide ergogenic benefit to athletes engaged in endurance exercise performance.

E. ENHANCED BUFFERING CAPACITY

Phosphate loading has also been suggested to enhance acid–base balance during intense exercise. In this regard, phosphate is an active participant in many physiological buffer systems[6] and is involved in acid–base balance within the plasma and in the cells.[2] For example, sodium phosphate (Na_2HPO_4) acts as a weak base, while sodium dihydrogen phosphate (NaH_2PO_4) is a weak acid. Phosphates may also be combined with other cations, such as potassium. The power of the phosphate buffer system is rather weak in the extracellular fluids. However, the phosphate buffer is very important in the intracellular fluids as its concentration is much greater.[6,16] This is particularly true with respect to the kidneys. During exercise, the decreased pH usually associated with the production of lactic acid may be mitigated to some degree by the phosphate buffer system. Because the decline in the force of maximal voluntary muscular contractions has been associated with increases in $H_2PO_4{}_-$,[40] increases in basic $HPO_4{}_-$ through phosphate loading could provide ergogenic value in a manner similar to that reported with sodium bicarbonate supplementation.[41] Theoretically, a phosphate-stimulated enhancement in buffering capacity may improve exercise capacity during high-intensity sprint performance or in events in which the athlete competes near the anaerobic threshold. In support of this concept, reports have indicated that phosphate loading decreases lactate levels during submaximal exercise[27] as well as increases anaerobic threshold during incremental maximal exercise.[8,39,42]

F. ENHANCED PSYCHOLOGICAL RESPONSES TO EXERCISE

Phosphate loading has also been suggested to modify psychological processes. Phospholipids such as sphingomyelin are important structural components of the brain and nervous tissues. The intracellular functions of phosphates previously noted could influence the central nervous system, thereby affecting psychological responses to exercise. In support of this hypothesis, Jain and others[33] reported that learning efficiency was significantly better in subjects who were supplemented with phosphate compared to a placebo group. Consequently, phosphate loading may alter psychological responses to exercise, potentially allowing the athlete to exercise at higher exercise intensities although perceiving similar psychological stress.

IV. ANALYSIS OF THE ERGOGENIC VALUE OF PHOSPHATE SUPPLEMENTATION

A. EARLY RESEARCH FINDINGS

Studies investigating the ergogenic value of phosphate supplementation date back to the 1920s. Early studies suggested that phosphate salt supplementation could be used to increase physical working capacity and prevent fatigue.[44,45] Some initial research was also conducted on lecithin or phosphatidylcholine. Lecithin (phosphatidylcholine) has been theorized to possess ergogenic qualities due to either its phosphate or choline content, the latter being involved in the formation of the neurotransmitter acetylcholine.[41,43] Atzler and Lehmann[46] reported improvements in both static and dynamic power as well as endurance exercise capacity following lecithin ingestion. In addition, Dennig[47] reported favorable effects of soya lecithin upon exercise performance. In analysis of this literature, Boje[48] discredited much of the research on lecithin but noted that many of the studies suggested an ergogenic effect of phosphates, concluding that phosphate supplementation could probably increase human work output.

A few additional studies conducted in the 1950s did not support an ergogenic effect of phosphates or lecithin. In a field study, Johnson and Black[49] reported that 1 g of sodium phosphate administered to champion high-school cross-country runners 2.5 hr prior to competing in a 1.5-mi race did not affect run performance times. In addition, Staton[50] reported that 14 days of soya lecithin supplementation did not significantly affect grip strength. On the other hand, Keller and Kraut[51] reported that athletic performance in a diverse number of events (ranging from a 1500-m run to swimming distances of 100 to 1500 m) was enhanced by the ingestion of sodium phosphate an hour prior to competition. Consequently, early research findings suggested that the ergogenic effects of phosphate supplementation were equivocal.

B. CONTEMPORARY RESEARCH FINDINGS
1. Basic Research

Much of the contemporary research on phosphates has emanated from medical investigations attempting to identify the regulatory role of phosphate in erythrocytic and cellular metabolism. Anaerobic glycolysis is the primary metabolic pathway for synthesis of ATP in the mature erythrocyte.[6,52] Therefore, the rate of glycolysis in the erythrocyte cytoplasm and subsequent synthesis of ATP is essential in order to maintain normal red cell metabolism. Numerous studies in the late 1960s and early 1970s reported that intracellular phosphate is an important regulator of glycolysis in the mature erythrocyte.[19,21,22,52–60] The increased glycolytic activity has been demonstrated to be due to the influence of phosphate on the regulatory enzymes PFK[19,62] and G-3-P.[62,63] Additionally, inorganic phosphate is a required substrate and/or important cofactor in numerous metabolic pathways including glycolysis, ammoniagenesis, glycogenolysis, deamination of adenine nucleotides, and the hexose monophosphate shunt.[64,65] Consequently, increasing the availability of extracellular and intracellular phosphate may affect metabolism in a variety of ways.

For example, Brazy and colleagues[66,67] reported that varying concentrations of intracellular phosphate in the isolated tubules of rabbit renal cortex significantly influenced oxidative capacity. Moreover, addition of succinate, citrate, and malate in the phosphate-free medium preserved the rate of mitochondrial respiration, while the addition of these substrates to phosphate-treated medium accelerated mitochondrial respiration. The authors suggested that a decline in extracellular phosphate reduces the availability of specific metabolic substrates to the mitochondria, thereby limiting mitochondrial oxidative capacity. However, increasing extracellular phosphate enhances mitochondrial oxidative capacity. More recent nuclear magnetic resonance studies indicate that cellular inorganic phosphate content in canine proximal tubules is regulated by sodium-dependent and -independent transport mechanisms.[68] In addition, ATP content was found to be directly proportional to the cellular inorganic phosphate content over a physiological range.[68]

Collectively, basic research studies suggest that intracellular concentrations of inorganic phosphate are affected by extracellular phosphate concentrations and sodium-dependent phosphate transport mechanisms. Extracellular and intracellular phosphate concentrations are integrally involved in intracellular metabolism through an influence on glycolytic and tricarboxylic acid intermediates. Furthermore, the metabolic pathways for intracellular metabolism depend on and/or compete for inorganic phosphate regulating the rate of cellular metabolism. While the specific effects of variations of extracellular and intracellular phosphate concentrations on oxidative metabolism in skeletal muscle remain unclear, basic research findings support the hypothesis that alterations in extracellular and intracellular availability of phosphorus may affect oxidative metabolism and thereby exercise performance.

2. Exercise-Related Studies

A number of contemporary studies have investigated the effects of sodium and/or calcium phosphate supplementation on exercise capacity. The following discussion examines the primary studies which have evaluated the effects of sodium and/or calcium phosphate supplementation on exercise performance. This discussion is followed by an overall analysis of the literature in an attempt to draw some conclusions regarding the ergogenic value of phosphate supplementation.

a. Studies Reporting an Ergogenic Benefit

Much of the contemporary interest in phosphate supplementation as a potential ergogenic aid emanated from a report by Cade and associates in the early 1980s.[27]

In this study, ten trained male subjects ($\dot{V}O_2$max 56.2 ml/kg/min) were familiarized with the experimental protocol and performed a preliminary control testing session consisting of submaximal and incremental maximal exercise tests. The control session was followed 2 weeks later with a series of three randomly assigned supplementation trials (4 g/day of sodium phosphate or a placebo for 3 days) performed 1 week apart. The supplementation trials were then followed 2 to 3 weeks later by performing a final control session. Results revealed that phosphate loading significantly increased resting serum phosphate (1.17 to 1.22 mmol/l) and red cell 2,3-DPG levels (13.00 to 13.92 mg/g hemoglobin). In addition, phosphate loading decreased submaximal lactate while increasing maximal oxygen uptake from 6 to 12% depending on the order of administration of supplementation trials. The greatest increase in maximal oxygen uptake occurred in subjects ingesting sodium phosphate for two consecutive testing trials. These findings provided the first evidence from a well-controlled contemporary study that sodium phosphate supplementation may enhance exercise capacity in well-trained athletes.

Farber and co-workers[29] investigated the effects of acute and chronic phosphate loading on oxygen affinity of hemoglobin, red cell 2,3-DPG, P_{50} responses, and cardiovascular responses to exercise in six normal subjects. Subjects were administered either 20 mg/kg/day of dibasic sodium phosphate orally followed by infusion of 1.5 l of 10% fructose with 0.28 mmol/kg/hr of phosphate over a 3-hr period or the fructose–phosphate infusion without prior dibasic sodium phosphate ingestion. Cardiopulmonary measures were obtained prior to and following performing an incremental cycle ergometry test. Results revealed that the sum of 2,3-DPG and arterial ATP and P_{50} responses was significantly higher after both infusion periods regardless of whether phosphate was ingested prior to the infusion. In addition, while oxygen uptake responses were similar at each work load among test trials, cardiac index was significantly lower as P_{50} levels were increased with phosphate. The authors suggested that phosphate loading stimulated 2,3-DPG synthesis, facilitating a shift in the oxyhemoglobin curve as evident by the changes in ATP and 2,3-DPG as well as P_{50} responses.

In a follow-up study, Farber and co-workers[28] investigated the effects of phosphate-infused hyperphosphatemia on exercise compliance in hypoxemic chronic obstructive pulmonary disease (COPD) patients. In this study, nine COPD patients performed a 3-min cycling exercise bout at approximately 60% of the subjects' maximal functional capacity while administered 2 to 3 l/min of supplemental oxygen. The subjects were then infused 1.5 l of a 10% fructose and sodium phosphate (2.28 mmol/kg/hr) solution over a 3-hr period. This protocol was replicated 24 and 48 hr later. Results revealed that although cycling work loads were identical between trials, significant increases in exercise arteriovenous oxygen difference and oxygen extraction expressed as a percent of arterial oxygen flow were found following phosphate infusion. These data suggest that phosphate infusion enhances arteriovenous oxygen difference and peripheral extraction of oxygen in COPD patients. Interestingly, this response could not be attributed to changes in hemoglobin–oxygen affinity as had been previously reported[29] because P_{50} data were unchanged following phosphate infusion. The researchers concluded that phosphate administration may be beneficial in hypoxemic states where adequate tissue oxygenation cannot be achieved.

Kreider and associates[8] investigated the effects of sodium phosphate supplementation on maximal oxygen uptake, ventilatory anaerobic threshold, and 5-mi run performance in elite male runners. In this study, seven elite runners ($\dot{V}O_2$max 73.9 ± 6.3 ml/kg/min) participated in a placebo, double-blind, crossover experiment. Subjects were randomly assigned to ingest either 4 g/day of sodium phosphate or a glucose placebo for 6 days. On the third day of supplementation, the subjects performed either an incremental maximal exercise test or 5-mi treadmill performance run for time. On the sixth day of supplementation, the subjects then performed the remaining maximal test or performance run. Subjects observed a 14-day washout period and repeated the experiment after ingesting the alternate supplement.

Results demonstrated that resting serum phosphate values in the placebo maximal and performance trials were mildly hyperphosphatemic (1.41 ± 0.2 and 1.27 ± 0.3 mmol/l, respectively). Nevertheless, sodium phosphate supplementation significantly increased resting and postexercise serum phosphate levels by 7 to 12%, respectively. In addition, sodium phosphate supplementation resulted in a 9% increase in maximal oxygen uptake (73.9 ± 5 to 80.3 ± 4 ml/kg/min) and a 12% increase in ventilatory anaerobic threshold (58.0 ± 4 to 64.8 ± 2 ml/kg/min). During the 5-mi performance run, phosphate loading resulted in an 11.8-sec nonsignificant ($p = 0.14$) decrease in performance time (26.8 ± 1 to 26.6 ± 1 min) and a nonsignificant ($p = 0.07$) 2.52-sec decrease in average mile split time (5.361 ± 0.3 to 5.326 ± 0.2 min). However, mean oxygen uptake during the run was significantly lower in the phosphate-supplemented trial, suggesting an enhanced physiological efficiency during the performance run which would theoretically be of ergogenic value.

In a similar study, Stewart and colleagues[69] investigated the effects of sodium phosphate ingestion on maximal oxygen uptake, time to exhaustion, serum 2,3-DPG, and serum phosphate in eight trained male cyclists. The subjects performed one control maximal cycle ergometry test. In a double-blind, randomized manner and crossover manner, subjects were administered a placebo or 3.6 g/day of sodium phosphate for 3 days prior to performing a second maximal exercise test. Subjects then observed a 7-day washout period and began supplementation with the alternate supplement prior to performing a final maximal exercise test. Results revealed no significant alterations in resting serum phosphate or 2,3-DPG levels. However, postexercise 2,3-DPG levels were significantly higher in the phosphate trial. Furthermore, maximal oxygen uptake was significantly increased by 11% (control 48.5 ± 9, placebo 47.8 ± 9, phosphate 53.4 ± 6 ml/kg/min) and time to exhaustion was increased by 20% (control 9.9 ± 3, placebo 10.6 ± 3, phosphate 12.3 ± 3 min). In addition, although the subjects performed significantly more work in the phosphate trial, postmaximal exercise lactate values were slightly lower than control and placebo responses (control 12.5 ± 2, placebo 13.0 ± 3, phosphate 12.2 ± 2 mmol/l). These findings indicate that sodium phosphate supplementation may enhance exercise capacity by increasing maximal oxygen uptake possibly by facilitating an increase in 2,3-DPG and/or providing a greater buffering capacity.

Kreider and co-workers[39] conducted the most extensive study to date to evaluate the ergogenic value of phosphate loading. In this study, six highly trained male cyclists ($\dot{V}O_2$max 69.3 ± 12 ml/kg/min) participated in a placebo, double-blind, crossover study to determine the effects of sodium phosphate loading on metabolic and myocardial adaptations to maximal exercise and 40-km time trial performance. Subjects ingested either 4 g/day of tribasic sodium phosphate or a glucose placebo for 5 days. On the fourth day, subjects performed either an incremental maximal cycling test or a 40-km simulated time trial performed under controlled laboratory conditions using the subjects' racing bicycles attached to a computerized race simulator. Subjects performed the remaining performance test on the subsequent day of the investigation. Subjects observed a 14-day washout period and repeated the testing protocol with the alternate supplement regimen.

Analysis of maximal test results revealed that phosphate loading significantly increased premax serum phosphate levels (17%), maximal oxygen uptake (9%), minute ventilation (8%), ventilatory anaerobic threshold (10%), glucose (23%), free fatty acids (23%), echocardiographically determined mean ejection fraction (4%), and myocardial fractional shortening (8%). During the 40-km time trial, phosphate loading significantly increased mean power output (17%), oxygen uptake (18%), ventilation (15%), heart rate (8%), ejection fraction (13%), and fractional shortening (24%), resulting in an 8% reduction in performance time. Although the etiology of improved myocardial responses to exercise remains to be determined, these findings provide strong evidence that sodium phosphate supplementation provides ergogenic value to highly trained athletes.

b. Studies Reporting No Ergogenic Benefit

Not all studies evaluating the effects of phosphate loading have reported ergogenic value. For example, Duffy and Conlee[70] evaluated the effects of acute and chronic ingestion of a commercially available supplement containing sodium and potassium phosphate on leg power and high-intensity run performance. In this study, 11 untrained males participated in a placebo, double-blind, crossover experiment. Subjects ingested three phosphate-containing capsules (each containing 387 mg sodium phosphate, 27.5 mg tribasic potassium phosphate, and 30 mg vitamin C) or a placebo 60 min prior to performance assessment during the acute phase of ingestion. One week later, subjects began ingesting nine phosphate-containing capsules (3.7 g/day of sodium or potassium phosphate) or a placebo for 6 days. A 1-day washout period was observed and the subjects repeated the 6-day supplementation regimen with the alternate supplement. Results revealed no significant differences in endurance run time to exhaustion following acute or chronic ingestion of the phosphate capsules. Further, no significant differences were observed following acute or chronic phosphate supplementation in 1 min of leg extension power. Consequently, the authors concluded that phosphate supplementation possessed no ergogenic value in high-intensity exercise events lasting 1 to 3 min in duration.

In another paper, Bredle and co-workers[7] investigated the effects of calcium phosphate supplementation on maximal exercise tolerance and endurance capacity in 11 moderately trained males. In this study, subjects performed a preliminary control maximal treadmill test. Subjects were then randomly and blindly administered capsules containing 5.7 g/day of inorganic phosphate, 7.3 g/day of calcium, and 73 μm/day of vitamin C or a similar placebo containing 5.7 g/day of carbonate in place of the phosphate. Subjects ingested the supplements for 4 days. On the third day of supplementation, subjects performed a maximal treadmill test. On the fourth day of supplementation, subjects performed an endurance run to exhaustion at 70% of $\dot{V}O_2$max. Results revealed that calcium phosphate ingestion significantly increased serum phosphate levels on the fourth day of loading by 35% while not affecting 2,3-DPG, P_{50}, pH, and plasma bicarbonate levels. Additionally, no significant differences were observed in maximal oxygen uptake or run time to exhaustion. However, there was some evidence ($p < 0.07$) that cardiac output was lower (6%) while stroke volume was significantly higher (5%) at the 10-min mark into the exercise bout following phosphate loading. These findings indicate that calcium phosphate supplementation may increase serum phosphorus levels and influence cardiovascular function during endurance exercise. However, calcium phosphate supplementation does not enhance maximal exercise or endurance exercise performance.

Mannix and associates[71] investigated the effects of a single dose of calcium phosphate on submaximal exercise performance in ten untrained males. Subjects performed a preliminary maximal cycle ergometry test. The subjects were then blindly and randomly administered either a single dose of dicalcium phosphate (129 mmol of phosphorus, 5.0 g of calcium, and 50 μg of vitamin C) or a flour placebo. In addition, 500 ml of fluid containing 10% glucose was consumed 1 hr after ingestion of the dicalcium phosphate supplement and 500 ml of an artificially sweetened fluid was consumed 1 hr after ingestion of the placebo. Subjects then rested for 2 hr prior to performing a 30-min submaximal exercise bout at 61% of $\dot{V}O_2$max. Following the exercise bout, the subjects rested for 15 min and then performed a 10-min exercise bout at 57% of $\dot{V}O_2$max followed by a 10-min passive recovery. Subjects observed a 7-day washout period and repeated the testing procedures with the alternate supplement regimen.

Results revealed that the single dose of dicalcium phosphate and glucose significantly increased ($p < 0.05$) pre-exercise serum phosphate levels (13%), 2,3-DPG levels (11%), red cell ATP levels (5%), and P_{50} responses (4%). Serum phosphate, 2,3-DPG levels, and red cell ATP levels remained significantly elevated throughout the exercise session in response to phosphate loading. In addition, plasma pH levels were significantly lower in the phosphate–glucose trial following exercise. However, no significant differences were observed between placebo and phosphate trials in oxygen uptake, cardiac output, stroke volume, heart rate, arteriovenous oxygen difference, or oxygen deficit parameters. Consequently, the researchers concluded that although the dicalcium phosphate–glucose supplement promoted physiologically beneficial alterations, these adaptations did not induce an ergogenic enhancement in cardiovascular responses to exercise.

Kraemer and colleagues[72] investigated the effects of ingesting a commercially available supplement containing sodium phosphate, potassium bicarbonate, and carnosine on repetitive sprint performance and 2,3-DPG concentrations. In this study, ten trained and ten untrained cyclists were administered either a placebo or the multibuffer supplement (4 g/day of sodium phosphate, 0.8 g/day of potassium bicarbonate, 50 mg/day of L-carnosine) for 3.5 days. Subjects then performed four 30-sec cycle ergometer maximal effort sprints separated by a 2-min rest recovery. Subjects then observed a 14-day washout period and repeated the experiment following 3.5 days of ingesting the remaining supplement. Results revealed that multibuffer supplementation increased postexercise 2,3-DPG levels and the ratio of 2,3-DPG/hemoglobin in the trained cyclists. Further, acute recovery of peak power was enhanced in these subjects following phosphate loading. However, no significant differences were observed in acid–base status or repetitive sprint power output. These findings suggest that although this supplement promoted significant increases in 2,3-DPG and enhanced recovery of peak power, multibuffer supplementation provided no ergogenic benefit to repetitive sprint performance.

Finally, Galloway and associates[73] investigated the effects of acute calcium phosphate supplementation on submaximal and maximal exercise capacity in untrained and trained subjects. Subjects were divided into trained and untrained groups and participated in a double-blind, randomized, crossover experiment. Subjects ingested either a placebo or 22 g/day of dibasic calcium phosphate 90 min prior to performing a 20-min submaximal cycle ergometry exercise bout at 70% of peak oxygen uptake. Subjects then observed a 30-min rest followed by performing an incremental maximal exercise test to exhaustion. Subjects observed a 7-day washout period and repeated the experiment, ingesting the remaining supplement 90 min prior to exercise. Results revealed no significant differences among groups in 2,3-DPG, oxygen uptake, or plasma lactate. The researchers concluded that acute ingestion of calcium phosphate 90 min prior to submaximal and maximal exercise does not provide ergogenic benefit.

c. Analysis of the Ergogenic Value of Phosphate Supplementation

Although a cursory analysis of studies investigating the ergogenic value of phosphate supplementation would suggest equivocal results, critical analysis of these studies indicates that phosphate supplementation may be more or less ergogenic depending on several factors. First, the type and dosage of phosphate appear to impact the ergogenic value of phosphate supplementation. In this regard, most studies that have reported enhanced physiological adaptations and/or improved exercise capacity following phosphate supplementation have used 3 to 4 g/day of sodium phosphate for 3 to 6 days.[8,26,28–30,36,39,42,69,72] Studies that have used calcium phosphate[7,70,71,73] and/or single-dose acute supplementation protocols[70,71,73] have generally found no ergogenic value and/or limited physiological effects of phosphate loading.

Second, several of the studies which reported no ergogenic benefit employed crossover experimental trials with less than a 14-day washout period.[70,71,73] Cade and colleagues[27] indicated that a minimum of a 14-day washout period was necessary between repeated trials in order to negate any residual effects of phosphate supplementation. Consequently, it is possible that results in studies that employed brief washout periods (i.e., 1 to 7 days) may have been masked by a residual influence of phosphate supplementation.

Third, it appears that sodium phosphate supplementation (3 to 4 g/day for 3 to 4 days) may be more or less ergogenic depending on the type of exercise task evaluated. In this regard, most studies suggest that sodium phosphate supplementation may enhance aerobic capacity[8,26,39,75] and/or anaerobic threshold.[8,39] In addition, several studies indicate that phosphate supplementation may enhance cardiovascular responses to exercise.[8,26,28–30,36,39,42,69,72] However, sodium and/or calcium phosphate supplementation appears to have little ergogenic value during isokinetic and/or high-intensity intermittent exercise.[70,72] These findings suggest that the potential ergogenic value of sodium phosphate supplementation may be for endurance rather than nonendurance exercise. Finally, although a number of studies have been conducted to evaluate the effects of phosphate supplementation on exercise capacity, the experimental methods and procedures employed vary. Consequently, it is possible that differences in the experimental methods and procedures may account for some of the differences observed.

In analyzing the literature, it is clear that there is a significant body of basic research supporting the potential ergogenic value of phosphate supplementation. Although additional applied research is necessary with athletes in particular, most studies investigating the effects of sodium phosphate supplementation (3 to 4 g/day for 3 to 4 days) on maximal aerobic capacity and/or endurance exercise performance have reported ergogenic benefit.[8,26,28–30,36,39,42,69,72] The improved exercise capacity has been attributed to enhanced metabolic efficiency, improved myocardial responses to exercise, a phosphate-stimulated increase in 2,3-DPG levels, and/or enhanced peripheral extraction of oxygen.[8,26,28–30,36,39,42,69,72] On the other hand, it appears that acute and/or chronic calcium phosphate supplementation provides little ergogenic value.[7,70,71,73]

V. SUMMARY

Analysis of well-controlled contemporary research tends to support the hypothesis that short-term supplementation of phosphate (particularly sodium phosphate) may alter various physiological parameters which may affect endurance exercise performance. In this regard, in a variety of conditions and subject populations, phosphate loading has been reported to (1) elevate extracellular and intracellular phosphate concentrations[7,8,27–29,31,37–39,69,71,72] promoting a phosphate-stimulated glycolysis,[14,65–68] (2) attenuate anaerobic threshold,[8,27,39,42,69] (3) increase the availability of phosphate for oxidative phosphorylation and creatine phosphate synthesis,[18,68] (4) promote 2,3-DPG synthesis,[7,27–31,69,71,72] (5) affect myocardial and cardiovascular responses to exercise,[7,28–30,37,39] (6) increase peripheral extraction of oxygen,[7,28] (7) increase maximal oxygen uptake,[8,27,39,69] and (8) improve endurance exercise performance and/or efficiency.[8,37,39]

Although these findings are promising, it should be noted that not all studies report ergogenic benefit of phosphate loading possibly due to differences in the type and amount of phosphate ingested, the experimental design and procedures employed, and the type of exercise evaluated. Moreover, the specific mechanisms of action remain to be fully understood. Additional research is necessary to evaluate the effects of phosphate loading in various asymptomatic and symptomatic populations under varying exercise conditions. In addition, research should investigate the ergogenic value of phosphate loading for athletes engaged in a variety of athletic events.

ACKNOWLEDGMENTS

The author would like to thank the many subjects, students, research assistants, and colleagues at Old Dominion University and The University of Memphis who have contributed to studies investigating the ergogenic value of phosphate supplementation. The author would also like to thank Melvin Williams, Ph.D., FACSM, for his valuable insight and contributions to this chapter.

REFERENCES

1. Kreider, R.B., Phosphate loading and exercise performance, *J. Appl. Nutr.*, 44, 29–49, 1992.
2. Avioli, L., Calcium and phosphorus, in *Modern Nutrition in Health and Disease*, Shils, M. and Young, V. Eds., Lea & Febiger, Philadelphia, 1988, 254–288.
3. DHHS/USDA, Nutrition Monitoring in the United States: A Progress Report from the Joint Nutrition Monitoring Evaluation Committee, Department of Health and Human Services Publication Number (PHS) 86-1225, National Center for Health Statistics, Public Health Service, U.S. Department of Health and Human Services, Hyattsville, MD, 1986.
4. National Research Council, *Diet and Health*, National Academy Press, Washington, D.C., 1989.
5. National Research Council, *Recommended Dietary Allowances*, National Academy Press, Washington, D.C., 1989.
6. Guyton, A., *Textbook of Medical Physiology*, 8th ed., W.B. Saunders, Philadelphia, 1990, 6.
7. Bredle, D., Stager, J., Brechue, W., and Farber, M., Phosphate supplementation, cardiovascular function, and exercise performance in humans, *J. Appl. Physiol.*, 65, 1821–1826, 1988.
8. Kreider, R.B., Miller, G.W., Williams, M.H., Somma, C.T., and Nasser, T., Effects of phosphate loading on oxygen uptake, ventilatory anaerobic threshold, and run performance, *Med. Sci. Sports Exercise*, 22, 250–255, 1990.
9. Ljunghall, S., Joborn, H., Rastad, J., and Akerstrom, G., Plasma potassium and phosphate concentrations — influence by adrenaline infusion, beta-blockade and physical exercise, *Acta Med. Scand.*, 221, 83–93, 1987.

10. Dale, G., Fleetwood, J., Weddell, A., and Ellis, R., Fitness, unfitness, and phosphate, *Br. Med. J.*, 294, 939, 1987.

11. Dale, G., Fleetwood, J., Inkster, J., and Sainsbury. J., Profound hypophosphataemia in patients collapsing after a "fun run," *Br. Med. J.*, 292, 447–448, 1986.

12. Wilkie, D., Profound hypophosphatemia in patients collapsing after a "fun run," *Br. Med. J.*, 292, 692, 1986.

13. McCully, K., Argov, Z., Boden, B., Brown, R., Bank, W., and Chance, B., Detection of muscle injury in humans with 31-p magnetic resonance spectroscopy, *Muscle Nerve*, 11, 212–216, 1988.

14. Brazy, P. and Mandel, J., Does the availability of inorganic phosphate regulate cellular oxidative metabolism? *News Physiol. Sci.*, 1, 100–103, 1986.

15. Rasmussen, H., The cycling of calcium as an intracellular messenger, *Sci. Am.*, 261, 66–73, 1989.

16. Stryer, L., *Biochemistry*, W.H. Freeman, New York, 1988.

17. Benesch, R. and Benesch, R.E., Intracellular organic phosphates as regulators of oxygen release by haemoglobin, *Nature*, 221, 618, 1969.

18. Chasiotis, D., Role of cyclic AMP and inorganic phosphate in the regulation of muscle glycogenolysis during exercise, *Med. Sci. Sports Exercise*, 20, 545–550, 1988.

19. Eaton, J., Brewer, G., and Grover, E., Role of red cell 2,3-diphosphoglycerate in the adaptation of man to altitude, *J. Lab. Clin. Med.*, 73, 603, 1969.

20. Lenfant, C., Torrance, J., English, E., Finch, C., Reynafarje, C., Romos, J., and Faura, J., Effect of altitude on oxygen-binding by hemoglobin and organic phosphate levels, *J. Clin. Invest.*, 47, 2652, 1968.

21. Rose, I., Warms, J., and O'Connell, E., Role of inorganic phosphates in stimulating glucose utilization of human red blood cells, *Biochem. Biophys. Res. Commun.*, 15, 33–37, 1964.

22. Tsuboi, K. and Fukunaga, K., Inorganic phosphate and enhanced glucose degradation by intact erythrocytes, *J. Biol. Chem.*, 240, 2806–2810, 1965.

23. Hirvonen, J., Rehunen, S., Rusko, H., and Harkonen, M., Breakdown of high-energy phosphate compounds and lactate accumulation during short supramaximal exercise, *Eur. J. Appl. Physiol.*, 56, 253–259, 1987.

24. Miller, R., Giannini, D., Milner-Brown, H., Layzer, R., Koretsky, A., Hooper, D., and Weiner, M., Effects of fatiguing exercise on high energy phosphates, force, and EMG: evidence for three phases of recovery, *Muscle Nerve*, 10, 810–827, 1987.

25. Tesch, P., Colliander, E., and Kaiser, P., Muscle metabolism during intense, heavy-resistance exercise, *Eur. J. Appl. Physiol.*, 55, 362–366, 1986.

26. Lenfant, C., Torrance, C., Woodson, R., Jacobs, P., and Finch, C., Role of organic phosphates in the adaptation of man to hypoxia, *Fed. Proc.*, 29, 1115–1117, 1970.

27. Cade, R., Conte, M., Zauner, C., Mars, D., Peterson, J., Lunne, D., Hommen, N., and Packer, D., Effects of phosphate loading on 2,3-diphosphoglycerate and maximal oxygen uptake, *Med. Sci. Sports Exercise*, 16, 263–268, 1984.

28. Farber, M., Carlone, S., Palange, P., Serra, P., Paoletti, V., and Fineberg, N., Effect of inorganic phosphate in hypoxemic chronic obstructive lung disease patients during exercise, *Chest*, 92, 310–312, 1987.

29. Farber, M., Sullivan, T., Fineberg, N., Carlone, S., and Manfredi, F., Effect of decreased O_2 affinity of hemoglobin on work performance during exercise in healthy humans, *J. Lab. Clin. Med.*, 104, 166–175, 1984.

30. Cade, R., Privette, M., and Lunne, D., Effect of phosphate on 2,3-DPG, O_2 tension and hematocrit in patients on chronic hemodialysis, *Kidney Int.*, 16, 919, 1979.

31. Gibby, O.M., Veale, K.E.A., Hayes, T.M., Jones, J.G., and Wardrop, C.A.J., Oxygen availability from blood and the effect of phosphate replacement on erythrocyte 2,3-diphosphoglycerate and haemoglobin–oxygen affinity in diabetic ketoacidosis, *Diabetologia*, 15, 381–385, 1978.

32. Brain, M. and Card, R., Effect of inorganic phosphate on red cell metabolism — in vitro and in vivo studies, in *Hemoglobin and Red Cell Structure and Function*, Brewer, G., Ed., Plenum Press, New York, 1972, 88–124.

33. Jain, S., Effect of phosphate supplementation on oxygen delivery at high altitude, *Int. J. Biometeorol.,* 31, 249, 1987.
34. Fuller, T.J., Nichols, W.W., Brenner, B.J., and Peterson, J.C., Reversible depression in myocardial performance in dogs with experimental phosphorus deficiency, *J. Clin. Invest.,* 62, 1194, 1978.
35. Darsee, J.R. and Nutter, D.O., Reversible severe congestive cardiomyopathy in three cases of hypophosphatemia, *Ann. Intern. Med.,* 89, 867, 1978.
36. Stoff, J.S., Phosphate homeostasis and hypophosphatemia, *Am. J. Med.,* 72, 489–495, 1982.
37. Lunne, D., Zauner, C., Cade, R., Wright, T., and Conte, M., Effect of phosphate loading on RBC 2,3-DPG, cardiac output, and oxygen utilization at rest and during vigorous exercise, *Clin. Res.,* 28, 810, 1990.
38. Moore, L. and Brewer, G., Beneficial effect of rightward hemoglobin–oxygen dissociation curve for short-term high-altitude adaptation, *J. Lab. Clin. Med.,* 98, 145–154, 1981.
39. Kreider, R.B., Miller, G.W., Schenck, D., Cortes, C.W., Miriel, V., Somma, C.T., Rowland, P., Turner, C., and Hill, D., Effects of phosphate loading on metabolic and myocardial responses to maximal and endurance exercise, *Int. J. Sport Nutr.,* 2, 20–47, 1992.
40. Miller, R., Boska, M., Moussavi, R., Carson, P., and Weiner, M., 31P nuclear magnetic resonance studies of high energy phosphates and pH in human muscle fatigue: comparison of aerobic and anaerobic exercise, *J. Clin. Invest.,* 81, 1190–1196, 1988.
41. Williams, M.H., Drugs and sports performance, in *Sports Medicine,* Ryan, A. and Allman, F., Eds., Academic Press, New York, 1989.
42. Miller, G.W., Kreider, R.B., Schenck, D., Cortes, C.W., Miriel, V., and Crosson, D., Effects of phosphate loading on anaerobic threshold, *Med. Sci. Sports Exercise,* 23, S35, 1991.
43. Williams, M.H., *Nutritional Aspects of Human Physical and Athletic Performance,* Charles C Thomas, Springfield, IL, 1985.
44. Embden, G., Grafe, E., and Schmitz, E., Uber Steigerung der Leistungsfahigkeit durch Phosphazufuhr, *Z. Physiol. Chem.,* 113, 67, 1921.
45. Riabuschinsky, N., The effect of phosphate on work and respiratory exchange, *Z. Dtsch. Gesamte Exp. Med.,* 72, 20–31, 1930.
46. Atzler, E. and Lehmann, G., Die Wirkung von Lecithin auf Arbeitsstoffwechsel und Leistungsfahigkeit, *Arbeitsphysiologie,* 9, 76–93, 1935.
47. Dennig, H., Uber Steigerung der korperlichen Leistungsfahigkeit durch Eingriffe in den Sauerbasenhaushalt, *Dtsch. Med. Wochenschr.,* 63, 733–736, 1937.
48. Boje, O., Doping: a study of the means employed to raise the level of performance in sport, *League Nations Bull. Health Organ.,* 8, 439–469, 1939.
49. Johnson, W. and Black, D., Comparison of effects of certain blood alkalinizers and glucose upon competitive endurance performance, *J. Appl. Physiol.,* 5, 577–578, 1953.
50. Staton, W., The influence of soya lecithin on muscular strength, *Res. Q. Am. Assoc. Health Phys. Educ.,* 22, 201–207, 1951.
51. Keller, W. and Kraut, H., Work and nutrition, *World Rev. Nutr. Diet.,* 3, 65–81, 1959.
52. Lictman, M., Miller, D., Cohen, J., and Waterhouse, C., Reduced red cell glycolysis, 2,3-diphosphoglycerate and adenosine triphosphate concentration, and increased hemoglobin–oxygen affinity caused by hypophosphatemia, *Ann. Intern. Med.,* 74, 562–568, 1971.
53. Lictman, M., Miller, D., and Freeman, R., Erythrocyte adenosine triphosphate depletion during hypophosphatemia in a uremic patient, *N. Engl. J. Med.,* 280, 240–244, 1969.
54. Lictman, M. and Miller, D., Erythrocyte glycolysis, adenosine triphosphate and 2,3-diphosphoglycerate concentration and adenosine hydrolysis in uremic patients: relationship to extracellular phosphate, *J. Lab. Clin. Med.,* 76, 267–279, 1970.
55. Benesch, R. and Benesch, R.E., The effect of organic phosphates from human erythrocyte on allosteric properties of hemoglobin, *Biochem. Biophys. Res. Commun.,* 26, 162, 1967.
56. Benesch, R. and Benesch, R.E., Reciprocal binding of oxygen and diphosphoglycerate by human hemoglobin, *Proc. Natl. Acad. Sci. U.S.A.,* 59, 52, 1968.
57. Chanutin, A. and Curnish, R., Effect of organic and inorganic phosphates on oxygen equilibrium and human erythrocytes, *Arch. Biochem. Biophys.,* 121, 96–102, 1967.

58. Eaton, J., Brewer, G., Schlitz, J., and Sing, C., Variation in 2,3-diphosphoglycerate and ATP levels in human erythrocytes and effects on oxygen transport, in *Red Cell Metabolism and Function*, Brewer, G., Ed., Plenum Press, New York, 1970, 147–166.
59. Kawai, M., Guth, K., Winnikes, K., Haist, C., and Ruegg, J., The effect of inorganic phosphate on ATP hydrolysis rate and the tension transients in chemically skinned rabbit psoas fibers, *Eur. J. Appl. Physiol.*, 408, 109, 1987.
60. Nakoa, K., Direct relationship of adenosine triphosphate level and in vivo viability of erythrocytes, *Nature*, 197, 877–878, 1962.
61. Piiper, J., Di Prampero, P., and Cerretelli, P., Oxygen debt and high-energy phosphates in gastrocnemius muscle of the dog, *Am. J. Physiol.*, 215, 523–531, 1968.
62. Rose, Z., Enzymes controlling 2,3-diphosphoglycerate in human erythrocytes, *Fed. Proc.*, 29, 1105, 1970.
63. Rose, Z. and Liebowitz, J., 2,3-Diphosphoglycerate phosphatase from human erythrocytes: general procedures and activation anions, *J. Biol. Chem.*, 245, 3232, 1970.
64. Sestoft, L. and Bartels, P., Regulation of metabolism by inorganic phosphate, in *Short-Term Regulation of Liver Metabolism*, Hue, L. and Van de Were, G., Eds., North-Holland, Amsterdam, 1981.
65. Koobs, D., Phosphate mediation of the Crabtree and Pasteur effects, *Science*, 178, 127–133, 1972.
66. Brazy, P., Mandel, S., Gullans. S., and Soltoff, S., Interactions between phosphate and oxidative metabolism in proximal renal tubules, *Am. J. Physiol.*, 247, 575–581, 1984.
67. Brazy, P., Gullans. S., Mandel, L., and Dennis. V., Metabolic requirements for inorganic phosphate by the rabbit proximal tubule: evidence for a Crabtree effect, *J. Clin. Invest.*, 70, 53–62, 1982.
68. Chobanian, M.C., Anderson, M.E., and Brazy, P.C., An NMR study of cellular phosphates and membrane transport in renal proximal tubules, *Am. J. Physiol.*, 268, F375–384, 1995.
69. Stewart, I., McNaughton, L., Davies, P., and Tristram, S., Phosphate loading and the effects of VO_{2max} in trained cyclists, *Res Q.*, 61, 80–84, 1990.
70. Duffy, D. and Conlee, R., Effects of phosphate loading on leg power and high intensity treadmill exercise, *Med. Sci. Sport Exercise*, 18, 674–677, 1986.
71. Mannix, E.T., Stager, J.M., Harris, A., and Farber, M.O., Oxygen delivery and cardiac output during exercise following oral phosphate–glucose, *Med. Sci. Sport Exercise*, 22, 341–347, 1990.
72. Kraemer, W.J., Gordon, S.E., Lynch, J.M., Pop, M.E., and Clark, K.L., Effects of multibuffer supplementation on acid–base balance and 2,3-diphosphoglycerate following repetitive anaerobic exercise, *Int. J. Sport Nutr.*, 5, 300–314, 1995.
73. Galloway, S.D., Tremblay, M.S., Sexsmith, J.R., and Roberts, C.J., The effects of acute phosphate supplementation in subjects of different aerobic fitness levels, *Eur. J. Appl. Physiol.*, 72, 224–230, 1996.

Chapter **4**

MAGNESIUM IN EXERCISE AND SPORT

Lorraine R. Brilla
V. Patteson Lombardi

CONTENTS

0-8493-8196-7/99/$0.00+$.50
© 1999 by CRC Press LLC

I. INTRODUCTION

The primary goals of this chapter are to review research on magnesium (Mg) status, to examine the roles of Mg in skeletal muscle and energy production, and to succinctly present a current digest on the influence of Mg on exercise. Directions for future research are also presented.

Mg is crucial to many physical and chemical processes essential for optimal growth, health, and life itself. Mg is an activator of entire classes of enzymes, including those which guide the production of adenosine triphosphate (ATP). Mg is required for maintaining the shape and function of nuclear and mitochondrial deoxyribonucleic acid (DNA), ribonucleic acid (RNA), and ribosomes, protein-synthesizing factories. Thus, Mg is essential for transcription of genes and translation and regulation of proteins. Mg is also required for optimal functioning of the immediate (ATP–phosphocreatine), nonoxidative (glycolytic), and oxidative (aerobic) energy systems. It is clear that because Mg is required for muscle protein formation and regulation and all forms of energy transduction,[1-7] it is vitally important in aerobic and anaerobic exercise. However, because the dynamics of Mg homeostasis are rather poorly understood[8] and relatively few studies have examined the role of Mg in exercise, the precise role of Mg remains unclear.

II. MAGNESIUM STATUS

There is no consensus regarding the measurement of Mg status, which cannot be defined completely by a single measurement. It may be technically difficult to determine true Mg deficiency, which is classified as *marginal,* likely due to inadequate dietary intake and/or stress, or *profound,* which is secondary to factors such as malabsorption and recently identified genetic factors.[9,10]

A detailed two-tiered classification of Mg deficiency has been proposed.[11] There are three subcategories for stage I, all associated with normal serum Mg and difficult to detect: latent, occult, and subclinical (Figure 1). These are differentiated by an *Mg load test.* In latent Mg deficiency, there is a greater than 25% but less than 50% excretion of the load. As in occult, the excretion of the load in subclinical deficiency exceeds 50%, but decreased Mg in erythrocytes is an added criterion. In stage II, a lower than normal serum Mg is found in all four subclasses: acute, chronic, extreme, and death due to severe depletion. Stage I deficiency occurs mainly in those who are physically active, and common signs and symptoms include neuromuscular irritability, lower extremity cramps, migraine headaches, pre-

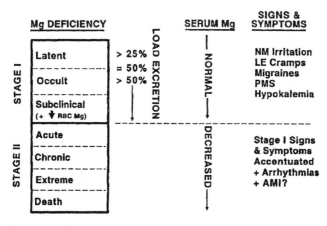

FIGURE 1 Magnesium deficiency classification criteria. (Adapted from Mansmann.[11,204])

menstrual syndrome, and hypokalemia. Those who are exposed to physical or psychological stress may also have a reduction in Mg.[3,12–20] Hypomagnesemia is most frequently acquired and secondary to inadequate dietary intake and increased urinary secretion, although it may be linked to medical abnormalities or iatrogenic agents such as thiazide diuretics and digitalis preparations.[21–23]

The concern with athletes is stage I or marginal Mg deficiency, as inherited Mg deficiencies are profound and usually present themselves early in an individual's life.[10] Most often, marginal deficiencies can be corrected simply by making wise food choices or by providing oral Mg supplements. It is not clear whether the additional Mg corrects the underlying deficiency state or possesses a unique pharmacological action. Mechanisms of action most likely involve normalizing or redistributing associated ions, including calcium and potassium, and/or enhancing phosphotransfer reactions.[5,24] Additional losses through urine and sweat can also contribute to a suboptimal Mg status,[25,26] although the level of dietary Mg needed for optimizing physical activity has not been established. Adrenergic effects of stress, both psychological and physical,[27] induce a shift of Mg from the intracellular to extracellular fluid space, which increases urinary output and depletes body stores.

A. DETERMINATION

Mg plays a vital role in maintaining the nervous, musculoskeletal, and cardiovascular systems, yet hypomagnesemia is likely the most underdiagnosed electrolyte deficiency.[28,29] Many factors may alter serum and urinary Mg, including acid–base balance, physical and mental stresses, and volume expansion. Serum Mg varies approximately 3% within and 7% between subjects, while urinary output varies more so, 26 to 36%.[30] Serum Mg is not included in routine screening, and a deficit can mimic other electrolyte imbalances.[29] Even if it is measured, serum Mg may be of limited prognostic value, because as little as 1% of the total body Mg may be present in the extracellular fluid compartment.[31] Serum values may not reflect tissue levels, as those with normal or marginal serum Mg levels may have low whole body, muscle, or bone Mg stores. Repeated measurements of serum Mg may be useful, with an intrasubject change of approximately 10% considered clinically significant. Urinary Mg excretion in steady-state, healthy individuals may reflect the Mg adequacy of the diet.[30] Muscle Mg has been suggested as a reliable way of measuring Mg status, but the invasive nature of a biopsy, subject discomfort, and cost must be considered. While methods for measuring intracellular Mg in muscle and leukocytes have been developed, their accuracy and usefulness require further verification.[31] Ion-selective electrodes exist, but their relevance to Mg metabolism is not clearly established.[30] Free Mg^{2+} concentration is important because it is the biologically active form, but practical, routine techniques for assessing it are not available.[32]

Mg infusion or *loading* may be the best way to determine true Mg deficiency. For this procedure, Mg is given intravenously and a 24-hr urine sample is collected to assess differences between input and output. Patients with a true Mg deficiency retain abnormally large amounts of the intravenous load,[29] with retention in excess of 20% considered pathological.[33] For example, patients with ischemic heart disease retain approximately one- to two-thirds of an Mg load compared to only 5% retention in controls. Running for about three-quarters of an hour just prior to loading may yield somewhat greater variability in Mg excretion, but infusion appears to be well tolerated by subjects, with only feelings of warmth or light headache reported.[33] There is an inverse relationship between load retention and skeletal muscle Mg.[34] Incorporating Mg load testing within double-blind, crossover supplementation studies will help clarify the effects of marginal Mg deficiency on exercise and sports performance.

Mg deficiencies may occur without overt signs and symptoms, which do not appear until extracellular levels have dropped to 1 meq/l (0.5 mmol/l) or less.[8] Significant Mg depletion can induce muscular weakness, irritability, tetany, bizarre facial and eye movements or twitches, confusion, hallucinations, convulsions, and cardiac arrhythmias.[6–8,22,35] Mg deficiency in infants and children can prevent normal growth and development. Mg is in great demand during pregnancy because it is needed to build the fetal skeleton.[36] It is apparent that using clinical end points, overt signs, or serum Mg may not be appropriate for detecting stage I marginal Mg deficiencies.[2,3,37] Serum Mg may not reflect whole muscle or intracellular stores; nearly half of patients with normal serum values have low muscle Mg.[38]

In contrast to Mg deficiency, excess oral Mg does not appear to induce symptoms of toxicity. Even large doses of Mg ingested in the form of laxative Epsom salts have not been associated with ill effects, except diarrhea.[22]

B. PREVALENCE OF DEFICIENCY

The average daily dietary consumption of Mg by adults in the U.S. is 76% of the Recommended Dietary Allowance (RDA) and has declined considerably from an estimated 410 mg/day since 1910.[39-43] Approximately 75% of the U.S. population obtains less than the Mg RDA, with about 40% consuming less than 70% of the recommended value.[39-43] Thus, based on dietary assessments alone, without even considering genetic predisposition, 75% of the population may be subjected to stage I (marginal) or stage II (frank) Mg deficiency.

A true dietary Mg deficiency exists when less than 70% of the RDA for Mg is obtained. Average or marginal Mg consumption may be further exaggerated by extreme activity or other severe physical or psychological stressors.[12-16,36] Some athletes obtain adequate dietary Mg,[44-49] but those who are most often weight-conscious, including gymnasts, ballerinas, and wrestlers, consume about two-thirds of the RDA,[50-52] a value similar to that of young untrained subjects initiating an exercise program.[53] Those individuals on low-energy diets should focus on obtaining Mg-dense foods,[54] but a lower than recommended Mg intake (~80% of RDA) may occur in those who are physically active, despite a relatively high kilocalorie intake (~3000 kcal/day).[55] Elite female marathoners[56] and collegiate cross-country runners,[57] female swimmers,[58] and female and male triathletes[60] may also consume considerably less than the RDA for Mg. Compared to female athletes, male athletes may have a greater dietary consumption of Mg but lower red cell Mg values.[58,59] Although further studies are certainly warranted, this may be due to erythrocyte sequestering of Mg to offset losses through menstruation or subtle differences between estrogen and testosterone on shuttling between mobile Mg storage pools.

C. DIETARY SOURCES AND AVAILABILITY

Mg is prevalent in many foods including legumes, dark green vegetables, seafoods, nuts, grains, and chocolate, with the most concentrated sources per serving found in spinach, oysters, sunflower seeds, and lima beans.[22] Despite widespread availability of Mg, surveys demonstrate that the RDA is rarely achieved.[61] There may be seasonal variations in Mg intake, with highs in the spring and summer and lows in the winter, likely influenced by the availability of fresh vegetables, seafood, legumes, nuts, and grains. The Mg RDA for a 15- to 18-year-old male is 400 mg/day, while that for a 15- to 18-year-old female is 300 mg/day. Adult females should obtain between 280 to 300 mg and adult males 350 mg/day. It is recommended that a pregnant female acquire 320 mg/day and a lactating female 355 mg/day during the first 6 months of lactation.

A high-fat diet impedes the absorption of Mg and may elevate body Mg requirements.[62-64] Because dietary fat consumed by Americans averages an estimated 37% of total kilocalories ingested,[65] which is 7% higher than recommended by a number of national organizations,[65-68] it is likely that most Americans are predisposed to marginal Mg deficiency.

While less is known about the effects of a high-protein diet on Mg absorption, strength-trained male athletes who consume well over double the RDA for protein do have an adequate dietary intake of Mg (about 135% of the RDA).[69] However, a high-protein diet may enhance the need for Mg,[70] which is required for the synthesis of gastrointestinal enzymes and proteolytic activity. A diet high in protein is not only common to strength-event athletes but is quite prevalent in the general U.S. population. Thus, despite daily intakes of Mg that meet or exceed the RDA, hyperproteinemia may make a large number of Americans, particularly strength-trained males, prone to stage I Mg deficiencies.

Together with carbohydrate, fat, and protein distributions in the diet, the ingestion of other minerals, particularly divalent cations, influences whole body Mg. Minerals are linked in a complex cascade, whereby an excess of one often depresses the absorption or bioavailability of another. For example, the ingestion of calcium reduces the bioavailability of Mg^{63} and iron.[22] Thus, a diet high in dairy products may act synergistically with other common dietary practices (e.g., low-carbohydrate, high-fat, high-protein meals) to reduce further whole body Mg stores.

Like other nutrients, Mg is easily lost from foods during processing. The downward trend in the consumption of Mg over the last century is likely due to the modern-day generation's greater reliance on processed foods. Also, agricultural practices and pollution factors may disrupt the Mg content of the soil. Mg deficiency in humans may be due to a decreased availability of Mg in the ecosystem.[71] The combination of acidic rains, emissions, and intensive use of soils may create an exchange of extractable aluminum and Mg. The consequence is insufficient Mg in the food chain. Further evidence for the significance of a decrease in environmental Mg is indicated by the lower Mg content of garden soils and water associated with high incidences of amyotrophic lateral sclerosis and Parkinson's disease.[72-75] An insufficiency of dietary Mg with aluminum load induced increases in aluminum and calcium concentrations in the nervous system and neurodegradation.[75] Tilling practices and leaching in the Mississippi River watershed have resulted in loss of soil Mg, and Mg content in American streams has decreased from about 24 mg/l in 1973 to 17 mg/l in 1995.[76] Because only about one-third of an adult's average daily Mg intake is absorbed by the small intestine,[8] seemingly marginal dietary deficiencies may be compounded substantially by these apparently global environmental factors.

D. SUPPLEMENTATION

In addition to often unusual dietary practices, it is common for athletes to rely upon supplements. Despite supplementation, nearly one-quarter of athletes may have Mg intakes below the RDA, with males obtaining about 90% and females about 75% of recommended values.[52,60] A daily multivitamin-mineral supplement[59] or Mg supplementation at 33% of the RDA for 3 months[77] may not alter athletes' blood Mg values. A dietary limit for Mg saturation may exist because urinary excretion rates of Mg may increase for up to nearly 4 months when strength-trained athletes take Mg supplements.[78] This lower saturation limit may be further defined by combining Mg load tests with Mg urinalyses in supplementation research. Acute Mg supplementation during 2 hr of endurance exercise does not alter the decline in plasma Mg.[79] Mg–aspartate salts have been used to improve endurance performance with conflicting results.[80,81] No effect of this salt is seen on force production in humans.[82]

Marginal Mg intake may be offset by exercise, which may enhance the absorption and therefore bioavailability of Mg.[83] Although it has been documented that physical activity induces decreases in specific body pools of Mg, such as plasma and perhaps bone,[16,84] it is still unclear as to how much regular physical activity may increase the body's need for Mg. In contrast to those who engage in restrictive dieting or rely on supplements, athletes who emphasize carbohydrate loading or vegetarianism may enhance their Mg status. For example, runners who consume a diet of approximately 3500 kcal, nearly two-thirds of which is carbohydrate, obtain almost double the RDA for Mg.[85] Provided enough calories are consumed, a vegetarian diet without supplementation may provide adequate to high levels of Mg.[86]

E. STRESS AND MAGNESIUM COMPARTMENTALIZATION

Mg deficiency may accentuate the adverse effects of exposure to acute or prolonged stress.[87] Long-term deficits in Mg intake may disrupt Mg homeostasis and induce a pathological positive feedback regenerative cycle.

Acute exercise in animals on normal diets without deficiencies or supplements decreases serum Mg, but the decline appears transient and returns to baseline during recovery.[88,89] Surprisingly, this recovery response seems to be more pronounced in male animals, perhaps due to the unique effects of testosterone versus estrogen on Mg homeostasis.[89] Animals fed Mg-deficient diets have depressed Mg in plasma, red cells, bone, and muscle, but the muscle decrease appears to be corrected by moderate to long-term endurance exercise.[84–88] Also, intermediate to chronic endurance training in animals appears to enhance the ability to recover to homeostasis when Mg deficiencies are induced, which implies that endurance exercise alters Mg balance and redistribution to tissue storage sites. Short-duration endurance exercise training may not alter serum Mg levels, but may create lower Mg in bone of female animals and erythrocytes of male animals. Again, gender differences are likely due to unique influences of androgenic versus estrogenic-type hormones on Mg homeostasis.

Supplementation may improve bone and plasma Mg, but may not alter Mg concentrations in soft connective tissues or relatively rapid turnover pools including skeletal muscle, kidney, red cells, and hepatocytes. Thus, apparently supplementation can enhance bone Mg content. Bone is a more rigid connective tissue storage site and appears to be relatively selfish in sequestering minerals compared to other less dense connective tissues (e.g., erythrocytes) with a more diffuse extracellular matrix. Compared to controls, chronically endurance-trained animals have lower Mg levels in muscle, liver, and red blood cells. Thus, animal studies indicate that marginal Mg deficiencies in specialized body compartments may occur in response to moderate to long-term endurance exercise training.[21,60]

Consistent, repeated, metabolic acidosis induced during high-intensity, chronic exercise sessions may work to redistribute Mg from soft tissues to plasma and foster a higher concentration of Mg excreted in urine.[56] Future studies should confirm this observation through Mg loading and urinalyses.

The results of human studies are somewhat consistent with those derived from animal research, although few have examined exercise training and Mg compartmentalization. Mg supplements given to adolescent female swimmers increase serum but not red blood cell Mg.[90] Moderately endurance-trained male athletes have higher serum Mg levels compared to controls matched for energy expenditure,[62] but erythrocyte Mg levels are lower in trained versus untrained males.[91] Compared to controls, moderately endurance-trained females have slightly lower serum Mg, while endurance-trained female athletes have substantially lower serum Mg[92,93] but higher red cell Mg.[74] Serum or plasma Mg may be entirely transient and in fact an inappropriate measure, providing little if any information about Mg homeostasis in trained individuals. Elite male and female athletes may have similar resting serum Mg values compared to untrained subjects,[94] and acute endurance competition may or may not alter serum Mg levels.[95] The effect on muscle Mg in athletes is unknown. Supplements may help correct but not normalize reduced muscle Mg in patients treated with diuretics.[96] Certainly, there is much work to be done to help clarify the effects of exercise and stress on Mg homeostasis. Future studies should (1) identify the form of exercise involved, (2) ensure that subjects are indeed in a resting state (at least 48 hr postexercise when examining the influence of chronic training), (3) rely upon Mg loading and urinalyses, (4) measure Mg content in a variety of body compartments simultaneously, and (5) focus on clarifying female and male differences.

III. METABOLISM

Physical activity requires greater energy production to meet the increased needs of working muscle. In maximal muscular exercise in well-trained athletes, overall metabolic heat production can increase 20-fold above baseline during aerobic training and up to 50-fold above baseline during short bursts of anaerobic activity.[97,98] All energy for muscle contraction comes from the hydrolysis of ATP, which involves the cleavage of high-energy phosphate bonds by the enzymatic addition of water.[99] All known adenosine triphosphatase (ATPase) reactions require Mg for ATP hydrolysis.[100,101] In skeletal muscle, Mg must be attached to ATP before the thick-filament myosin ATPase can hydrolyze ATP. Mg is also essential for the activity of the calcium–Mg ATPase enzyme, which pumps calcium back into the sarcoplasmic reticulum (SR) to induce relaxation. Thus, in order for skeletal muscle contraction to proceed normally, adequate levels of Mg are required.[102]

A. METABOLIC PATHWAYS

Creatine phosphokinase (CPK, also called creatine kinase) is a key enzyme in the formation of ATP by the immediate energy system. CPK is regulated by free Mg and hydrogen ion concentrations.[103] ATP is preferentially synthesized when Mg levels are high, while creatine phosphate is synthesized when Mg levels are low.[104,105]

Mg is an absolute requirement for over two-thirds of the enzymes involved in glycolysis, including phosphofructokinase, the key regulatory catalyst. Glucokinase catalyzes an essentially irreversible reaction in the very first step of glycolysis, producing glucose 6-phosphate from glucose, with the Mg^{2+} chelate of ATP (Mg^{2+}–ATP^{4-}) as the actual substrate. If not for the positive effector activity of the Mg chelate and inorganic phosphate, the glucokinase reaction would proceed at only 5% of $\dot{V}_{max}$.[106] Mg is the only alkaline-earth metal that reacts with enolase.[107] Altered glucose homeostasis is influenced by Mg, through its effects on liver glycogen content, glucose disposal, and insulin sensitivity.[108–112]

Pyruvate dehydrogenase contains a number of proteins and coenzymes including thiamin pyrophosphate, which requires Mg for its synthesis.[106] Thus, Mg is essential for making a key catalytic cofactor of a multienzyme, which is poised as a regulatory switch between anaerobic and aerobic metabolism. Further, isocitrate dehydrogenase requires Mg for its activity and determines the overall rate of the citric acid cycle.[100,113]

Mg deficiency depresses key regulatory glycolytic and oxidative enzymes which are critical for energy production. Deficiency in animals is associated with red blood cell membrane disruption and mitochondrial disturbances and swelling.[45,114,115] These alterations in cell and organelle membrane function presumed to be caused by disturbances in lipid metabolism may adversely affect the transport of ions and nutrients and the bioenergetics of glycolytic and oxidative metabolism.[116–118]

Mg also influences ATP production both directly and indirectly by functioning in lipid metabolism. Fasting, cold exposure, and endurance exercise stimulate lipid mobilization through beta-adrenergic stimulation.[98,119–121] Beta-adrenergic stimulation increases the second messenger, cyclic adenosine monophosphate, which increases lipolysis and simultaneously decreases extracellular Mg. Extracellular Mg is sequestered by adipocytes and chelated by free fatty acids. Sodium nicotinate, a derivative of the reduced coenzyme NADH, which has an antilipolytic action, inhibits the production of nonesterified fatty acids and ketone bodies and prevents hypomagnesemia.[121] Hypomagnesemia has been detected in subjects who engage in continuous exercise for longer than 1 hr.[16,20,122] Adrenergic outflow, which stimulates lipolysis and induces an influx of Mg into adipocytes, may partially account for this exercise-associated reduction in serum Mg, yet this may not be the case, as 2 hr of endurance exercise with supplemental glucose does not alter plasma Mg but damps increases in free fatty acids.[79] The fatty acid–glucose–Mg connection as well as other indirect mechanisms require further investigation.

Dietary Mg deficiency decreases plasma protein levels and overall growth in animals.[97,98] This depression may be caused by a direct or indirect inhibitory effect of Mg on (1) genes which code for protein-type hormones such as growth hormone or (2) mitogens like insulin-like growth factor-1 (IGF-1) which help modulate protein synthesis. IGF-1 is regulated by the divalent cations zinc and Mg.[122] Mg deficiency also affects sodium/potassium pump concentrations, which results in disturbances of electrolyte function and further affects muscle protein function.[95,104,105]

B. METABOLIC BY-PRODUCTS

In the past decade, it has been clearly demonstrated that strenuous physical exercise induces oxidative stress.[126–128] Proposed sources of oxidative stress include mitochondrial superoxide production and autoxidation of catecholamines. Severe or prolonged exercise can overwhelm antioxidant defenses, as evidenced by direct measurements of antioxidants such as glutathione. Free-radical-induced damage in muscle may be one of a multitude of factors which lead to fatigue during exercise.[129] In heart dysfunction, cardiac tissue mineral contents of calcium, copper, and iron are reduced, and in Mg deficiency, iron-, copper-, and aluminum-induced oxidations are heightened.[130–138] At high concentrations, Mg may inhibit lipid peroxidation directly, but in low concentrations may deplete glutathione and potentiate lipid peroxidation.[138] Antioxidants like vitamin E may offer significant protection against the oxidative stress aggravated by Mg deficiency;[132] however, oxidative damage is not the direct result of a decreased vitamin E status.[134] Humans have reduced Mg and a tendency for increases in oxidative stress after 40 min of running.[139] Glutathione is higher following aerobic training with an increase in superoxide dismutase activity, typically depressed in Mg deficiency.[140] Certainly, additional exercise research, examining a range of subjects from young to old and normal to pathological, is needed to clarify the role of Mg in resistance to oxidative damage.

IV. TARGET TISSUE: MUSCLE

Mg plays important roles in muscular contraction/relaxation, the maintenance of energy, and electrochemical equilibrium, given its diverse association with phosphate compounds, structural and enzymatic proteins, intracellular organelles, and cytoskeletal components in muscle. Electron-probe analyses demonstrate that approximately 20% of whole muscle Mg is bound to ATP (Mg^{2+}–ATP) in frogs, with most of the remaining amounts stored in creatine phosphate and the calcium-sensor protein parvalbumin.[141] Within the sarcoplasm, some Mg is bound to troponin, myosin light chains, and F-actin.[142-144] Mg in the SR is bound to the calcium pump ATPase, parvalbumin, and calmodulin.[143]

The energy requirement of exercise increases the demand for Mg because it is required for the mechanochemical transduction of ATP hydrolysis.[101] Mg anchors adenosine diphosphate (ADP) at the myosin active site.[145] The myosin head is an actin-activated, Mg-dependent ATPase.[146] Mg ion can chelate or bind to one of two sites on the ATP molecule: between the first and second or second and third phosphate. Thus, Mg must be absolutely essential for regulating the entire contractile cycle including (1) ATP binding to the nucleotide-binding pocket on the myosin head, (2) inorganic phosphate release and power stroke initiation, (3) stabilizing bound ADP within the transient intermediate configuration of the myosin head, (4) ADP release from the myosin head, and (5) binding of a fresh ATP molecule to the myosin head nucleotide pocket to dislodge myosin from actin. Mg also helps calcium regulate troponin and functions in the calcium–Mg ATPase enzyme responsible for SR calcium uptake to effect relaxation. Clearly, the direct and indirect effects of Mg, as well as its functions which are synergistic and antagonistic to calcium and other divalent cations, require considerable further study.

A. DETAILED FUNCTIONS

Mg is needed to ensure high-energy activation of the myosin head, which contains an ATPase enzyme, as well as the subsequent interaction of the myosin head with the actin binding site. Without Mg attached to ATP, the myosin ATPase cannot hydrolyze the ATP,[102] and no energy would be available for cross-bridge cycling. This absolute requirement of Mg for cross-bridge cycling makes it absolutely essential for the performance of all physical activities.

The interaction of calcium with the regulatory protein troponin primarily determines whether or not a muscle fiber contracts or relaxes. Pure troponin C, the calcium-binding unit of troponin, has six divalent cationic binding sites. Two of the binding sites have an exclusive affinity for calcium and two bind Mg, while the remaining two bind with either ion.[106,147,148] Mg alters the conformational state of troponin to inhibit the interaction of myosin and actin during contraction; this underlies the depressant effect of shortening.[143] The transient decrease in muscle force during shortening is enhanced by increased Mg.

An essential Mg ATPase reaction in pumps is used to concentrate calcium in the SR. The transport of calcium by the SR is Mg dependent.[149-155] Relatively fast phosphorylation of SR calcium ATPase is attributed to an Mg-dependent accelerating effect of ATP on the isomerization of ATPase.[156,157] Increases in Mg stimulate the SR active transport system for calcium.[154]

Mitochondria produce most of the ATP needed for exercise; a proton-motive force is used to generate ATP. ATP is synthesized by an inner mitochondrial membrane enzyme complex called ATP synthase, also known as F_0F_1, or H^+–ATPase.[100] ATP synthase, like all ATPase enzymes, requires Mg for its activation. Skeletal muscle mitochondria also have a highly active, energy-dependent, Mg transport system.[158] The mitochondrial potassium–hydrogen ion exchanger which helps to regulate mitochondrial matrix volume is inhibited by Mg.[114] The mitochondrial potassium–hydrogen ion exchanger which helps to regulate mitochondrial matrix volume and ion distribution is inhibited by Mg.[114] Hindering this exchanger could depress the inner to outer mitochondrial membrane proton gradient and inhibit synthase production of ATP. With extreme Mg deficiency, there is severe mitochondrial swelling[45,115] together with disruption of the SR membrane. Alterations in membrane permeability and stability could disturb not only simple ion movement across membranes[118,159] but also macromolecular transport, cell sensitivity to extracellular signaling molecules such as hormones and neurotransmitters, and overall cell viability. These roles of Mg bear significant implications for exercise performance.

Each of the 20 building-block amino acids must be picked up and carried by a unique transfer ribonucleic acid (tRNA) to ribosomes, where the synthesis of all proteins, including structural and enzymatic muscle proteins, takes place. The single enzyme aminoacyl-tRNA synthetase, which catalyzes the linkage of the tRNA with a specific amino acid, requires Mg for its activity.[106] Thus, Mg not only is required for the hydrolysis of ATP so that muscle contraction can proceed normally but also is essential for the building of crucial regulatory and contractile muscle proteins. Inadequate amounts of Mg will compromise muscle building and subsequent contractions[109] and limit the performance of both anaerobic and aerobic activities. Additionally, the roles of Mg in linking amino acids to tRNA and in ribosomal protein production imply that it is an important limiting factor in recovery from intense exercise and in repair and healing of damaged muscle.

B. FORCE PRODUCTION AND PATHOLOGY

Mg inadequacy causes decreased absolute and relative force production and muscle hyperexcitability, reflected by spasms, cramps, and even tetany, in chronic or severe Mg deficiency.[69,160,161] Mg deficiency in animal muscles causes a marked tension reduction for both single-twitch and tetanus contractions and significantly prolongs half-relaxation time.[160] These decrements are attributed to irreversible skeletal muscle myopathy including fiber swelling, sarcomere cytoskeletal striatal disruption, swollen and vacuolated mitochondria, and ultimately reduced muscle mass.

In clinical studies, maximal voluntary contraction of the quadriceps is positively correlated with muscle and serum Mg.[161] Hypomagnesemic patients have lower isometric strength in a variety of muscles.[161–163] Healthy subjects who are supplemented with Mg and engage in strength training have significantly greater gains in torque production compared to nonsupplemented strength-trained controls.[53] Mg may augment force production through its regulation of protein synthesis, a process which is highly sensitive to available Mg.[165,167] Severe Mg depletion induces conformational changes in ribosomes with subsequent rhabdomyolysis.[115,165] The entire flow of information from the nucleus to the cytoplasm within all cells, including myocytes — from transcription of DNA to RNA to translation or protein synthesis at the ribosome — depends upon optimal Mg availability.[166,167]

Muscle potassium and muscle Mg share nearly 40% common variance.[168] The powerful association is likely due to the action of Mg on the ATPase sodium–potassium pump[24,95,125,170] and the mitochondrial potassium–hydrogen ion exchanger. Mg deficiency impairs the ability of muscle to replenish potassium and also increases blood urea nitrogen (BUN) production.[28,38,120] BUN elevations may represent high protein intake, metabolic acidosis, or catabolic states associated with increased muscle breakdown, dehydration, or renal dysfunction. Ammonia is formed by muscles during exercise and may require Mg for clearance and adequate metabolism to urea, because several enzymes involved in this process are dependent upon Mg salts.[174] Inadequate Mg and potassium and increased urea may increase the likelihood of contractures or a slower response to relaxation and ultimately reduce force production.

Inadequate Mg is implicated in fibromyalgia and chronic pain syndromes.[171–173] The symptoms of fibromyalgia mimic those associated with low Mg: sleep irregularities, anxiety, fatigue, muscle spasms and jerking, stiffness, aching, and pain associated with rhabdomyolysis. Mg in combination with a complete therapy program reduces pain and trigger point involvement and enhances function. It is postulated that fibromyalgia patients have an Mg deficiency despite normal plasma Mg.

Many of the prominent signs and symptoms of Mg deficiency involve alterations in neuromuscular control including cramps, spasms or tremors, fasciculations, myoclonus, tetanus, seizures, and muscle weakness.[35,108,175–178] At least 20 to 30% of alcoholics demonstrate Mg deficiency as measured by serum, and a greater number are classified as Mg deficient based on muscle assessments.[163,164] Mg supplementation (15 mmol/day) in alcoholics increases strength significantly without an intervening strength program and also improves liver function and the status of potassium and other electrolytes.[163] Skeletal muscle myopathy resulting from Mg deficiency is similar to the myopathy described in alcoholism.[159,160,162] The underlying mechanisms contributing to hypomagnesemic-induced myopathy include the role of Mg in muscle cellular bioenergetics, excitation–contraction coupling, and functional integrity of the cell membrane.[159]

One pathophysiological attribute of muscle highly sensitive to Mg levels is *spasmophilia,* a condition in which the motor nerves show an unusual sensitivity to mechanical or electrical stimulation and patients demonstrate an uncontrollable tendency for spasms, tetany, and convulsions. This is similar to a form of epilepsy except with more prominent features demonstrated in the peripheral nervous system. When hypomagnesemia is induced in animals, tetany and contractures are observed.[149,150] Mg is still heavily concentrated in the terminal cisternae despite an increased permeability of the SR membrane to Mg during tetanus.[136]

Hypomagnesemia may depress the functioning of *desaturase,* which plays a crucial role in fatty acid metabolism and maintenance of cell membrane function and fluidity.[181] Transient contractures, spasms, and cramps during high-intensity sports performance may be induced or augmented by low levels of Mg.[182] Poor dietary Mg intake, or an enhanced Mg requirement, or changes in fatty acid metabolism induced by exercise training may promote a form of spasmophilia, which certainly would markedly impair sports performance.

There are inherited disorders that may result in severe Mg deficiency associated with disordered renal tubular reabsorption of Mg.[10,183] Hypomagnesemic tetany is one form of inherited derangement in Mg metabolism involving an isolated defect in carrier-mediated intestinal Mg transport. Hypomagnesemic tetany symptoms, including painful muscle spasms, carpopedal spasms, rhythmic blinking, shaking hands, impaired speech, and agitation, may be resistant to treatment with calcium and potassium but alleviated by Mg.[10,188] Multiple case reports solidify the Mg deficiency–spasmophilia symptom connections[178,182,184–191] and include carpopedal cramps in a female tennis player,[178] gastrocnemius spasms and pervasive muscle soreness in a male military recruit,[152] posterior thigh cramping in a paraplegic patient,[153] and spontaneous tetany with subsequent arrhythmias.[187] In all cases, the symptoms were alleviated by Mg supplementation.

Poor eating habits, an active lifestyle with enhanced fluid loss due to sweating, and contractures potentially induced by prior neuronal disruption may cause a negative Mg balance, which if perpetuated could result in deficiency. The combined effects of a poor diet and enhanced physical effort have been recognized by the South African Armed Forces, and an Mg supplement is prescribed prophylactically.[184] Even though it is difficult to study Mg and spasmophilias in a prospective manner, case reports support the contention that Mg can reduce the potential for muscle spasms and cramps.

Patients with severe tetanus and persistent autonomic dysfunction improve symptoms with adjunct Mg therapy and have decreased amplitude electromyographic (EMG) tracings in hand muscles following infusion of Mg.[187,189] Heightened EMG activity is also associated with Mg deficiency in patients with suspected spasmophilia, and Mg supplementation is recommended for therapeutic treatment in these cases.

Mg excess increases the alkalinity of the cytosol and augments cross-bridge cycling, which could enhance buffering capacity as well as muscle contractile strength and endurance for both anaerobic and aerobic exercises.[35,142] However, although overdosing is extremely rare, excessive Mg may induce toxicity[22] and may depress muscle activity, as indicated by reduced neuromuscular junctional end-plate potential amplitudes.[35,146]

EMG and Mg findings are intriguing when combined with a recent hypothesis on the etiology of muscle cramps during exercise.[192] Although the origin is poorly understood, exercise-associated skeletal muscle cramps are defined as painful, spas-modic, involuntary contractions during or immediately after physical activity. Elec-trolyte, metabolic end-product, and dehydration theories have been proposed to explain the cause of muscle cramps. Because EMG activity increases during cramp-ing and spasms in runners, and decreased amplitude of the EMG baseline is well correlated with recovery, some have theorized that cramps are caused by sustained abnormal reflex activity, secondary to muscle fatigue. Neural excitability including spasms, cramps, hyperarousal, hyperventilation, and asthenia is associated with abnormal levels of Mg and irregular electroencephalography.[27] Mg salts may im-prove symptoms. There is no question that the role of Mg in preventing exercise-induced muscle cramps is a fertile area for study.

Integrins are transmembrane heterodimers, which are crucially important re-ceptor proteins because they determine the binding and response of cells to the extracellular matrix.[99] The binding of integrins to their ligands depends upon the presence of divalent cations, Mg or calcium, depending on the particular integrin. Thus the roles of Mg and calcium appear to be expanding endlessly; they are not limited to bone homeostasis, neurotransmission, and skeletal muscle contraction and relaxation, but also include interactive effects among cells including cell mi-gration, growth, and development. Therefore, the function of Mg in skeletal muscle is more important than once presumed and probably includes broad regulation of myocytes within tissues, formation of satellite cells, hypertrophy, and hyperplasia. It is obvious that regulation of integrins by Mg together with calcium provides even more evidence of the dual importance of these ions in exercise performance and adaptation.

V. EXERCISE

Decreases in plasma Mg were first reported in humans in the 1970s after a marathon, cross-country skiing, or ergometer work.[17,20,193–196] The roles Mg plays in basic body functions, and especially the striking effects of Mg on the neuromus-cular system and in energy production, has renewed interest in Mg and exercise effects. This observation is readily evident upon perusal of Table 1. This summary table represents the primarily English-language articles on Mg and exercise from the 1970s to the present. Review articles that include sections on Mg are not included in the table.[19,60,65,197,198,219,227,236,238,240,241,243,254,256,259]

Research has shown a link between low Mg levels and impaired endurance exercise (physical activity of a continuous nature that lasts one or more hours).[199,201,202,219] Mg deficiencies may also depress performance in strength events.[69,161] The working hypothesis is that suboptimal Mg status leads to a dec-rement in exercise work output and sports performance. For the purposes of clas-sification, suboptimal is defined as less than 100% of the RDA, or less than 4 mg/ kg body weight per day. Some argue that 6 mg/kg body weight per day is needed

TABLE 1 Magnesium and Exercise Research Summary

Author	Sport or Activity	Major Findings[a]	Comments
Anderson et al. (1991)[205] n = 8	Leg exercise; immersion	NS U-Mg due to carbohydrate loading	Humans
Beals and Manore (1998)[206] n = 24 experimental n = 24 control	Various female athletes	Diet deficiencies were ameliorated by supplement practices; Mg normal	Cross-sectional study on female athletes with subclinical eating disorders
Bell et al. (1988)[255] n = 28	Weight training	U-Mg excretion higher in trained	≥1 year exercise; age-matched controls
Beller et al. (1975)[17] n = 8	Walking (90 min)	↓ S-Mg not explained by sweat Mg	Heat study
Brilla and Gunter (1995)[245] n = 32	Running	↑ time to exhaustion in humans postsupplementation	Supplementation study
Brilla and Haley (1992)[53] n = 26	Weight training	↑ strength gains with Mg supplement	Training study
Brilla and Lombardi (1987)[220] n = 32	Swimming	↑ cholesterol with ↓ D-Mg ameliorated by exercise	Animals
Brilla et al. (1989)[84] n = 32	Swimming	Slowly exchanging pools: ↓ Mg with ↓ Mg diet; exercise: ↑ skeletal muscle Mg versus controls	Animals
Buchman et al. (1998)[199] n = 26	Marathon	Significant ↓ S-Mg and ↓ U-Mg; authors speculate on ↑ muscle demand for Mg	Pre/postrace results
Caddell et al. (1986)[221] n = 84	Shock-tetany	Massive ↑ catecholamines in ↓ D-Mg	Animals
Casoni et al. (1990)[222] n = 11 experimental n = 30 control	25-km run	Athletes ↓ Mg with physical stress	Pre/postrace results

Study	Exercise	Result	Comments
Chadda et al. (1985)[223] n = 59	Max aerobic test	No significant change in Mg homeostasis	Patients
Cohen and Zimmerman (1978)[193] n = 18	Marathon runners	Highly significant ↓ S-Mg postmarathon race	Early report on ↓ S-Mg with strenuous exercise
Conn et al. (1988)[224] n = 22	Swimming, max aerobic capacity	P-Mg correlation with max aerobic capacity, r = +0.42	Not true in females
Cordova et al. (1990)[208] n = 60	Swimming	Mg only changed after swim to exhaustion	Animal study; exhaustive exercise
Cordova et al. (1992)[248] n = 40	Swimming	Exercise and hypoxia both affect Mg homeostasis	Animals; various tissue samples
Cordova et al. (1994)[47] n = 12	Ergometer tests	NS S-Mg but ↑ E-Mg after high-intensity exercise tests	Multiple high-intensity exercise
Crespo et al. (1995)[94] n = 18 runners n = 22 controls	Marathon runners	No difference in baseline Mg between elite marathon runners and control	Comparison study using prerace values compared to sedentary controls
de Haan et al. (1985)[82] n = 20 humans	Weight training	Force and local endurance not enhanced by Mg Asp	Animal and human
Deuster and Singh (1993)[79] n = 10	Running, 120 min	↓ P-Mg to lowest value at 120 min; glucose–electrolyte solution diminishes ↑ FFA → why ↓ P-Mg?	Supplementation study; replacement during run; unknown mechanism for ↓ P-Mg with smaller ↑ FFA
Deuster et al. (1986)[56] n = 13	Sprint intervals	Transient shift of Mg; ↑ U-Mg loss	90% aerobic max to exhaustion
Dolev et al. (1992)[200] n = 73	Physical training	12-week physical training program for military recruits yielded ↓ mononuclear cells-Mg; reduction in exchangeable Mg body stores; ↑ S-Mg related to rhabdomyolysis	Training study

TABLE 1   Magnesium and Exercise Research Summary (continued)

Author	Sport or Activity	Major Findings[a]	Comments
Fitzherbert (1982)[225]	Running	Effect of ↓ Mg in water, food on competition	Synopsis
Fogelhohm et al. (1992)[46] n = 21 experimental n = 18 control	Fitness training	S-Mg was similar between groups	Long-term exercise: 24 weeks
Fogelhohm (1992)[209] n = 427 experimental n = 150 control	Various	S-Mg highest in moderately trained athlete; authors conclude that sports training does not have a negative effect on biochemical indices of Mg	Survey of multiple data collections
Fogelhohm et al. (1993)[252]	Weight class sports: wrestling, judo	D-Mg intake below recommendation during weight loss procedures; no impaired performance in anaerobic tests over 3 weeks	Short-term study on ↓ Mg diet in anaerobic sports
Franck et al. (1991)[226] n = 56	Physical training	PE class for 8 weeks, two to three sessions per week; ↓ S-Mg after 4 weeks, S-Mg returned to normal after 8 weeks; reactive ↑ parathyroid hormone	Bone and physical activity
Franz et al. (1985)[122] n = 1	Marathon	↓ Mg postrace; related to ↑ plasma FFA	Case study
Golf et al. (1984)[228] n = 9	1-hr ergometer	Mg supplement → lowers aldosterone, and cortisol ↑ with exercise; E-Mg ↓ with exercise; NS: U-Mg	Measured serum, urine, and sweat
Golf et al. (1989)[247] n = 14	Rowing	Improved lactate elimination following two bouts of 6 min of rowing in 5-hr period	Small cases supplement study
Gullestad et al. (1992)[163] n = 49	Strength	Significant increase in hand grip strength in alcoholics on ↑ Mg supplementation	Supplementation study; 6 weeks no training
Helbig et al. (1989)[258] n = 27	Body building	Prophylactic use of Mg to ameliorate spasms and cramps	Supplement study

Reference	Mode	Findings	Comments
Imaki et al. (1995)[93] n = 36	Bicycle ergometer	Train on ergometer at 30 to 40% of $\dot{V}O_2$max, three times per week for 6 weeks; slight, nonsignificant ↓ S-Mg	Training study to follow changes in S-Mg
Joborn et al. (1985)[229] n = 10 (ergometer) n = 5 (strength)	Ergometer to max; 1-hr ergometer; strength	Short term → ↑ P-Mg; long term → ↓ P-Mg; adrenergic infusion → ↓ Mg	Five-part comprehensive study
Koivisto et al. (1992)[210] n = 16 triathletes n = 26 skiers	Triathlon, 75-km cross-country skiing	Compared diabetics to healthy controls in long-duration exercise; consistent ↓ S-Mg	Two separate studies reported
Laires and Alves (1991)[230] n = 8 experimental n = 10 control	Swimming	After exercise → ↓ P-Mg; more pronounced in swimming than control	Blood and urine samples; swimmers at higher intensity than controls
Laires et al. (1989)[231] n = 17	Swimming	↓ endurance capacity	Animal study
Lijnen et al. (1988)[18] n = 23	Marathon	↓ E-Mg and S-Mg after marathon; propose mechanism for Mg to enter adipocyte	Compartmental shifts
Liu et al. (1983)[178] n = 1	Tennis	Frank hypomagnesemia with carpopedal spasms following 6 hr exercise	Case study
Ljunghall et al. (1987)[232] n = 10	Ergometer to max	Altered acid-base balance, adrenergic stimulation, and compartmental shifts of K, follows Mg change	Only K measured directly
Ljunghall et al. (1988)[233] n = 17	Field exercise	NS: S-Mg; ↑ parathyroid hormone	Military exercise; winter
Lowney et al. (1988)[201]	Running	↓ endurance capacity; ↓ plasma insulin with ↓ D-Mg; ↑ tissue calcium	Animal study; four levels of D-Mg
Lowney et al. (1990)[202] n = 24	Walking/running	Reduced endurance capacity in ↓ D-Mg; no change in 2,3-DPG; Mg via water alleviates negative response	Animals

TABLE 1 Magnesium and Exercise Research Summary (continued)

Author	Sport or Activity	Major Findings[a]	Comments
Lukaski et al. (1983)[234] n = 44 trained n = 20 control	Max aerobic test	P-Mg correlated to max aerobic capacity in trained only	Max test
Lukaski et al. (1996)[281] n = 10	Swimming	Competitive swim athletes; females had ↑ E-Mg and superoxide dismutase activity compared to males; S-Mg was similar; D-Mg was 269 mg/day for females and 393 mg/day for males	Training study, varsity athletes
Madsen et al. (1993)[266] n = 9	Detraining	Muscle Mg ↑ postexhaustive exercise; ↑ Mg inhibits Ca^{++} release from SR	Detraining study
Manore et al. (1989)[235] n = 10	Running, 30 min	↓ S-Mg, ↑ E-Mg, ↓ haptoglobin	10-km race pace
Meacham et al. (1994)[92] n = 17 experimental n = 11 controls	Various	Boron supplementation increased Mg in all subjects; highest Mg in sedentary group	One-year study
Monteiro et al. (1997)[140] n = 16	Aerobic training	Normal S-Mg and ↓ E-Mg after 16-week training program	Training study; Down syndrome sample
Navas and Cordova (1996)[88] n = 40	Swimming	Training (3 weeks, 5 days/week) ↓ Mg in liver, muscle, RBCs; supplementation ↑ S-Mg, bone	Training and supplementation effects on body pools; an animal study
Navas et al. (1997)[89] n = 120	Swimming	Compartmental changes; ↓ Mg in bone and E-Mg; S-Mg level depended on exercise situation: rest, exercise, recovery	Animal study; training; discriminant analysis of Mg pools
Newhouse et al. (1993)[211] n = 111	Runners	Effect of Fe supplements on Mg; may ↓ S-Mg	Supplementation study

Study	Exercise	Results	Comments
Olha et al. (1982)[237] n = 5 trained n = 5 control	Ergometer to max	Both groups ↓ S-Mg after exercise; most pronounced in trained, 6.7% versus 2.4%; may be related to greater amount of work to reach max (↑ mitochondrial Mg in rats)	Trained versus untrained
Powell and Tucker (1991)[57] n = 10	Cross-country runners	<U.S. RDA standards for Mg; running 40 to 50 mi/week; Fe supplementation has no effect on Mg	Two-week study
Rama et al. (1993)[213] n = 7	100-km race	↑ S-Mg; pre/postrace; ↑ attributed to ↓ renal function	Competition changes
Rasmussen et al. (1998)[212] n = 9	Bicycle test	i.v. 10 mmol MgCl; 3-week crossover resulted in NS for maximal work capacity between placebo and Mg	Short-term study periods
Rayssiguier et al. (1990)[4]	Various	Physical exercise is a factor leading to ↓ Mg	Proposed mechanism
Refsum et al. (1973)[195] n = 16	Cross-country skiing 70 km, 90 km	Transient ↓ S-Mg values immediately postrace	Compartmental shifts
Resina et al. (1994)[214] n = 11	Marathon training	↓ blood Mg; negative correlation between E-Mg and 2,3-DPG	Training study
Rose et al. (1970)[20] n = 8	Marathon	↓ S-Mg postrace	First study on sport and Mg
Rowe (1992)[215]	Endurance exercise	↓ Mg and catecholamine action on cerebrovascular system	Hypothesis developed from previous data reports
Singh et al. (1992)[55] n = 11 experimental n = 11 control	Physically active	NS effect of high-potency vitamin–mineral supplement on blood Mg over 12-week period	Short-term pre/poststudy
Stendig-Lindberg (1992)[216] n = 15	Hiking	↓ Mg postexercise; proposed cerebrovascular effects	Humans; extended follow-up
Stendig-Lindberg and Rudy (1983)[161]	Weight training	MVC in quadriceps related to S-Mg	↓ S-Mg by alcoholism

TABLE 1 Magnesium and Exercise Research Summary (continued)

Author	Sport or Activity	Major Findings[a]	Comments
Stendig-Lindberg et al. (1987)[16] n = 20	120-km hike	↓ S-Mg posthike; persisted for 3 months; ↑ S-Mg past 24 hr may be due to exertional rhabdomyolysis on loss of membrane integrity	Recovery follow-up
Tate et al. (1978)[194]	Running	Mitochondria accumulate Mg during acute exercise; maintain membrane integrity and offset effects of exercise Ca^{++} uptake	Animal study
Tate et al. (1982)[242] n = 8 (each group)	Swimming	Matched pairs; Mg inhibits Ca uptake in mitochondria, greater in control than exercise group	Animal study
Tibes et al. (1974)[196] n = 15	Ergometer	During control and work, S-Mg was lower in trained than untrained; pattern similar to acidosis without exercise	Not corrected for hemoconcentration
van Rensburg et al. (1986)[217] n = 23	Triathlon	↓ Mg; pre/postrace	Competition changes
Verde et al. (1982)[257] n = 8	Running	Mg concentration decreased as sweat flow increased	Heat study
Yeh and Aloia (1991)[83] n = 10 (each group)	Not described	Mg absorption and retention higher in exercise groups than sedentary or immobilization	Absorption study

[a] S-Mg = serum magnesium, NS = no significant difference, E-Mg = erythrocyte magnesium, P-Mg = plasma magnesium, Mg Asp = magnesium aspartate, U-Mg = urinary magnesium, FFA = free fatty acids, K = potassium, 2,3-DPG = 2,3-diphosphoglycerate, D-Mg = dietary magnesium, MVC = maximal voluntary contraction.

for Mg balance.[197,203] Balance is achieved not only through gastrointestinal absorption but through sweat loss, cellular redistribution, and renal excretion in particular.[32,204] Given the pervasive role of Mg in the production of energy in skeletal muscle and other body systems, it is logical that both anaerobic and aerobic exercise performance could be altered dramatically by dietary practices and the subsequent availability of Mg. Exercise itself may differentially affect Mg absorption and metabolic Mg requirement.

Appraisal of the role of Mg in exercise must be done with respect to the type of activity and whether the focus is on primary Mg deficiency due to reduced intake or Mg depletion due to dysfunctional metabolism. Also, the extent to which exercise affects the Mg requirement is unknown.

A. AEROBIC

Strenuous endurance activity has received the most attention with respect to Mg influence.[4,16,18–20,69,79,84,93,122,161,174,178,194–196,199,200,205–244] Consistency is demonstrated in the expression of hypomagnesemia in response to aerobic exercise. There are some reports to the contrary when replete athletes are further supplemented with Mg,[96] but there are few training studies[140,209] or inclusion of females.[140,209] Intensity of exercise was not monitored in many studies; however, duration was consistently reported. Mg deficiency decreased endurance time when animals[202,219] or humans[245] were run to exhaustion. Increases in physical working capacity may result from Mg supplementation; however, baseline Mg status was not well-defined across studies.

Changes in membrane fluidity may cause erythrocytes to become fragile, disturb electrolyte balances, and hinder uptake of nutrients and removal of metabolic waste products.[4,6,116,202,246,247] All of these factors may contribute to fatigue. Aberrations in fuel production may also contribute to reduced exercise capacity. This is attributed to the partial uncoupling of oxidative phosphorylation noted in hypomagnesemia which results in reduced ADP/O_2 ratio, increased O_2 uptake for ADP phosphorylation, and an increased O_2 need without a corresponding increase in ATP production.[4,103,248] This Mg-mediated mechanism also has implications for improved running economy, which has been noted in some Mg supplementation studies,[239,248] but more recently was not supported in a study on two sports drinks, one supplemented with Mg.[249] An additional mechanism may support a role for Mg in endurance exercise: sympathetic activation releases epinephrine, and it is inactivated in the liver and kidneys by the enzyme catechol-*O*-methyltransferase. As with all methyltransferases, this requires Mg for its effective action.[106] When released during exercise, epinephrine activates adenylate cyclase in liver and muscle to trigger the cyclic adenosine monophosphate (cAMP) cascade. This cascade greatly amplifies the relatively weak epinephrine signal and stimulates glycogen breakdown, making more glucose available for use by the active muscle. Mg complexed with ATP ($2Mg^{2+}$–ATP) binds to the catalytic subunit of a protein kinase enzyme, preventing its activation by cAMP and inhibiting the release of glucose.[100] Thus,

Mg is used both extracellularly, to turn off a major hormonal signal, and intracellularly, to limit the amplification of that signal. During endurance exercise, this specific, dual, fine-tuning action of Mg may help to preserve glucose and foster the transition from predominately sugar to fat metabolism in production of ATP in muscle.

Mg enhancement of endurance performance is contrasted with extended exercise bouts which may contribute to a decrement of Mg,[199,201,216] resulting in a positive feedback amplification/regenerative cycle.[215] The cycle mechanism is related to removal of free Mg ions by chelation with catecholamine-induced free fatty acids. The lowered Mg increases release of catecholamines. Hypoxia would provoke continuation of the cycle. In contrast, Mg supplementation was related to lower aldosterone and cortisol in 1-hr ergometer exercise.[229] The additional Mg may ameliorate the hyperadrenocorticolism noted during stress exposure by other researchers.[250]

The Mg responses of trained individuals versus sedentary controls to a bout of exercise[196,223,238] or to a maximal graded exercise test have been compared.[225,235] In the exercise bouts, the trained individuals had lower plasma Mg at rest compared to the sedentary groups and expressed a greater Mg reduction to exercise, which may be partially related to their ability to achieve higher work loads. These studies demonstrate lower Mg status in trained individuals at rest, which is exacerbated by a subsequent exercise bout. With respect to maximal oxygen consumption ($\dot{V}O_2$max), there were significant correlations of $\dot{V}O_2$max and resting plasma Mg in trained runners and swimmers, with discrepant results in sedentary subjects.[234,244] Physically active individuals demonstrate a tighter relationship with indicators of Mg status and flux; however, further study is warranted. Improvements in various cardiorespiratory parameters have been described following Mg supplementation in athletes,[239,242,248] although no change was noted in a patient sample.[224] The changes included increased physical working capacity[242] and decreased heart rate, systolic blood pressure, $\dot{V}_e$, and $\dot{V}O_2$, with no significant improvement in final work load.[239,248] Mg supplementation reduces release of cortisol during exercise, which may account for the lower heart rates at similar work loads that have been noted.[229,248] In a 90% $\dot{V}O_2$max run to exhaustion, time increased from 11 to 12 min in the supplementation treatment compared to placebo, with reductions in $\dot{V}_e$ and $\dot{V}O_2$ at the final stage.[245] In animals made to swim to exhaustion, increased Mg content was reported in serum, gastrocnemius muscle, and liver; when the exercise to exhaustion was coupled with environmentally induced hypoxia, Mg was reduced in serum, gastrocnemius, and liver.[248] The relationship between Mg status and maximal exercise testing responses, including exercise-induced hypoxia, requires further study.

In the endurance studies, Mg was measured in erythrocytes or other tissues, such as bone, muscle, liver, and kidney.[84,219,251] Muscle levels of Mg are fairly intractable. It would be expected that Mg would leak out of the intracellular compartment of muscle because of the muscle membrane damage associated with strenuous exercise as indicated by elevated plasma CPK and lactate dehydrogenase levels associated with exertional rhabdomyolysis.[16,122,252] However, it has been demonstrated in both animal and human studies that muscle Mg is well maintained during exercise.[84,247,251,253] Low serum Mg has been observed in overtrained athletes.[254] In a 100-km race, serum Mg was elevated and was attributed to depressed renal function related to the event.[213] However, this is an area with little research and therefore no consensus.

B. ANAEROBIC

Few studies report on Mg and anaerobic exercise. Anaerobic, or high-intensity, exhaustive exercise and Mg studies generally demonstrate hypermagnesemia immediately postexercise.[69,82,161,229,230,248,251,255–259] The observed increased plasma Mg may be attributed to decreased plasma volume associated with strenuous exercise and increased effluent of Mg into the vascular pool.[230] Also, the accompanying metabolic acidosis may increase tissue release of Mg into the bloodstream.[260] Postexercise diminution of Mg is related to intensity of exercise: more severe in trained athletes immediately after strenuous effort, delayed after moderate exercise, and not evident following mild exercise.[197] Much more research is needed to further study the body Mg response to high-intensity, exhaustive exercise.

A positive relationship exists between Mg status and strength,[69,161] and Mg levels may be reduced due to strength training.[78] Mg supplementation may have anabolic effects, first noted in early growth studies in animals. Mg supplements enhance gains due to strength training independent of changes in body weight or body fat,[69] provided the treatment is sustained for more than a few weeks.[82] A supporting mechanism for anabolic effects may be the role of Mg in expression of activity of IGF-1. Liver is the major site of IGF-1 synthesis. In animal studies, both zinc and Mg deficiencies have been implicated in diminished IGF-1, while no changes in growth hormone were noted.[123] Low Mg levels and their implications on IGF-1 require further elucidation. The mechanisms involved in strength may be related to the role of Mg in protein synthesis and muscle physiology parameters already discussed, again with possible effect of energy production. It is apparent that more studies are needed to examine the role of Mg in strength and power events.

Mg supplements decrease neuromuscular excitability such as spasms and cramps.[178,258] Prophylactic use of Mg supplements minimizes spasms and cramps in bodybuilders.[258] Beneficial effects in the treatment of spasmophilia have been noted previously. Further work is needed to develop a consensus on what criteria are needed for effective Mg supplementation.

C. FATIGUE

Chronic fatigue in athletes is considered a common phenomenon.[261] There are no direct studies of Mg and fatigue in exercise and sports performance. There are studies on Mg in chronic fatigue syndrome,[171] human immunodeficiency viral disease,[262] and surgical/postoperative fatigue.[263] The effect of fatigue and low Mg is diminished performance, specifically, depressed endurance,[201,202] where contributing mechanisms are the role of Mg on enzymatic action and cellular control through membrane actions affecting the intracellular environment. Reduced Mg directly results in a reduction of muscle potassium.[95,125,169] The concomitant rise in sodium may reduce membrane excitability. Therefore, contractility of muscle is reduced. Both reduced Mg and elevated intracellular sodium may favor cellular accumulation of calcium.[264,265] Evidence suggests that muscle cellular injury may occur as a consequence of abnormal accumulation of intracellular calcium. Additionally, Mg might contribute to fatigue during endurance exercise by inhibiting calcium release from the SR.[266]

The abnormal potassium compartmentalization and resulting physiological aberrations may be related to altered potassium entry and/or exit from the cell. Mg is key to both processes. Reduced numbers of sodium–potassium pumps seen in Mg deficiency may have implications in premature fatigue from the rise in intracellular sodium which contributes to reduced membrane excitability and therefore contractility of muscle.[265] The concentration of sodium–potassium pumps determines the maximum muscle cell uptake of potassium. Reduced Mg and increased sodium also favor accumulation of calcium,[267] which is furthered implicated in early onset of fatigue. Additionally, Mg may directly affect ion channels or alter membrane surface charge. When cellular Mg levels are normal, potassium efflux decreases by inhibition of Mg-sensitive potassium channels;[268] rectifier potassium channels are very sensitive to intracellular Mg concentration. Overall, the potassium efflux seen with diminished Mg may induce premature muscle fatigue. Further studies on a possible role of Mg as a primary or secondary factor in accelerated fatigue are warranted.

D. ADAPTATION

Few researchers have examined the role of Mg or other cations in adaptation to exercise.[16,84,88–89] Mg is lost in sweat at about the same level in trained and untrained persons,[17] contrary to other major ions, which are conserved in body fluids with training. Exercisers had a lower level of serum Mg, which was still reduced even 3 months after they began a training program.[16] Endurance exercise may reduce plasma and bone Mg, but may exert a protective effect in skeletal muscle in order to maintain homeostatic balance of intramuscular Mg and ATP.[84] Low serum Mg has been observed in overtrained and in trained endurance athletes.[253,254] Additional Mg losses in hypomagnesemic subjects may occur due to the cumulative effects of overtraining.

The depression in Mg after endurance exercise is likely transient, although it may persist for months after exceedingly strenuous prolonged activity. Hypomagnesemia may persist due to consistently engaging in physical activity, which boosts Mg requirements and enhances Mg losses.[16,224] Mg losses in hypomagnesemia occur due to accumulative effects through such mechanisms as sweat production;[17,254] decreased renal-concentrating mechanism as influenced by aldosterone and ADH;[229,251] other hormonal changes related to stress and systemic antioxidant capacity;[250,269] increased lactic acid affecting bone resorption and subsequent hypermagnesuria;[83,233] the stressor of exercise increases release of catecholamines, which is associated with hypermagnesuria;[229,248,256] and the observed hypermagnesuria is correlated with high-intensity performance and the extent of lactate production and excess postexercise oxygen consumption.[4,257] Excess postexercise oxygen consumption is affected by both intensity and duration of exercise or the overall volume of exercise.

Plasma Mg is well maintained and is not the best index of overall Mg status, with possible exceptions in acute conditions of a single bout of endurance exercise or a prolonged exhaustive exercise routine. In some endurance studies, Mg was measured in erythrocytes or other tissues, bone, muscle, liver, and kidney.[84,88–89,202] Endurance exercise may reduce plasma and bone Mg, but seems to exert a protective effect in skeletal muscle in order to maintain homeostatic balance of intramuscular Mg and ATP.[84] Muscle Mg is well maintained during exercise regardless of Mg intake,[84,244,251] although there are some contradicting reports.[89]

The proposed mechanisms for exercise-induced hypomagnesemia are primarily compartmental shifts,[18,84,88,89,195,229,257] with some contribution from sweat production and urinary loss.[17,30,33,34,78,83,259] It is hypothesized that Mg enters muscle and adipose tissue and is removed from bone. The role of Mg in muscle is to maintain the integrity of muscle function and contribute to the energy demands as a cofactor for enzymes and as an ion important to the resonance bonds of ATP. The Mg action in adipose tissue is to form salt complexes with the free fatty acids released in lipolysis.[18,122] This mechanism is postulated as one of the main contributors to hypomagnesemia observed in endurance exercise. However, a glucose–electrolyte supplementation study has demonstrated that serum Mg still decreases despite blunted mobilized fatty acid levels, which infers that an additional contributing mechanism is acting to reduce serum Mg.[79] Mg may be critical to the glucose transfer to muscle and maintenance of membrane integrity to facilitate oxidative metabolism,[194,219,237,243,247,248] thereby enhancing physical working capacity.[224,234] To some degree, Mg may also enter erythrocytes to act as a cofactor in glycolysis and contribute to the production of 2,3-diphosphoglycerate, thereby facilitating oxygen delivery by hemoglobin.[219,234,235] Other roles for Mg include involvement in the hexose monophosphate shunt, production of NADPH, and facilitating glutathione-reductase coenzyme, which protects hemoglobin, enzymes, and membranes against oxidative damage.[129–140,222]

Anaerobic, or high-intensity, exhaustive exercise and Mg have been studied, and these studies generally demonstrate hypermagnesemia immediately postexercise.[82,161,229,247,255,258,259] Increases in urinary Mg with and without Mg loading have been observed. Thus, there is a leakage to plasma, with no renal adaptation that may serve to exacerbate Mg loss in anaerobic exercise.

Adaptation of Mg metabolism to a regular training program is an area with a paucity of research. Long-term studies are necessary to identify body-conserving mechanisms or to elucidate any additional intake needs in exercising individuals.

VI. RECOMMENDATIONS: MAGNESIUM AND EXERCISE

Mg maintains an intimate association with the body's common energy currency, ATP. By way of this intrinsic link, Mg maintains important and pervasive roles in (a) creation of ATP and the regulation of its metabolism and (b) the use of ATP for (1) molecular synthesis of muscle proteins and all biological enzymes, (2) the mechanical work of muscle contraction as well as relaxation, and (3) pumping ions and developing concentration gradients needed for controlling cell volumes and for muscle cell contraction and nerve cell transmission. Mg is required for cellular integrity related to energetics, ionic milieu, and membrane fluidity associated with phospholipid changes. Mg is also critical for growth and optimal functioning of all body systems, especially the nervous, muscular, endocrine, and cardiovascular systems.

Marginal primary Mg deficit is postulated to affect 15 to 20% of the population. Mg requirements should be considered in relative rather than absolute amounts due to the requirements correlated with mesological (mainly diet and exercise) and constitutional conditioning factors.[270] Mg balance studies are warranted, especially in conjunction with exercise, because a synopsis of clinical balance studies indicates that 6 mg/kg body weight per day is needed for equilibrium.[270] Research studies with present methodology may not be able to detect small changes that would be critical to competitive performance.[49,207] Long-term consequences of compromised status, even marginally, are not known. Exercise studies have reported supplementation of <1 year, typically <6 months.

A. DIET

Hard water and mineral water may be important contributors to Mg intake. High fat, sugar, and alcohol decrease bioavailability of Mg. There has been a decline in U.S. Mg intake from 410 mg equivalent, 5+ mg/kg/day, in 1922, with the latest large population figures showing a mean intake of 250 mg in 1975.[11] However, the possible increase required by increased metabolism has not been identified.[270] Up to 8 mg/kg/day has been used with minimal side effects in individuals with normal renal function.[53] With oral Mg, loose stools will develop before any significant accumulation of Mg occurs. In the occurrence of loose stools, the dose can be split throughout the day instead of a single dose with good acclimation.

Vegetarian diets generally contain an abundance of Mg.[270] Physically active individuals usually consume more dietary energy; therefore they should also have a greater intake of Mg, if the diet is balanced. Some researchers have suggested that the hypomagnesemia connected with exercise involvement implies that the diet of the athlete must be supplemented with Mg.[16,20,199,222] Absorption of Mg is approximately 30% of intake. There is a report of exercise training adaptation on increased Mg absorption of unknown mechanism, perhaps improvement of transport systems, and retention of Mg.[83] Metabolic depletion that may be associated with exercise potentially aggravates marginal Mg intake. Diet choices must be scrupulously made and supplementation may be warranted.

B. EXERCISE

The physiological consequences of hypomagnesemia on physical performance have not been firmly established.[4,19] Impaired endurance exercise performance is noted, with Mg recovery variable depending on duration and extent of exercise.[16,201,202,213,230,231] Additionally, low plasma Mg is implicated in spasms and cramps.[161,175–178,182–187,189] Mg supplementation has been shown to affect performance by improved aerobic capacity, economy, and increases in strength, although much more research is required to elucidate metabolic and performance implications of Mg loading. Some of these effects may be related to alleviating a true Mg deficiency or suboptimal intake. An optimal intake for exercise has not been determined, although balance studies indicate that 6 mg/kg/day is needed[270] and exercise may elevate that amount; 8 mg/kg/day has been used with nonexistent side effects.[83,245] Any extended exercise or overtraining, whether of aerobic or anaerobic mode, requires careful attention to potential Mg loss. Prophylactic addition of Mg to the diet or prudent supplementation may be imminent.

There are surges of biochemicals into the circulation that have a profound effect on Mg: catecholamines, glucocorticoids, glucose, and alcohol.[11,250] Some are intimately involved in the body's response to exercise. Acute or chronic stress is implicated in elevation of catecholamines, glucocorticoids, and glucose. Catecholamines affect both the binding of Mg with free fatty acid salts and the redistribution of Mg from extracellular to intracellular pools, or perhaps membrane activity, especially with second messengers.[84,88,89,273] It has also been well established that stress reduces body Mg.[27,203,273–275] Hyperglucocorticism has been implicated in muscle atrophy and immunosuppression.[250] Mg deficit may have a role in expression of hyperglucocorticism. This condition may mimic some of the attributes seen in overload training. The onset may be precipitated by the Mg deficit-and-stress vicious cycle. More specific studies are definitely justified to explore these topics.

C. ENVIRONMENT

Rarely have true environmental conditions which influence Mg status been reported. Attributes of environment that may affect Mg are temperature, both cold[119,203] and heat[16,17] stress, and altitude, related to hypoxic effects.[276,277] All conditions exacerbate the body's need for Mg. Environmental stress and physical activity may be superimposed and create a greater requirement for Mg. These areas require caution on the part of the individual to ensure Mg adequacy in the nutrient density of his or her diet, perhaps supplemented with a high Mg water source.[270] Well-controlled studies should examine the combined effects of exercise and environmental stressors on Mg status.

VII. SUGGESTIONS FOR FUTURE RESEARCH

Mg research has been limited by technical difficulties in measurement,[278,279] but recently the availability of a suitable radioisotope for Mg and reliable means of measuring free intracellular Mg have been advanced.[279] Development of ionized selective electrodes and particle-induced X-ray transmission[278,279] may rekindle efforts to expand studies on Mg and exercise.

Research criteria[11] adapted to establish Mg efficacy in exercise include consistency of the association via epidemiologic, animal, biochemical, and related clinical studies; *strength* of any associations; *specificity* related to Mg; *degree of exposure,* such as normomagnesemia Mg deficiency versus clinical hypomagnesemia; and *biological credibility,* the reasonable mechanism that may account for the observation. Some research issues for consideration in Mg and exercise research, as adapted from a broader presentation on study of nutrition and sport,[280] are presented in Table 2.

The pathological effects of Mg deficiencies have been broadly established. Research on the effects of Mg on exercise performance, while not conclusive, does provide a framework for developing models for predicting the effects of Mg on

TABLE 2   Research Considerations for Magnesium and Exercise Studies

Subjects	Sex
	Genetics
	Current physiological state
	Compliance issues with humans
Diet	Macronutrient distribution and caloric adequacy
	Diuretic drinks (caffeine, alcohol)
	Nutrient density
	Nutrient bioavailability/interactions: cation antagonists and differing absorption rates
Exercise training	Volume of training: intensity, duration, frequency
	Distribution of training sessions
	Mode
Environment	Heat: sweat losses, tissue redistribution
	Cold: catecholamine secretion, tissue redistribution
	Altitude: hypoxia influence
Study criteria	Control (blinded, groupings)
	Adequate power
	Longitudinal versus cross-sectional
	• Technological advances to measure ionic form, precision, reproducibility
	• Functional versus static measurements
	• Appropriate statistical usage
	• Key points are supported by data and literature
	• Speculations and conclusions are relevant to data

Adapted from Bucci.[280]

sports performance. To verify proposed models, future studies should examine the acute and chronic effects of Mg on the performance of anaerobic and aerobic exercises by untrained and trained animals and human subjects. In examining the influence of Mg on exercise performance, researchers should implement double-blind, placebo-controlled, if possible, crossover designs and provide a clear distinction between supramaximal and adequate Mg status and marginal and severe Mg deficiency. Mg load testing is recommended, as it is likely the only definitive way to determine whether or not subjects are Mg deficient until further technology is established. Dynamic functional outcomes versus static measurements have been proposed.[281]

Given that an estimated one-third of the Mg ingested is absorbed by way of the small intestine, it is likely that large doses of at least two times the RDA will be necessary to induce significant treatment effects. These levels of Mg may be obtained from the diet through wise food choices, while higher doses may be achieved through supplementation. However, because divalent cations bind competitively in the small intestine, larger supplemental doses of Mg may induce subsequent deficiencies among antagonist cations and therefore have disadvantages which are yet unknown. For example, pharmacological doses of Mg may induce calcium deficiencies and may predispose endurance-trained athletes to bone mineral deficiency. Researchers should measure the levels of antagonistic divalent cations such as calcium and zinc. This will help to establish more clearly both the advantages and disadvantages of Mg supplementation.

There have been inconsistencies in experimental protocol on exercise and Mg, especially in quantifying work intensity, frequency, and duration. These inconsistencies need to be methodically addressed so results of the studies may be substantiated or refuted through future research. Appraisal of the role of Mg in physical activity must be done with respect to the type of activity and whether the focus is on Mg deficiency effects due to reduced intake or Mg depletion effects due to dysfunctional metabolism. The relationship between Mg status and maximal exercise testing responses, including exercise-induced hypoxia, requires further study, as does the implied enhanced economy in tests to exhaustion.

The pervasive roles of Mg at all levels of organization — nuclear, organelle, membrane, and extracellular matrix — and in all phases of ATP generation and utilization, from ion pumping to muscle contraction and relaxation, make for an exciting research area certain to expand within the next few decades. Only by collaboration of researchers in exercise physiology, biomechanics, molecular biology, chemistry, and genetics will this unique ion and its role in exercise, sports performance, and adaptation begin to be understood.

VIII. SUMMARY

The integral involvement of Mg in exercise is salient because of the association of Mg with all phosphotransfer reactions, among other essential physiological mechanisms. Chronic exercise results in diminished pools of Mg, while acute intense exercise may elicit transient hypermagnesemia and hypermagnesuria. An optimal level of Mg for exercise is unknown. Supplementation has had positive benefits in many studies, while some studies demonstrate that Mg-replete subjects have no ergogenic effect from additional Mg. Indeed, Mg, like other minerals, has untoward effects in large doses that would negatively affect physical performance. Mg and exercise presents an intriguing field of study, although precision of Mg status may have been hampered methodologically. Technological advances being made should facilitate further studies.

REFERENCES

1. Classen, H.G., Speich, M., Schimatschek, H.F., and Rattanatayarom, W., Functional role of magnesium in vivo, in *Magnesium 1993*, Golf, S., Dralle, D., and Vecchiet, L., Eds., John Libbey & Company, London, 1993, 13.
2. Durlach, J., *Magnesium in Clinical Practice*, John Libbey & Company, London, 1988.
3. Kubena, K.S. and Durlach, J., Historical review of the effects of marginal intake of magnesium in chronic experimental magnesium deficiency, *Magnesium Res.*, 3, 219, 1990.
4. Rayssiguier, Y., Guezennec, C.Y., and Durlach, J., New experimental and clinical data on the relationship between magnesium and sport, *Magnesium Res.*, 3, 93, 1990.
5. Rude, R.K., Magnesium metabolism and deficiency, *Endocr. Metab. Clin. N. Am.*, 22(2), 377, 1993.
6. Wacker, W.E.C. and Parisi, A.F., Magnesium metabolism, *N. Engl. J. Med.*, 28, 712, 1968.
7. Wester, P.O., Magnesium, *Am. J. Clin. Nutr.*, 45, 1305, 1987.
8. Woo, J. and Cannon, D.C., Metabolic intermediates and inorganic ions, in *Clinical Diagnosis and Management by Laboratory Methods*, 17th ed., Henry, J.B., Ed., W.B. Saunders, Philadelphia, 1984.
9. Durlach, J., Bac, P., Durlach, V., Bara, M., and Guiet-Bara, A., Neurotic, neuromuscular, and autonomic nervous form of magnesium imbalance, *Magnesium Res.*, 10, 169, 1997.
10. Ramage, I.J., Ray, M., Patron, R.D., Logan, R.W., and Beattie, T.J., Hypomagnesemic tetany, *J. Clin. Pathol.*, 49, 343, 1996.
11. Mansmann, H.C., Consider magnesium homeostasis. III. Cytochrome P450 enzymes and drug toxicity, *Pediatr. Asthma Allergy Immunol.*, 8, 7, 1994.
12. Altura, B.M., Altura, B.T., Gebrewold, A., Ising, H., and Günther, T., Noise-induced hypertension and magnesium in rats: relationship to microcirculation and calcium, *J. Appl. Physiol.*, 72, 194, 1992.
13. Classen, H.G., Stress and magnesium, *Artery*, 9, 182, 1981.
14. Henrotte, J.G., Type A behavior and magnesium metabolism, *Magnesium*, 5, 201, 1986.
15. Ising, H., Interaction of noise-induced stress and Mg decrease, *Artery*, 9, 205, 1981.
16. Stendig-Lindberg, G., Shapiro, Y., Epstein, Y., Galun, E., Schonberger, E., Graff, E., and Wacker, W.E.C., Changes in serum magnesium concentration after strenuous exercise, *J. Am. Coll. Nutr.*, 6, 35, 1987.
17. Beller, G.A., Maher, J.T., Hartley, L.H., Bass, D.E., and Wacker, W.E.C., Changes in serum and sweat magnesium levels during work in the heat, *Aviat. Space Environ. Med.*, 46, 709, 1975.
18. Lijnen, P., Hespel, P., Fagard, R., Lysens, R., Vanden Eynde, E., and Amery, A., Erythrocyte, plasma and urinary magnesium in men before and after a marathon, *Eur. J. Appl. Physiol.*, 58, 252, 1988.
19. McDonald, R. and Keen, C.L., Iron, zinc and magnesium nutrition and athletic performance, *Sports Med.*, 5, 171, 1988.
20. Rose, L.I., Carroll, D.R., Lowe, S.L., Peterson, E.W., and Cooper, K.H., Serum electrolyte changes after marathon running, *J. Appl. Physiol.*, 29, 449, 1970.

21. Berklehammer, C. and Bear, R.A., A clinical approach to common electrolyte problems. 4. Hypomagnesemia, *Can. Med. Assoc. J.,* 132, 360, 1985.
22. Sizer, F.S. and Whitney, E.N., *Nutrition: Concepts and Controversies,* 7th ed., West/Wadsworth Publishing, Minneapolis–St. Paul, 1997.
23. Holifield, B., Magnesium deficiency and ventricular ectopy, *Am. J. Cardiol.,* 63, 22G, 1989.
24. McLean, R.M., Magnesium and its therapeutic uses: a review, *Am. J. Med.,* 96, 63, 1994.
25. Brotherhood, J.R., Nutrition and sports performance, *Sports Med.,* 1, 350, 1984.
26. Lukaski, H.C., Micronutrients (magnesium, zinc, copper): are mineral supplements needed for athletes, *Int. J. Sport Nutr.,* 5, S74, 1995.
27. Galland, L., Magnesium, stress and neuropsychiatric disorders, *Magnesium Trace Elem.,* 10, 287, 1991.
28. Whang, R., Morosi, H.J., Rodgers, D., and Reyes, R., The influence of sustained magnesium deficiency on muscle potassium repletion, *J. Lab. Clin. Med.,* 70, 895, 1967.
29. Cerrato, P.L., Nutrition support: don't overlook this mineral deficiency, *RN,* 55, 61, 1992.
30. Djurhuus, M.S., Gram, J., Hyltoft Petersen, P., Klitgaard, N.A.H., Bollerslev, J., and Beck-Nielsen, H., Biological variation of serum and urinary magnesium in apparently healthy males, *Scand. J. Clin. Lab. Invest.,* 55, 549, 1995.
31. Olson, R.E., Ed., Magnesium deficiency and ischemic heart disease, *Nutr. Rev.,* 46, 311, 1988.
32. Quamme, G.A., Laboratory evaluation of magnesium status, *Clin. Lab. Med.,* 13, 209, 1993.
33. Gullestad, L., Midtvedt, L., Dolva, O., Norseth, J., and Kjekshus, J., The magnesium loading test: reference values in healthy subjects, *Scand. J. Clin. Lab. Invest.,* 54, 23, 1994.
34. Holm, C.N., Jepsen, J.M., Sjogaard, G., and Hessob, I.A., A magnesium load test in the diagnosis of magnesium deficiency, *Clin. Nutr.,* 41, 301, 1987.
35. Rude, R.K. and Singer, F.R., Magnesium deficiency and excess, *Annu. Rev. Med.,* 32, 245, 1981.
36. Whitney, E.N. and Rolfes, S.R., *Understanding Nutrition,* 7th ed., West/Wadsworth Publishing, Minneapolis–St. Paul, 1997.
37. Fisher, P.W.F., Giroux, A., L'Abbe, M.R., and Nera, E.A., The effects of moderate magnesium deficiency in the rat, *Nutr. Rep. Int.,* 24, 993, 1981.
38. Fiaccadori, E., Del Canale, S., Coffrini, E., Melej, R., Vitali, P., Guariglia, A., and Borghetti, A., Muscle and serum magnesium in pulmonary intensive care unit patients, *Crit. Care Med.,* 16, 751, 1988.
39. Pao, E.M. and Mickle, S.J., Problem nutrients in the United States, *Food Technol.,* 35, 58, 1981.
40. Lowenstein, F.W. and Stanton, M.F., Serum magnesium levels in the United States, 1971–1974, *J. Am. Coll. Nutr.,* 5, 399, 1986.
41. Marier, J.R., Quantitative factors regarding magnesium status in the modern-day world, *Magnesium,* 1, 3, 1982.
42. Marier, J.R., Magnesium content of the food supply in the modern-day world, *Magnesium,* 5, 1, 1986.
43. Morgan, K.J., Stampley, G.L., Zabik, M.E., and Fischer, D.R., Magnesium and calcium dietary intakes of the U.S. population, *J. Am. Coll. Nutr.,* 4, 195, 1985.
44. Clarkson, P.M., Minerals: exercise performance and supplementation in athletes, *J. Sports Sci.,* 9, 91, 1991.
45. Bazzarre, T.L., Scarpino, A., Sigmon, R., Marquart, L.F., Wu, S.L., and Izurieta, M., Vitamin-mineral supplement use and nutritional status of athletes, *J. Am. Coll. Nutr.,* 12, 162, 1993.
46. Fogelholm, G.M., Himberg, J.J, Alopaeus, K., Gref, C.G., Laasko, J.T., Lehto, J.J., and Mussalo-Rauhamaa, H., Dietary and biochemical indices of nutritional status in male athletes and controls, *J. Am. Coll. Nutr.,* 11, 181, 1992.
47. Cordova, A., Navas, F.J., Gomez-Carraminana, M., and Rodriquez, H., Evaluation of Mg intake in elite sportsmen, *Magnesium Bull.,* 16, 59, 1994.
48. Kleiner, S.M., Bazzarre, T.L., and Ainsworth, B.E., Nutritional status of nationally ranked elite bodybuilders, *Int. J. Sport Nutr.,* 4, 54, 1994.
49. Clarkson, P.M., Micronutrients and exercise: antioxidants and minerals, *J. Sports Sci.,* 13, S11, 1995.

50. Benson, J., Gillien, D.M., Bourdet, K., and Loosli, A.R., Inadequate nutrition and chronic calorie restriction in adolescent ballerinas, *Physician Sportsmed.*, 13, 79, 1985.
51. Loosli, A.R., Benson, J., Gillien, D.M., and Bourdet, K., Nutrition habits and knowledge in competitive adolescent female gymnasts, *Physician Sportsmed.*, 8, 118, 1986.
52. Steen, S.N. and McKinney, S., Nutrition assessment of college wrestlers, *Physician Sportsmed.*, 14, 101, 1986.
53. Brilla, L.R. and Haley, T.F., Effect of magnesium supplementation on strength training in humans, *J. Am. Coll. Nutr.*, 11, 326, 1992.
54. Economos, C.D., Bortz, S.S., and Nelson, M.E., Nutritional practices of elite athletes: practical recommendations, *Sports Med.*, 16, 381, 1993.
55. Singh, A., Moses, F.M., and Deuster, P.A., Vitamin and mineral status in physically active men: effects of a high-potency supplement, *Am. J. Clin. Nutr.*, 55, 1, 1992.
56. Deuster, P.A., Kyle, S.B., Moser, P.B., Vigersky, R.A., Singh, A., and Schoonmaker, E.B., Nutritional survey of highly trained women runners, *Am. J. Clin. Nutr.*, 44, 954, 1986.
57. Powell, P.D. and Tucker, A., Iron supplementation and running performance in female cross country runners, *Int. J. Sports Med.*, 12, 462, 1991.
58. Lukaski, H.C., Siders, W.A., Hoverson, B.S., and Gallagher, S.K., Iron, copper, magnesium, and zinc status as predictors of swimming performance, *Int. J. Sports Med.*, 17, 535, 1996.
59. Telford, R.D., Catchpole, E.A., Deakin, V., McLeay, A.C., and Plank, A.W., The effect of 7 to 8 months of vitamin/mineral supplementation on the vitamin and mineral status of athletes, *Int. J. Sport Nutr.*, 2, 123, 1992.
60. Worme, J.D., Doubt, T.J., Singh, A., Ryan, C.J., Moses, F.M., and Deuster, P.A., Dietary patterns, gastrointestinal complaints, and nutrition knowledge of recreational triathletes, *Am. J. Clin. Nutr.*, 51, 690, 1990.
61. Williams, M.H., Vitamin and mineral supplements to athletes: do they help? *Clin. Sports Med.*, 3, 623, 1984.
62. Vitale, J.J., White, P.L., Nakamura, M., Hegsted, D.M., Zamcheck, N., and Hellerstein, E.E., Interrelationships between experimental hypercholesteremia, magnesium requirement, and experimental atherosclerosis, *J. Exp. Med.*, 106, 757, 1957.
63. Holtmeier, H.J. and Kuhn, M., Problems of nutritional intake of calcium and magnesium and their possible influence on coronary disease, *Magnesium Health Dis.*, 73, 671, 1980.
64. Kubena, K.S., Landman, W.A., and Carpenter, Z.L., Suboptimal intake of magnesium in rats: effects during growth and gestation, *Nutr. Res.*, 3, 385, 1983.
65. Report from the Executive Director, 1992–93, HD705BS, American Institute for Cancer Research, Washington, D.C., 1993.
66. *Dietary Guidelines for Americans,* American Heart Association, Dallas, Texas, 1985.
67. United States Senate Select Committee on Nutrition and Human Needs, Dietary Goals for the United States, U.S. Government Printing Office, Washington, D.C., 1977.
68. National Research Council, Committee on Diet and Health of the Food and Nutrition Board, National Academy of Sciences Report. Diet and health: implications for reducing chronic disease risk, *Nutr. Rev.*, 47, 142, 1989.
69. Lombardi, V.P. and Taffe, D.R., Do all modes of exercise minimize cardiovascular disease risk? *The Physiologist*, 35, 183, 1992.
70. Bunce, G.E., Reeves, P.G., Oba, T.S., and Sauberlich, H.E., Influence of dietary protein level on the magnesium requirement, *J. Nutr.*, 79, 220, 1963.
71. Golf, S.W., Biochemistry of magnesium in man, in *Magnesium 1993*, Golf, S., Dralle, D., and Vecchiet, L., Eds., John Libbey and Co., London, 1993, 31.
72. Yasui, M., Ota, K., and Yoshida, M., Effects of low calcium and magnesium dietary intake on the CNS tissues of rats and calcium–magnesium related disorders in amyotrophic lateral sclerosis in the Kii Peninsula of Japan, *Magnesium Res.*, 10, 39, 1997.
73. Yasui, M., Yase, Y., Kihira, T., Adachi, K., and Suzuki, Y., Magnesium and calcium contents in CNS tissues of amyotrophic lateral sclerosis patients from the Kii Peninsula of Japan, *Eur. Neurol.*, 32, 95, 1992.

74. Yasui, M., Yase, Y., Ota, K., Mukoyama, M., and Adachi, K., High aluminum deposition in the CNS of patients with amyotrophic lateral sclerosis from the Kii Peninsula of Japan: two case reports, *Neurotoxicology*, 12, 277, 1991.

75. Mitani, K., Relationship between neurological diseases due to aluminum load, especially amyotrophic lateral sclerosis and magnesium status, *Magnesium Res.*, 5, 203, 1992.

76. CDC Epi-Info from the USGS National Stream Water Quality Monitoring Network, http://www.execpc.com/~magnesium/.

77. Weight, L.M., Noakes, T.D., Labadarios, D., Graves, J., Jacobs, P., and Berman, P.A., Vitamin and mineral status of trained athletes including the effects of supplementation, *Am. J. Clin. Nutr.*, 47, 186, 1988.

78. Beuker, F., Classen, H.G., and Helbig, H.J., Biokinetics of magnesium supplementation during strength training in popular athletes, *Magnesium Res.*, 3, 308, 1990.

79. Deuster, P.A. and Singh, A., Responses of plasma magnesium and other cations to fluid replacement during exercise, *J. Am. Coll. Nutr.*, 12, 286, 1993.

80. Maughan, R.J. and Sadler, D.J.M., The effects of oral administration of salts of aspartic acid on the metabolic response to prolonged exhausting exercise in man, *Int. J. Sports Med.*, 4, 119, 1983.

81. Wesson, M., McNaughton, L., Davies, P., and Tristram, S., Effects of oral administration of aspartic acid salts on the endurance capacity of trained athletes, *Res. Q. Exercise Sport*, 59, 234, 1988.

82. de Haan, A., van Doorn, J.E., and Wesstra, H.G., Effects of potassium + magnesium aspartate on muscle metabolism and force development during short intensive static exercise, *Int. J. Sports Med.*, 6, 44, 1985.

83. Yeh, J.K. and Aloia, J.F., Effect of physical activity on the metabolism of magnesium in the rat, *J. Am. Coll. Nutr.*, 10, 487, 1991.

84. Brilla, L.R., Fredrickson, J.H., and Lombardi, V.P., Effect of hypomagnesemia and exercise on slowly exchanging pools of magnesium, *Metabolism*, 38, 797, 1989.

85. Fogelholm, M., Tikkanen, H., Näveri, H., and Härkönen, M., High-carbohydrate diet for long distance runners: a practical viewpoint, *Br. J. Sports Med.*, 23, 94, 1989.

86. Kramer, L.B., Osis, D., Coffey, J., and Spencer, H., Mineral and trace element content of vegetarian diets, *J. Am. Coll. Nutr.*, 3, 3, 1984.

87. Wirell, M.P., Wester, P.O., and Stegmayr, B.G., Nutritional dose of magnesium in hypertensive patients on beta blockers lowers systolic blood pressure: a double-blind, cross-over study, *J. Intern. Med.*, 236, 189, 1994.

88. Navas, F.J. and Cordova, A., Effect of magnesium supplementation and training on magnesium tissue distribution in rats, *Biol. Trace Elem. Res.*, 53, 137, 1996.

89. Navas, F.J., Martin, F., and Cordova, A., Compartmental shifts of calcium and magnesium as a result of swimming and swimming training in rats, *Med. Sci. Sports Exercise*, 29, 882, 1997.

90. Ruddel, H., Werner, C., and Ising, H., Impact of magnesium supplementation on performance data in young swimmers, *Magnesium Res.*, 3, 103, 1990.

91. Abbasciano, V., Levato, F., and Reali, M.G., Reduction of erythrocyte magnesium concentration in heterozygote beta-thalassemic subjects and in normal subjects submitted to physical stress, *Magnesium Res.*, 1, 213, 1988.

92. Meacham, S.L., Taper, J., and Volpe, S.L., Effects of boron supplementation on bone mineral density and dietary, blood, and urinary calcium, phosphorus, magnesium, and boron in female athletes, *Environ. Health Perspect.*, 102, 79, 1994.

93. Imaki, M., Hara, T., Yoshida, Y., Ohguri, M., Tanada, S., and Yamasaki, M., Effect of light exercise on serum magnesium in human subjects, *J. Jpn. Soc. Magnesium Res.*, 14, 7, 1995.

94. Crespo, R., Relea, P., Lozano, D., Macarro-Sanchez, M., Usabiaga, J., Villa, L.F., and Rico, H., Biochemical markers of nutrition in elite-marathon runners, *J. Sports Med. Phys. Fitness*, 35, 268, 1995.

95. Terblanche, S., Noakes, T.D., Dennis, S.C., Marais, D., and Eckert, M., Failure of magnesium supplementation to influence marathon running performance or recovery in Mg-replete subjects, *Int. J. Sport Nutr.*, 2, 154, 1992.

96. Dorup, I., Skajaa, K., and Thybo, N.K., Oral magnesium supplementation restores the concentrations of magnesium, potassium, and sodium–potassium pumps in skeletal muscle of patients receiving diuretic treatment, *J. Intern. Med.,* 233, 117, 1993.

97. Guyton, A.C. and Hall, J.E., *Textbook of Medical Physiology,* 9th ed., W.B. Saunders, Philadelphia, 1996.

98. Powers, S.K. and Howley, E.T., *Exercise Physiology: Theory and Application to Fitness and Performance,* Wm. C. Brown, Dubuque, IA, 1997.

99. Alberts, B., Bray, D., Lewis, J., Raff, M., Roberts, K., and Watson, J., *Molecular Biology of the Cell,* 3rd ed., Garland Publishing, New York, 1994.

100. Stryer, L., *Biochemistry,* 3rd ed., W.H. Freeman, New York, 1988.

101. Miki, M., Wahl, P., and Auchet, J., Fluorescence anisotropy of labeled F-actin: influence of divalent cations on the interaction between F-actin and myosin heads, *Biochemistry,* 21, 3661, 1982.

102. Sherwood, L., *Human Physiology: From Cells to Systems,* 2nd ed., West Publishing, St. Paul, 1993.

103. Garfinkel, L. and Garfinkel, D., Magnesium regulation of the glycolytic pathway and the enzymes involved, *Magnesium,* 4, 60, 1985.

104. Saks, V.A., Chernousova, G.B., Gukovsky, D.E., Smirnov, V.N., and Chazov, E., Studies of energy transport in heart cells, *Dur. J. Biochem.,* 57, 273, 1975.

105. Aikawa, J.K., *Magnesium: Its Biological Significance,* CRC Press, Boca Raton, FL, 1981.

106. White, A., Handler, P., Smith, E.L., Hill, R.L., and Lehman, I.R., *Principles of Biochemistry,* 6th ed., McGraw-Hill, New York, 1978.

107. Wold, F. and Ballou, C.E., Studies on the enzyme enolase, *J. Biol. Chem.,* 227, 301, 1957.

108. Abbott, L.G. and Rude, R.K., Clinical manifestations of magnesium deficiency, *Miner. Electrolyte Metab.,* 19, 314, 1993.

109. Fahim, F.A., Morcos, N.Y.S., and Esmat, A.Y., Effects of dietary magnesium and/or manganese variables on the growth rate and metabolism of mice, *Ann. Nutr. Metab.,* 34, 183, 1990.

110. Nadler, J.L., Buchanan, T., Natarajan, R., Antonipillai, I., Bergman, R., and Rude, R.K., Magnesium deficiency produces insulin resistance and increased thromboxane synthesis, *Hypertension,* 21, 1024, 1993.

111. Preuss, H.G., Effects of glucose/insulin perturbations on aging and chronic disorders of aging: the evidence, *J. Am. Coll. Nutr.,* 16, 397, 1997.

112. White, J.R. and Campbell, R.K., Magnesium and diabetes: a review, *Ann. Pharmacother.,* 27, 775, 1993.

113. Lehninger, A.L., *Biochemistry: The Molecular Basis of Cell Structure and Function,* 2nd ed., Worth Publishers, New York, 1975.

114. Nakashima, R.A., Dordick, R.S., and Garlid, K.D., On the relative roles of Ca^{2+} and Mg^{2+} in regulating the endogenous K^+/H^+ exchanger of rat liver mitochondria, *J. Biol. Chem.,* 257, 12540, 1982.

115. Robeson, B.L., Martin, W.G., and Friedman, M.H., A biochemical and ultrastructural study of skeletal muscle from rats fed a magnesium-deficient diet, *J. Nutr.,* 110, 2078, 1980.

116. Heaton, F.W. and Elie, J.P., Metabolic activity of liver mitochondria from magnesium-deficient rats, *Magnesium,* 3, 21, 1984.

117. Elin, R.J., Utter, A., Tan, H.K., and Corash, L., Effect of magnesium deficiency on erythrocyte aging in rats, *Am. J. Pathol.,* 100, 765, 1980.

118. Tongyai, S., Rayssiguier, Y., Motta, C., Gueux, E., Maurois, P., and Heaton, F.W., Mechanism of increased erythrocyte membrane fluidity during magnesium deficiency in weanling rats, *Am. J. Physiol.,* 257, C270, 1989.

119. Heroux, O., Peter, D., and Heggtveit, A., Long-term effect of suboptimal dietary magnesium on magnesium and calcium contents of organs, on cold tolerance and on lifespan, and its pathological consequences in rats, *J. Nutr.,* 107, 1640, 1977.

120. Grace, N.D. and O'Dell, B.L., Effect of magnesium deficiency on the distribution of water and cations in the muscle of the guinea pig, *J. Nutr.,* 100, 45, 1970.

121. Rayssiguier, Y. and Larvor, P., Hypomagnesemia following stimulation of lipolysis in ewes: effects of cold exposure and fasting, *Magnesium Health Dis.,* 9, 67, 1980.
122. Franz, K.B., Ruddel, H., Todd, G.L., Dorheim, T.A., Buell, J.C., and Eliot, R., Physiologic changes during a marathon, with special reference to magnesium, *J. Am. Coll. Nutr.,* 4, 187, 1985.
123. Dorup, I., Flyvbjerg, A., Everts, M.E., and Clausen, T., Role of insulin-like growth factor 1 and growth hormone in growth inhibition induced by magnesium and zinc deficiencies, *Br. J. Nutr.,* 66, 505, 1991.
124. Solomon, R., The relationship between disorders of K^+ and Mg^{+2} homeostasis, *Semin. Nephrol.,* 3, 253, 1987.
125. Dorup, I., Effects of K^+, Mg^{+2} deficiency and adrenal steroids on Na^+,K^+-pump concentration in skeletal muscle, *Acta Physiol. Scand.,* 156, 305, 1996.
126. Kretzschmar, M. and Muller, D., Aging, training and exercise: a review of effects on plasma glutathione and lipid peroxides, *Sports Med.,* 15, 196, 1993.
127. Sen, C.K., Oxidants and antioxidants in exercise, *J. Appl. Physiol.,* 79, 675, 1995.
128. Packer, L., Oxidants, antioxidant nutrients and the athlete, *J. Sports Sci.,* 15, 353, 1997.
129. Vendetti, P. and Di Meo, S., Antioxidants, tissue damage, and endurance in trained and untrained young male rats, *Arch. Biochem. Biophys.,* 331, 63, 1996.
130. Dickens, B.F., Weglicki, W.B., Li, Y.S., and Mak, I.T., Magnesium deficiency in vitro enhances free radical-induced intracellular oxidation and cytotoxicity in endothelial cells, *FEBS,* 311, 187, 1992.
131. Freedman, A.M., Mak, I.T., Stafford, R.E., Dickens, B.F., Cassidy, M.M., Muesing, R.A., and Weglicki, W.B., Erythrocytes from magnesium-deficient hamsters display an enhanced susceptibility to oxidative stress, *Am. J. Physiol.,* 262, C1371, 1992.
132. Kramer, J.H., Misik, V., and Weglicki, W.B., Magnesium-deficiency potentiates free radical production associated with postischemic injury to rat hearts: vitamin E affords protection, *Free Rad. Biol. Med.,* 16, 713, 1994.
133. Calviello, G., Ricci, P., Lauro, L., Palozza, P., and Cittadini, A., Mg deficiency induces mineral content changes and oxidative stress in rats, *Biochem. Mol. Biol. Int.,* 32, 903, 1994.
134. Gueux, E., Azais-Braesco, V., Bussiere, L., Grolier, P., Mazur, A., and Rayssiguier, Effect of magnesium deficiency on triacylglycerol-rich lipoprotein and tissue susceptibility to peroxidation in relation to vitamin E content, *Br. J. Nutr.,* 74, 849, 1995.
135. Kumar, B.P. and Shivakumar, K., Depressed antioxidant defense in rat heart in experimental magnesium deficiency. Implications for the pathogenesis of myocardial lesions, *Biol. Trace Elem. Res.,* 60, 139, 1997.
136. Shivakumar, K. and Kumar, B.P., Magnesium deficiency enhances oxidative stress and collagen synthesis in vivo in the aorta of rats, *Int. J. Biochem. Cell Biol.,* 29, 1273, 1997.
137. Chugh, S.N., Kolley, T., Kakkar, R., Chugh, K., and Sharma, A., A critical evaluation of antiperoxidant effect of intravenous magnesium in acute aluminum phosphide poisoning, *Magnesium Res.,* 10, 225, 1997.
138. Regan, R.F., Jasper, E., Guo, Y., and Panter, S.S., The effect of magnesium on oxidative neuronal injury in vitro, *J. Neurochem.,* 70, 77, 1998.
139. Laires, M.J., Madeira, F., Sergio, J., Colaco, C., Vaz, C., Felisberto, G.M., Neto, I., Breitenfeld, L., Bicho, M., and Manso, C., Preliminary study of the relationship between plasma and erythrocyte magnesium variations and some circulating pro-oxidant and antioxidant indices in a standardized physical effort, *Magnesium Res.,* 6, 233, 1993.
140. Monteiro, C.P., Varela, A., Pinto, M., Neves, J., Felisberto, G.M., Vaz, C., Bicho, M.P., and Laires, M.J., Effect of an aerobic training on magnesium, trace elements and antioxidant systems in a Down syndrome population, *Magnesium Res.,* 10, 65, 1997.
141. Maughan, D., Diffusible Mg in frog skeletal muscle cells, *Biophys. J.,* 43, 75, 1983.
142. Ekelund, M.C. and Edman, K.A.P., Shortening induced deactivation of skinned fibres of frog and mouse striated muscle, *Acta Physiol. Scand.,* 116, 189, 1982.

143. Lopez, J.R., Alamo, L., Caputo, C., Vergara, J., and DiPolo, R., Direct measurement of intracellular free magnesium in frog skeletal muscle using magnesium-selective microelectrodes, *Biochim. Biophys.*, 804, 1, 1974.

144. Kitazawa, T., Shuman, H., and Somlyo, A.P., Calcium and magnesium binding to thin and thick filaments in skinned muscle fibres: electron probe analysis, *J. Muscle Res. Cell Motil.*, 3, 437, 1982.

145. Watterson, J.G., Foletta, D., Kunz, P.A., and Schaub, M.C., Interaction of ADP and magnesium with the active site of myosin subfragment-1 observed by reactivity changes of the critical thiols and by direct binding methods at low and high ionic strength, *Eur. J. Biochem.*, 131, 89, 1983.

146. Rayment, I., Holden, H., Whittaker, M., Yohn, C., Lorenz, M., Holmes, K., and Milligan, R., Structure of the actin–myosin complex and its implications for muscle contraction, *Science*, 261, 58, 1993.

147. Potter, J.D. and Gergely, J., The calcium and magnesium binding sites on troponin and their role in the regulation of myofibrillar adenosine triphosphatase, *J. Biol. Chem.*, 250, 4628, 1975.

148. Potter, J.D., Robertson, S.P., and Johnson, J.D., Magnesium and the regulation of muscle contraction, *Fed. Proc.*, 40, 2653, 1981.

149. Somlyo, A.V., Gonzalez-Serratos, H., Shuman, H., McClellan, G., and Somlyo, A.P., Calcium release and ionic changes in the sarcoplasmic reticulum of tetanized muscle: an electron-probe study, *J. Cell Biol.*, 90, 577, 1981.

150. Yoshioka, T. and Somlyo, A.P., Calcium and magnesium contents and volume of the terminal cisternae in caffeine-treated skeletal muscle, *J. Cell Biol.*, 99, 558, 1984.

151. Hasselbach, E., Fassold, E., Migala, A., and Rauch, B., Magnesium dependence of sarcoplasmic reticulum calcium transport, *Fed. Proc.*, 40, 2657, 1981.

152. Kovacs, L., Rios, E., and Schneider, M.F., Calcium transients and intramembrane charge movement in skeletal muscle fibres, *Nature*, 279, 391, 1979.

153. Morsy, F.A. and Shamoo, A.E., Trans-magnesium dependency of ATP-dependent calcium uptake into sarcoplasmic reticulum of skeletal muscle, *Magnesium*, 4, 182, 1985.

154. Stephenson, E.W., Magnesium effects on activation of skinned fibers from striated muscle, *Fed. Proc.*, 40, 2662, 1981.

155. Stephenson, E.W. and Podolsky, R.J., Regulation by magnesium of intracellular calcium movement in skinned muscle fibers, *J. Gen. Physiol.*, 69, 1, 1977.

156. Nakamura, J., The ADP- and Mg^{2+}-reactive calcium complex of the phosphoenzyme in skeletal sarcoplasmic reticulum Ca^{2+}-ATPase, *Biochim. Biophys.*, 723, 182, 1983.

157. Champeil, P., Gingold, M.P., and Guillain, F., Effect of magnesium on the calcium-dependent transient kinetics of sarcoplasmic reticulum ATPase, studied by stopped flow fluorescence and phosphorylation, *J. Biol. Chem.*, 258, 4453, 1983.

158. Somlyo, A.P. and Somlyo, A.V., Effects and subcellular distribution of magnesium in smooth and striated muscle, *Fed. Proc.*, 40, 2667, 1981.

159. Brautbar, N. and Carpenter, C., Skeletal myopathy and magnesium depletion: cellular mechanisms, *Magnesium*, 3, 57, 1984.

160. Sarkar, K., Parry, D.J., and Heggtveit, H.A., Skeletal myopathy in chronic magnesium depletion, *Magnesium Bull.*, 2, 108, 1981.

161. Stendig-Lindberg, G. and Rudy, N., Predictors of maximum voluntary contraction force of quadriceps muscles in man: ridge regression analysis, *Magnesium*, 2, 93, 1983.

162. Perkoff, G.T., Dioso, M.M., Bleisch, V., and Klinkerfuss, G., A spectrum of myopathy associated with alcoholism, *Ann. Intern. Med.*, 67, 481, 1967.

163. Gullestad, L., Dolva, L.O., Soyland, E., Manger, A.T., Falch, D., and Kjekshus, J., Oral magnesium supplementation improves metabolic variables and muscle strength in alcoholics, *Alcohol Clin. Exp. Res.*, 16, 986, 1992.

164. Lim, P. and Jacob, E., Magnesium status of alcoholic patient, *Metabolism*, 21, 1045, 1972.

165. Gunther, T., Functional compartmentation of intracellular magnesium, *Magnesium*, 5, 53, 1986.

166. Gunther, T., Averdunk, R., and Ising, H., Biochemical mechanisms in magnesium deficiency, *Magnesium Health Dis.*, 8, 57, 1980.

167. Cronin, R.E., Fluids and electrolytes, in *Magnesium Disorders,* Kokko, J.P. and Tannen, R.L., Eds., W.B. Saunders, Philadelphia, 1986, 502.

168. Sjogren, A., Floren, C., and Nilsson, A., Magnesium and potassium status in healthy subjects as assessed by analysis of magnesium and potassium in skeletal muscle biopsies and magnesium in mononuclear cells, *Magnesium,* 6, 91, 1987.

169. Dorup, I., Skajaa, K., and Thybo, N.K., Oral magnesium supplementation restores the concentrations of magnesium, potassium, and sodium–potassium pumps in skeletal muscle of patients receiving diuretic treatment, *J. Intern. Med.,* 233, 117, 1993.

170. Ravn, H.B. and Dorup, I., The concentration of sodium, potassium pumps in chronic obstructive lung disease (COLD) patients: the impact of magnesium depletion and steroid treatment, *J. Intern. Med.,* 241, 23, 1997.

171. Cox, I.M., Campell, M.J., and Dowson, D., Red blood cell magnesium and chronic fatigue syndrome, *Lancet,* 337, 757, 1991.

172. Eisinger, J., Plantamura, A., Marie, P.A., and Ayavou, T., Selenium and magnesium status in fibromyalgia, *Magnesium Res.,* 7, 285, 1994.

173. Russell, I.J., Michalek, J.E., Flechas, J.D., and Abraham, G.E., Treatment of fibromyalgia syndrome with Super Malic: a randomized, double blind, placebo controlled, crossover pilot study, *J. Rheumatol.,* 22, 953, 1995.

174. de Haan, A., van Doorn, J.E., and Wesstra, H.G., Effects of potassium + magnesium aspartate on muscle metabolism and force development during short intensive static exercise, *Int. J. Sports Med.,* 6, 44, 1985.

175. Abraham, G.E. and Lubran, M.M., Serum and red cell magnesium levels in patients with premenstrual tension, *Am. J. Clin. Nutr.,* 34, 2364, 1981.

176. Cronin, R.E., Ferguson, E.R., Shannon, W.A., and Knochel, J.P., Skeletal muscle injury after magnesium depletion in the dog, *Am. J. Physiol.,* 243, F113, 1982.

177. Lorkovic, H. and Rudd, R., Influence of divalent cations on potassium contracture duration in frog fibres, *Pflugers Arch.,* 398, 114, 1983.

178. Liu, L., Borowski, G., and Rose, L.I., Hypomagnesemia in a tennis player, *Physician Sportsmed.,* 11, 79, 1983.

179. Somlyo, A.V., Gonzalez-Serratos, H., Shuman, H., McClellan, G., and Somlyo, A.P., Calcium release and ionic changes in the sarcoplasmic reticulum of tetanized muscle: an electron-probe study, *J. Cell Biol.,* 90, 577, 1981.

180. Yoshioka, T. and Somlyo, A.P., Calcium and magnesium contents and volume of the terminal cisternae in caffeine-treated skeletal muscle, *J. Cell Biol.,* 99, 558, 1984.

181. Galland, L., Normocalcemic tetany and candidiasis, *Magnesium,* 4, 339, 1985.

182. Williamson, S.L., Johnson, R.W., Hudkins, P.G., and Strate, S.M., Exertional cramps: a prospective study of biochemical and anthropometric variables in bicycle riders, *Cycling Sci.,* 15, 1993.

183. Henrotte, J.G., Franck, G., Santarromana, M., Frances, H., Mouton, D., and Motta, R., Mice selected for low and high blood magnesium levels: a new model for stress studies, *Physiol. Behav.,* 61, 653, 1997.

184. Bilbey, D.G. and Prabhakaran, V.M., Muscle cramps and magnesium deficiency: case reports, *Can. Fam. Physician,* 42, 1348, 1996.

185. Clinton, C.W., Braude, B.M., and James, M.F.M., Painful muscle spasm reversed by magnesium sulphate, *S. Afr. Med. J.,* 68, 332, 1985.

186. Dahle, L.O., Berg, G., Hammar, M., Hurtig, M., and Larsson, L., The effect of oral magnesium substitution on pregnancy-induced leg cramps, *Am. J. Obstet. Gynecol.,* 173, 175, 1995.

187. James, M.F.M. and Wright, G.A., Tetany and myocardial arrhythmia due to hypomagnesemia, *S. Afr. Med. J.,* 69, 48, 1986.

188. Brucato, A., Bonati, M., Gaspari, F., Colussi, G., Giachetti, M., Zoppi, F., and Ruggerone, M.L., Tetany and rhabdomyolysis due to surreptitious furosemide — importance of Mg supplementation, *Clin. Toxicol.,* 31, 341, 1993.

189. Vizinova, H., Bartousek, J., and Bartek, J., Magnesium balance in patients with spasmophilia: relation to results of electromyography, *Cas. Lek. Cesk.,* 136, 448, 1997.

190. Hermans, C., Lefebvre, C., Devogelaer, J.P., and Lambert, M., Hypocalcaemia and chronic alcohol intoxication: transient hypoparathyroidism secondary to magnesium deficiency, *Clin. Rheumatol.,* 15, 193, 1996.

191. Siegal, T., Muscle cramps in the cancer patient: causes and treatment, *J. Pain Symptom. Manage.,* 6, 84, 1991.

192. Schwellnus, M.P., Derman, E.W., and Noakes, T.D., Aetiology of skeletal muscle "cramps" during exercise: a novel hypothesis, *J. Sports Sci.,* 15, 277, 1997.

193. Cohen, I. and Zimmerman, A.L., Changes in serum electrolyte levels during marathon running, *S. Afr. Med. J.,* 53, 12, 1978.

194. Tate, C.A., Bonner, H.W., and Leslie, S.W., Calcium uptake in skeletal muscle mitochondria: the effects of long-term chronic and acute exercise, *Eur. J. Appl. Physiol.,* 39, 117, 1978.

195. Refsum, H.E., Meen, H.D., and Stromme, S.B., Whole blood, serum and erythrocyte magnesium concentrations after repeated heavy exercise of long duration, *Scand. J. Clin. Lab. Invest.,* 32, 123, 1973.

196. Tibes, U., Hemmer, B., Schweigart, U., Boning, D., and Fotescu, D., Exercise acidosis as cause of electrolyte changes in femoral venous blood of trained and untrained man, *Pflugers Arch.,* 347, 145, 1974.

197. Dreosti, I.E., Magnesium status and health, *Nutr. Rev.,* 53, S23, 1995.

198. Clarkson, P.M. and Haymes, E.M., Exercise and mineral status of athletes: calcium, magnesium, phosphorus and iron, *Med. Sci. Sports Exercise,* 27, 831, 1995.

199. Buchman, A.L., Keen, C., Commisso, J., Kiliip, D., Ou, C.N., Rognerud, C.L., Dennis, K., and Dunn, J.K., The effect of a marathon run on plasma and urine mineral and metal concentrations, *J. Am. Coll. Nutr.,* 17, 124, 1998.

200. Dolev, E., Burstein, R., Wishnitzer, R., Lubin, F., Chetriet, A., Shefi, M., and Deuster, P.A., Longitudinal study of magnesium status of Israeli military recruits, *Magnesium Trace Elem.,* 10, 420, 1992.

201. Lowney, P., Gershwin, M.E., Hurley, L.S., Stern, J.S., and Keen, C.L., The effect of variable magnesium intake on potential factors influencing endurance capacity, *Biol. Trace Elem. Res.,* 16, 1, 1988.

202. Lowney, P., Stern, J.S., Gershwin, M.E., and Keen, C.L., Magnesium deficiency and blood 2,3 diphosphoglycerate concentrations in sedentary and exercised male Osborne–Mendel rats, *Metabolism,* 39, 788, 1990.

203. Seelig, M., Consequences of magnesium deficiency on the enhancement of stress reactions; preventive and therapeutic implications (a review), *J. Am. Coll. Nutr.,* 13, 429, 1994.

204. Mansmann, H.C., Consider magnesium homeostasis, *Pediatr. Asthma Allergy Immunol.,* 5, 273, 1991.

205. Anderson, R.A., Bryden, N.A., Polansky, M.M., and Thorp, J.W., Effects of carbohydrate loading and underwater exercise on circulating cortisol, insulin and urinary losses of chromium and zinc, *Eur. J. Appl. Physiol.,* 63, 146, 1991.

206. Beals, K.A. and Manore, M.M., Nutritional status of female athletes with subclinical eating disorders, *J. Am. Diet. Assoc.,* 98, 419, 1998.

207. Cordova, A., Gimenez, M., and Escanero, J.F., Changes of plasma zinc and copper at various times of swimming until exhaustion in the rat, *J. Trace Elem. Electrolytes Health Dis.,* 4, 189, 1990.

208. Cordova, A., Gimenez, M., and Escanero, J.F., Effect of swimming to exhaustion, at low temperatures, on serum Zn, Cu, Mg and Ca in rats, *Physiol. Behav.,* 48, 595, 1990.

209. Fogelholm, M., Micronutrient status in females during a 24-week fitness-type exercise program, *Ann. Nutr. Metab.,* 36, 209, 1992.

210. Koivisto, V.A., Sane, T., Fyhrquist, F., and Pelkonen, R., Fuel and fluid homeostasis during long-term exercise in healthy subjects and type I diabetic patients, *Diabetes Care,* 15, 1736, 1992.

211. Newhouse, I.J., Clement, D.B., and Lai, C., Effects of iron supplementation on serum copper, zinc, calcium, and magnesium levels in women, *Med. Sci. Sports Exercise,* 25, 562, 1993.

212. Rasmussen, H.S., Videbaek, R., Melchior, T., Aurup, P., Clintin, C., and Pedersen, N.T., Myocardial contractility and performance capacity after magnesium infusion in young healthy persons: a double-blind, placebo-controlled, cross-over study, *Clin. Cardiol.*, 11, 541, 1988.

213. Rama, R., Ibanez, J., Pages, T., Callis, A., and Palacios, L., Plasma and red blood cell magnesium levels and plasma creatine after a 100 km race, *Rev. Esp. Fisiol.*, 49, 43, 1993.

214. Resina, A., Brettoni, M., Gatteschi, L., Galvan, P., Orsi, F., and Rubenni, M.G., Changes in the concentrations of plasma and erythrocyte magnesium and of 2,3-diphosphoglycerate during a period of aerobic training, *Eur. J. Appl. Physiol.*, 68, 390, 1994.

215. Rowe, W.J., Extraordinary unremitting endurance exercise and permanent injury to normal heart, *Lancet*, 340, 712, 1992.

216. Stendig-Lindberg, G., Sudden death of athletes: is it due to long-term changes in serum magnesium, lipids, and blood sugar? *J. Basic Clin. Physiol. Pharmacol.*, 3, 153, 1992.

217. van Rensburg, J.P., Kielblock, A.J., and van der Linde, A., Physiologic and biochemical changes during a triathlon competition, *Int. J. Sports Med.*, 7, 1, 1986.

218. Whang, R., Electrolyte and water metabolism in sports activities, *Comp. Ther.*, 24, 5, 1998.

219. Binder, F., Huntzelmann, A., and Golf, S., Biochemical effects of magnesium on glucose metabolism during a sporting event in fencers, *Magnesium Res.*, 5, 160, 1992.

220. Brilla, L.R. and Lombardi, V.P., Variable response of serum magnesium and total cholesterol to different magnesium intakes and exercise levels in rats, *Magnesium*, 6, 205, 1987.

221. Caddell, J., Kupiecki, R., Proxmire, D.L., Satoh, P., and Hutchinson, B., Plasma catecholamines in acute magnesium deficiency in weanling rats, *J. Nutr.*, 116, 1896, 1986.

222. Casoni, I., Guglielmini, C., Graziano, L., Reali, M.G., Mazzotta, D., and Abbasciano, V., Changes of magnesium concentrations in endurance athletes, *Int. J. Sports Med.*, 11, 234, 1990.

223. Chadda, K.D., Cohen, J., Werner, B.M., and Gorfien, P., Observations on serum and red blood cell magnesium changes in treadmill exercise-induced cardiac ischemia, *J. Am. Coll. Nutr.*, 4, 157, 1985.

224. Conn, C.A., Schemmel, R.A., Smith, B.W., Ryder, E., Heusner, W.W., and Ku, P., Plasma and erythrocyte magnesium concentrations and correlations with maximum oxygen consumption in nine- to twelve-year-old competitive swimmers, *Magnesium*, 7, 27, 1988.

225. Fitzherbert, J., Magnesium: the vital ingredient? *Aust. Runner*, 2, 20, 1982.

226. Franck, H., Beuker, F., and Gurk, S., The effect of physical activity on bone turnover in young adults, *Exp. Clin. Endocrinol.*, 98, 42, 1991.

227. Golf, S., Graef, V., Happel, O., and Seim, K.E., Blood hemoglobin, erythrocytes, leukocytes, and hematocrit in physical exercise after magnesium supplementation, *J. Am. Coll. Nutr.*, 4, 393, 1985.

228. Golf, S., Happel, O., and Graef, V., Plasma aldosterone, cortisol and electrolyte concentrations in physical exercise after magnesium supplementation, *J. Clin. Chem. Clin. Biochem.*, 22, 717, 1984.

229. Joborn, H., Akerstrom, G., and Ljunghall, S., Effects of exogenous catecholamines and exercise on plasma magnesium concentrations, *Clin. Endocrinol.*, 23, 219, 1985.

230. Laires, M.J. and Alves, F., Changes in plasma, erythrocyte, and urinary magnesium with prolonged swimming exercise, *Magnesium Res.*, 4, 119, 1991.

231. Laires, M.J., Rayssiguier, Y., Guezennec, C.Y., and Alves, F., Effect of magnesium deficiency on exercise capacity in rats, *Magnesium Res.*, 2, 136, 1989.

232. Ljunghall, S., Joborn, H., Rastad, J., and Akerstrom, G., Plasma potassium and phosphate concentrations: influence by adrenaline infusion, β-blockade and physical exercise, *Acta Med. Scand.*, 221, 83, 1987.

233. Ljunghall, S., Joborn, H., Roxin, L., Skarfors, E.T., Wide, L.E., and Lithell, H.O., Increase in serum parathyroid hormone levels after prolonged physical exercise, *Med. Sci. Sports Exercise*, 20, 122, 1988.

234. Lukaski, H.C., Bolonchuk, W.W., Klevay, L.M., Milne, D.B., and Sandstead, H.H., Maximal oxygen consumption as related to magnesium, copper, and zinc nutriture, *Am. J. Clin. Nutr.*, 37, 407, 1983.

235. Manore, M.M., Wells, C.L., and Lehman, W.R., Blood magnesium and red blood cell hemolysis following exercise in female runners consuming adequate dietary magnesium, *Nutr. Rep. Int.*, 39, 787, 1989.

236. Munch, J., Golf, S.W., Graef, V., and Nowacki, P.E., Magnesium in the metabolism of high performance sportsmen, *Magnesium Res.*, 3, 307, 1990.

237. Olha, A.E., Klissouras, V., Sullivan, J.D., and Skoryna, S.C., Effect of exercise on concentration of elements in the serum, *J. Sports Med.*, 22, 414, 1982.

238. Ripari, P., Pieralisi, G., Giamberardino, M.A., Resina, A., and Vecchiet, L., Effects of magnesium pidolate on some cardiorespiratory submaximal effort parameters, *Magnesium Res.*, 2, 70, 1989.

239. Ruddel, P., Pratt, K., and Franz, K.B., Magnesium metabolism in subjects during aerobic endurance exercise, *J. Am. Coll. Nutr.*, 4, 347, 1985.

240. Smith, R.T., Miller-Ihli, N.J., Sunde, M.L., and Smith, E.L., Changes in bone magnesium content with exercise at two levels of dietary calcium intake, *J. Am. Coll. Nutr.*, 4, 392, 1985.

241. Steinacker, J.M., Grunert-Fuchs, M., Steininger, K., and Wodick, R.E., Effects of long-time-administration of magnesium on physical capacity, *Int. J. Sports Med.*, 8, 151, 1987.

242. Tate, C.A., Wolkowicz, P.E., and McMillin-Wood, J., Exercise-induced alternations of hepatic mitochondrial function, *Biochem. J.*, 208, 695, 1982.

243. Tiedt, H.J. and Grimm, M., Changes in serum magnesium over a prolonged period in young competitive athletes, *Magnesium Res.*, 5, 159, 1992.

244. Sjogaard, G., Electrolytes in slow and fast muscle fibers of humans at rest and with dynamic exercise, *Am. J. Physiol.*, 245, R25, 1983.

245. Brilla, L.R. and Gunter, K.B., Effect of magnesium supplementation on exercise time to exhaustion, *Med. Exercise Nutr. Health*, 4, 230, 1995.

246. Hespel, P., Lijnen, P., Fiocchi, R., Denys, B., Lissens, W., M'Buyamba-Kabangu, J., and Amery, A., Cationic concentrations and transmembrane fluxes in erythrocytes of humans during exercise, *J. Appl. Physiol.*, 61, 37, 1986.

247. Golf, S., Munch, J., Graef, V., Temme, H., Brustle, A., Roka, L., Beuther, G., Heinz, N., Buhl, C., and Nowacki, P.E., Effect of a 4-week magnesium supplementation on lactate elimination in competitive rowers during exhaustive simulated rowing, *Magnesium Res.*, 2, 71, 1989.

248. Cordova, A., Escanero, J.F., and Gimenez, M., Magnesium distribution in rats after maximal exercise in air and under hypoxic conditions, *Magnesium Res.*, 5, 23, 1992.

249. Marcuk, D. and Brilla, L.R., The effects of ergogenic aid supplementation on aerobic economy in competitive long-distance runners, *J. Am. Coll. Nutr.*, 15, 541, 1996.

250. Durlach, J., Dulach, V., Bac, P., Rayssiguier, Y., Bara, M. and Guiet-Bara, A., Magnesium and aging. II. Clinical data: aetiological mechanisms and pathophysiological consequences of magnesium deficit in the elderly, *Magnesium Res.*, 6, 379, 1993.

251. Costill, D.L., Cote, R., and Fink, W., Muscle water and electrolytes following varied levels of dehydration in man, *J. Appl. Physiol.*, 40, 6, 1976.

252. Fogelholm, G.M., Koskinin, R., Laasko, J., Rankinin, T., and Ruokonen, I., Gradual and rapid weight loss: effects on nutrition and performance in male athletes, *Med. Sci. Sports Exercise*, 25, 371, 1993.

253. Lehmann, M., Schnee, W., Scheu, R., Stockhausen, W., and Bachl, N., Decreased nocturnal catecholamine excretion: parameter for an overtraining syndrome in athletes? *Int. J. Sports Med.*, 13, 236, 1992.

254. Lehmann, M., Foster, C., and Keul, J., Overtraining in endurance athletes: a brief review, *Med. Sci. Sports Exercise*, 25, 854, 1993.

255. Bell, N.H., Godsen, R.N., Henry, D.P., Shary, J., and Epstein, S., The effects of muscle-building exercise on vitamin D and mineral metabolism, *J. Bone Miner. Res.*, 3, 369, 1988.

256. Golf, S., Kuhn, D., Zeblin, A., Graef, V., Temme, H., Roka, L., and Czeke, J., The role of magnesium in endogenous activation of fibrinolysis by local acidosis in dependence of predictive parameters of blood, *Magnesium Res.*, 2, 72, 1989.

257. Verde, T., Shephard, R.J., Corey, P., and Moore, R., Sweat composition in exercise and in heat, *J. Appl. Physiol.*, 53, 1540, 1982.

258. Helbig, J., Beuker, F., and Munz, T., Magnesium levels in body builders during the precompetition period, *Magnesium Res.*, 2, 69, 1989.

259. Mader, A., Hartmann, U., Fischer, H.G., Reinhards, G., Bohnerti, K.J., and Hollmann, W., Magnesium supplementation, magnesium excretion and general relation to training intensity and volume in elite rowers during high altitude training, *Magnesium Res.*, 3, 58, 1990.

260. Newman, J.C. and Amarsinham, J.L., The pathogenesis of eclampsia: the magnesium ischaemia hypothesis, *Med. Hypothesis*, 40, 250, 1993.

261. Derman, W., Schwellnus, M.P., Lambert, M.I., Emms, M., Sinclair-Smith, C., Kirby, P., and Noakes, T.D., The "worn-out athlete": a clinical approach to chronic fatigue in athletes, *J. Sports Sci.*, 15, 341, 1995.

262. Skurnick, J.H., Bogden, J.D., Baker, H., Kemp, F.W., Sheffet, A., Quattrone, G., and Louria, D.B., Micronutrient profiles in HIV-1-infected heterosexual adults, *J. Acquir. Defic. Syndr. Hum. Retrovirol.*, 12, 75, 1996.

263. Cordova, A., Variations of serum magnesium and zinc after surgery, and postoperative fatigue, *Magnesium Res.*, 8, 367, 1995.

264. Duan, C., Delp, M.D., Hayes, D.A., Delp, P.D., and Armstrong, R.B., Rat skeletal muscle mitochondrial $[Ca^{+2}]$ and injury from downhill walking, *J. Appl. Physiol.*, 68, 1241, 1990.

265. Knochel, J.P., Neuromuscular manifestations of electrolyte disorders, *Am. J. Med.*, 72, 521, 1982.

266. Madsen, K., Pedersen, P.K., Djurhuus, M.S., and Klitgaard, N.A., Effects of detraining on endurance capacity and metabolic changes during prolonged exhaustive exercise, *J. Appl. Physiol.*, 75, 1444, 1993.

267. Clausen, T., Everts, M.E., and Kjeldsen, K., Quantification of the maximum capacity for active sodium–potassium transport in rat skeletal muscle, *J. Physiol.*, 388, 163, 1987.

268. Agus, Z.S. and Morad, M., Modulation of cardiac ion channels by magnesium, *Annu. Rev. Physiol.*, 53, 299, 1991.

269. Konig, D., Keul, J., Northoff, H., and Berg, A., Rationale for a specific diet from the viewpoint of sports medicine and sports orthopedics: relation to stress reaction and regeneration, *Orthopade*, 26, 942, 1997.

270. Durlach, J., Recommended dietary amounts of magnesium: magnesium RDA, *Magnesium Res.*, 2, 195, 1989.

271. Shils, M.E., Magnesium, in *Modern Nutrition in Health and Disease*, 8th ed., Lea & Febiger, Philadelphia, 1994, 164.

272. Shils, M.E. and Rude, R.K., Deliberations and evaluations of the approaches, endpoints and paradigms for magnesium dietary recommendations, *J. Nutr.*, 126, 2398S, 1996.

273. Hansen, O. and Johansson, B.W., S-Mg does not change inversely to S-FFA during acute stress situations, *Angiology*, 40, 1011, 1989.

274. Amyard, N., Leyris, A., Monier, C., Frances, H., Boulu, R.G., and Henrotte, J.G., Brain catecholamines, serotonin and their metabolites in mice selected for low (MGL) and high (MGH) blood magnesium, *Magnesium Res.*, 8, 5, 1995.

275. Bac, P., Pages, N., Herrenknecht, C., and Teste, J.F., Inhibition of mouse-killing behavior in magnesium-deficient rats: effect of pharmacological doses of magnesium pidolate, magnesium aspartate, magnesium lactate, magnesium gluconate and magnesium chloride, *Magnesium Res.*, 8, 37, 1995.

276. Chatterji, J.C., Ohri, V.C., Chadha, K.S., Das, B.K., Akhtar, M., Tewari, S.C., Bhattacharji, P., and Wadhwa, A., Serum and urinary cation changes on acute induction to high altitude (3200 and 3771 metres), *Aviat. Space Environ. Med.*, 53, 576, 1982.

277. Mairbaurl, H., Oelz, O., and Bartsch, P., Interactions between Hb, Mg, DPG, and Cl determine change in Hb–O_2 affinity at high altitude, *J. Appl. Physiol.*, 74, 40, 1993.

278. Durlach, J., Present and future of magnesium research, *J. Jpn. Soc. Magnesium Res.*, 12, 113, 1993.

279. Ryan, M.P., Interrelationships of magnesium and potassium homeostasis, *Miner. Electrolyte Metab.*, 19, 290, 1993.
280. Bucci, L.R., Nutritional ergogenic aids, in *Nutrition in Exercise and Sport*, Hickson, J.F., Jr. and Wolinsky, I., Eds., CRC Press, Boca Raton, FL, 1989, chap. 7.
281. Lukaski, H.C. and Penland, J.G., Functional changes appropriate for determining mineral element requirements, *J. Nutr.*, 126, 2354S, 1996.

WATER AND ELECTROLYTES

Chapter 5

WATER IN EXERCISE AND SPORT

Paul N. Taylor
Ira Wolinsky
Dorothea J. Klimis

CONTENTS

0-8493-8196-7/99/$0.00+$.50
© 1999 by CRC Press LLC

I. INTRODUCTION

Biologists, nutritionists, and physiologists are in general agreement that water is a major necessity for life on earth and is the most important nutrient for the human body. We can live for weeks without eating, but will quickly die if deprived of water.[1] Water is an essential nutrient because our bodies cannot synthesize enough to replace the amounts lost in metabolism.[2] Yet many of us fail to appreciate the importance of water in our daily lives. Too often, a person (including athletes) will invest much time and effort in developing and following a prudent diet and a sound training regimen, but will fail to drink enough fluids to avoid dehydration. How many of us dismiss fatigue, lethargy, headache, or poor performance as only the consequence of an "off" day, never realizing that even mild dehydration causes decreased exercise performance? For all who exercise and/or participate in sports, whether at a recreational, amateur, or professional level, a willingness to commit to a strategy for optimum hydration is necessary to ensure peak performance and maintenance of health.

II. EUHYDRATION

Euhydration exists when water loss equals water intake,[3] and the total body water content is such that an individual is normally hydrated.[4] The total body water is distributed in biological "compartments," but there is a constant "flow" of water within and between these compartments.

A. PARTITIONING OF WATER

By weight, the human body is about 60% water, depending on age, gender, and fat content (in general, men have a higher body water content than women, because women tend to have a larger percentage of body fat than men); in both sexes, body water content is inversely proportional to age.[5] Within tissues, the water content varies as well, with more contained in blood (90%), for example, than in bone (25%).[6-8]

About 42 l of water is contained in an average 70-kg adult male and about 27.5 l in an average 55-kg adult female. For convenience, the body is usually divided into two major fluid compartments: the intracellular (containing 40 to 50% of total body water) and the extracellular (containing 50 to 60% of total body water).[9] The extracellular fluid compartment is further subdivided into the interstitial fluid compartment and the blood plasma.[5,8] Some authors describe a third fluid compartment, the transcellular, comprising such epithelial secretions as synovial and cerebrospinal fluids, ocular humor, and gastric secretions.[6,8] However, none of these transcellular fluids is known to be compromised during exercise.

B. WATER BALANCE

At rest, total body water content is generally constant despite the continuous flow within and between fluid compartments and exchange with the external environment. Although the actual volumes of water intake and loss vary from person to person and are affected by many variables (e.g., body composition, heat, humidity, gender), an average 2.1 (women) to 2.9 (men) l/day of water is exchanged. Ten percent of the usual daily "intake" of water results from cellular oxidative phosphorylation (i.e., it is synthesized by the body). The remaining 90% must come from external sources, 60% ingested as liquid and 30% from ingested food. The daily output, or loss, of water is comprised of urine excretion by the kidneys (60%), evaporation from respiration and skin diffusion (30%, termed "insensible" water loss), sweating (5%), and excretion of feces (5%).[1,5,8]

C. REQUIREMENTS FOR WATER

The Recommended Dietary Allowance (RDA) for water for adults at rest under average conditions of environmental exposure is 1 ml/kcal of energy expenditure,[2] or 2.2 l/day for women and 2.9 l/day for men.[8] Those who drink eight 8-oz (~1.9-l) glasses per day of water should easily meet the RDA (considering that most foods also contain water). The RDA may be safely increased to 1.5 ml/kcal to cover the variations in activity levels, sweating, and solute loads of active individuals.[2]

D. THE PHYSIOLOGICAL FUNCTIONS OF WATER

Water is found in all of the tissues of the body.[5] At the cellular level, water, as a component of the cytoplasm, provides the turgor necessary for structural firmness.[8]

Lubrication is a function of water that is of importance in exercise.[8] The synovial fluid surrounding the joints allows bones to move freely against each other.[7] Within muscles, the fluid of the sarcoplasm contains all of the constituents necessary for contraction and expansion,[10] facilitating the movement of actin and myosin filaments against each other.

Blood, lymph, gastric secretions, and urine are all examples of the role of water as a transport medium. Blood plasma, for example, serves as a transporter for a variety of substances.[7] Active muscles require oxygen, which is carried to the tissues by red blood cells. Likewise, nutrients necessary to muscle function, such as glucose and various fatty and amino acids, arrive via the bloodstream. As muscles work, they generate metabolic wastes such as carbon dioxide and lactic acid, which are transported away from the muscles by the plasma. Hormones which regulate the activity and metabolism of the working muscles are delivered to the tissues via the plasma. Blood also contains substances which act as buffering agents to maintain pH in the presence of lactate. Exercising muscles produce quantities of lactic and other organic acids from which hydrogen ions dissociate. The presence of excess hydrogen ions impairs performance by inhibiting muscle contractility and reducing the generation of adenosine triphosphatase.[7,10–12]

Water facilitates the cooling of the body as a necessary component of the thermoregulatory process. Guyton and Hall[13] describe heat loss from a human body at rest via three routes: conduction and evaporation (both influenced by air convection) and radiation. Provided body temperature is greater than that of its surroundings, most of the heat (78%) is lost by radiation and conduction. If the surrounding air temperature is greater than the body temperature, then the body gains heat by radiation and conduction, and evaporation becomes the sole route of heat loss.

At rest, a person loses 450 to 600 ml of water from the skin and lungs, which represents an insensible heat loss of 12 to 16 kcal/hr.[13] Should the body temperature begin to rise, this evaporation of diffused water cannot be adjusted. Rather, the rate of heat loss by evaporation can only be accelerated by an increase in the rate of sweating. In even moderately warm weather, copious amounts of water are lost by sweating, so much so that even individuals who consciously make an effort to maintain euhydration are not entirely successful. The voluntary intake of fluids rarely replaces more than about half of the water that is lost by sweating, leading to "involuntary" dehydration.[14,15] To make matters worse, most people do not voluntarily rehydrate adequately even when water is available, leading to "voluntary" dehydration.[16]

III. HYPOHYDRATION

Whenever water loss is greater than water intake, a body water deficit, or hypohydration, ensues (dehydration refers to the loss of body water).[4] The body is very sensitive to even small losses of water. Active individuals should take precautions to prevent losing more than 1 to 2% of body mass as water during periods of athletics, exercise, or work. Most of us are aware that water loss can be substantial in hot/dry and hot/humid environments, but activities in other environments (e.g., cold, water, high altitude) may also cause hypohydration.

A. EXERCISE IN THE HEAT

Most of us probably need to worry most about dehydration when exercising in hot/dry or hot/humid conditions. Much of the early research into human physiological adaptations to work in extremes of heat was summarized 50 years ago by Adolf and his colleagues,[17] in preparation for the conduct of war in the desert. Many recent insights have also come about as the result of military necessity,[18–23] as well as from research in the exercise and sports sciences.[24–30] Physiological responses to exercise in the heat include changes in cardiovascular function (a "competition" between active muscles and skin for blood supply, the muscles needing transported oxygen and the skin needing blood to facilitate heat loss), changes in energy pro-duction (increased oxygen uptake, resulting in increased rate of glycogenolysis and lactate production[31]), and changes in body fluid balance (renal and hormonal re-sponses,[32] increased sweating, reduced blood volume), some of which are discussed below.[33]

B. CHANGES IN WATER BALANCE DURING EXERCISE

The dangers of dehydration for endurance athletes were first reported almost 30 years ago[34] and are now almost universally accepted.[1,35-39] Performance begins to decline almost as soon as water loss is greater than water intake, although muscular strength and endurance may be unaffected.[40] For every 1% of body weight lost, plasma volume decreases by 2.5% and muscle water decreases by 1%, while rectal temperature increases 0.4 to 0.5°C.[36] Once the loss reaches 3%, physiological changes (e.g., decreased blood volume, decreased urinary output) occur, along with diminished physical performance and decreased endurance. A water loss of 9 to 12% of body weight can be fatal.[1]

If a person were to exercise without drinking any water for more than 30 min, water would still be added to the total-body water pool endogenously. First, me-tabolism increases as exercise intensity increases, enough so that about 100 to 150 ml/hr of water is produced. Second, muscle glycogenolysis liberates 3 to 4 g of water per gram of glycogen, which when added to the metabolic water increases total body water by about 600 to 650 ml/hr.[1,6]

Another consequence of increased metabolic rate during exercise is increased heat production, followed by increased sweating. At the same time, blood flow is shifted so that more blood is delivered to the skin surface for dissipation of heat, while less is delivered to the kidneys in an effort to conserve water. Therefore, even though the body "gains" 600 ml of water during the exercise session, the amount falls far short of the increased demand for water to dissipate heat. Accel-erated fluid losses occur primarily through the mechanisms of respiration and sweating. The amount of water lost in respiration is closely related to the expen-diture of energy[41] and can be as high as 75 ml/hr, while the amount of sweat produced, around 1.5 l/hr, is also related to energy expenditure but is affected by other factors, such as environmental temperature, body size, and an individual's unique metabolic rate. For an endurance athlete exercising in extremes of heat and humidity, sweat loss may approach 3 l/hr.[1]

C. CHANGES IN PLASMA DURING EXERCISE

During exercise there is considerable activity in the circulatory system, where there is always an exchange of gases (O_2, CO_2), electrolytes, nutrients, and water between the blood and the interstitial fluids. Under normal circumstances, the amount of fluid leaving the capillaries is nearly equal to the amount of fluid returning ("the

Starling equilibrium").[42] On a daily basis, then, the net filtration, or the amount of fluid that escapes to the interstitium and must be returned to the circulation via the lymphatic system, amounts to about 2 ml/min or 2 to 3 l/day.[43]

During exercise, blood pressure rises to ensure that adequate blood flow reaches the active muscles. The resulting increase in hydrostatic pressure forces fluid out of the capillaries and into the interstitium, while at the same time the osmotic pressure in the muscle cells themselves increases, tending to pull water out of the interstitial fluid and capillaries.[6,44] Most of the fluid that is lost this way comes from the plasma during the first few minutes of intense exercise, and the amount lost varies according to the hydration status of the individual[45] and the intensity of the exercise,[6,44] in the range of 10 to 20% of the plasma volume.[44,46] Reduced plasma volume is temporary, returning to ambient levels soon after the exercise session ends. However, during long-term exercise sessions, the loss of plasma volume may affect performance by two mechanisms. First, if blood viscosity increases sufficiently (hematocrit >60%), oxygen transport may be compromised[44] at the same time that the oxygen-carrying capacity per unit of blood is increased (due to an increase in hemoglobin concentration).[6,44] Second, in order to cool the body, some blood is diverted from the active muscles to the skin. A diminished ability to regulate body temperature often accompanies a decrease in plasma volume (less blood is available to be diverted to the skin), but there is evidence to indicate that an increase in plasma osmolality has more of an effect on thermoregulation than does plasma volume alone.[47]

As for the "lost" fluid, except for the volume lost as sweat, it may be found in the interstitial spaces surrounding the active muscles, either in direct contact with the muscles or in the subcutaneous spaces.[6] Provided an effective hydration regimen has been followed, there seem to be no long-term deleterious plasma volume deficits associated with exercise.

D. EXERCISE IN ENVIRONMENTAL EXTREMES OTHER THAN HEAT

1. Exercise in the Cold

Exercise in the cold presents unique challenges to participants. As long as one is aware of the need to monitor hydration status in cold weather and pays attention to fluid intake, body fluid balance can be maintained.[48] Freund and Young[49] explain how the fluid status of an individual in a cold environment can be affected in a number of ways. First, exposure to cold increases urine flow concomitant with decreased plasma volume, although this diuretic effect is variable and the mechanism(s) of the diuresis remains undefined. Second, as the metabolic rate increases in the cold, respiratory water loss increases, perhaps by as much as 340 ml/day due to the cold air alone. Sweat losses can be substantial if the exerciser is wearing heavy clothing, with metabolic rate increasing 10 to 20% during exercise. Finally, fluid intake may be reduced in cold weather. Whereas cold fluids are usually indicated for rehydration in mild to hot environments, the same fluids consumed in a cold environment can have the unwanted effect of chilling an individual to uncomfortable or even dangerous levels. Therefore, the temperature of fluids consumed in cold environments should be between 25 and 30°C to avoid unwanted physiological changes.[50] In conditions of extreme cold, when freezing of fluids or water-containing foods may be expected, it is wise to carry fluids in vacuum bottles if there will be no easy access to a warm environment.

2. Exercise in the Water

Many a swimmer has assumed that because the body is surrounded by water, there is no sweat produced during the exercise and therefore no need to drink to stay hydrated.[39] In reality, swimmers may lose up to 1.5 l/hr of fluid without ever perceiving the loss,[51] and there is evidence that over time, swimmers develop measurable differences in regional body sweat responses compared to dry ground exercisers.[52,53] Furthermore, there is evidence that immersion in water promotes diuresis,[54] reduces the thirst sensation in hypohydrated swimmers,[55] and that fluid and electrolyte metabolism and blood circulation are affected differently in swimmers compared to land exercisers.[56] Swimmers and other water sports enthusiasts, therefore, must pay as much attention to hydration as any other athlete.

3. Exercise at High Altitude

The popularity of high-altitude, four-season resorts has increased substantially in the last 50 years. Such areas are located from about 1200 m elevation in the eastern United States to about 3500 m elevation in the West. Mountain hikers and climbers routinely reach those altitudes, and many venture much higher. Those who exercise at high altitude, especially for long periods of time, must be aware of some aspects of hydration that are not experienced at lower levels.

Wilmore and Costill[57] explain conditions at altitude that affect exercise. At sea level, barometric pressure (P_b) is about 760 mmHg and the partial pressure of oxygen (PO_2) is 159.2 mmHg. As one ventures higher, both values decline, so that at 1000 m elevation, P_b is about 674 mmHg and PO_2 is 141.2 mmHg; at 4000 m, P_b is about 462 mmHg and PO_2 is 96.9 mmHg. The air at altitude still contains the same 20.93% oxygen as it contains at sea level, but it is more difficult to breathe (i.e., a greater volume of air must be ventilated at altitude because the air is less dense). The effect of increased ventilation at altitude is the same as hyperventilation at sea level: respiratory alkalosis. Maximal oxygen uptake ($\dot{V}O_2$max) decreases by about 11% for every 1000-m increase in elevation above 1600 m, which translates into seriously diminished capacity for physical exercise.

Along with the respiratory stress imposed by altitude, there are other changes occurring.[58,59] Hypoxia at elevation induces weight loss, first due to loss of water and later due to malnutrition.[60] The total body water loss, which partially manifests itself as diuresis in 3 to 4 days, includes both decreases in plasma volume[57] and decreases in intra- and extravascular fluid volumes and is a physiological response to hypoxemia.[61] Along with the fluid loss, sodium-regulating hormones are affected,[62] leading to natriuresis,[61,62] and there seems to be a measurable fluid shift to the upper body.[63] Alpine guides recognized increased urine output as a sign of altitude adaptation, whereas those who could not adapt suffered water retention and mountain sickness.[61,64,65]

Compounding all of these effects, individuals exercising at altitude may also experience increased respiratory water loss and be subject to the same consequences of wearing heavy clothing as those exercising in the cold. Reduced appetite and thirst are also common with exposure to hypoxia, so that fluid intake is voluntarily reduced.

IV. HYPERHYDRATION

The term "hyperhydration" is used clinically to indicate a state of abnormally increased water content of the body.[9] In the literature of exercise and sports sciences, hyperhydration describes pre-exercise "fluid bulking" (i.e., drinking large volumes of water or other fluids before exercising) to forestall dehydration. Hyperhydration may also describe the expanded fluid volumes (both intra- and extravascular) of endurance-trained athletes,[66] in whom higher capillary filtration rates[67] and hypervolemia have been noted. A simpler definition of hyperhydration is water loss is less than water intake.

The prevailing opinion today is that hyperhydration before exercise is beneficial. Individuals may hyperhydrate by drinking extra fluids 1 to 2 days before undertaking an intense activity (e.g., running a marathon race) and by drinking 250 to 600 ml of cold water or sports beverage 10 to 20 min[6,8,36,39,45,47,51,68–71] up to 2 hr[72] before starting an activity (whether intense or not). These strategies are devised to delay the onset of dehydration, to increase sweating, and to modulate the expected rise in body core temperature.

Some have shown that it is possible to hyperhydrate athletes for up to 2 days by providing glycerol (2.9 to 3.1 g/kg/day) in the hydration fluid.[73] The benefits of glycerol-induced hyperhydration include elevated sweat rate, lower rectal temperature (indicative of a lower body core temperature), and no changes in fluid electrolytes or blood parameters.[74] These benefits seem to accrue only if the glycerol-containing beverage is consumed before the exercise session begins,[75] and hyperhydration at a lesser glycerol content (1.2 g/kg lean body mass) closer to the time of exercise (1 hr) appears to provide no improvement over water alone.[76]

There seem to be no adverse effects associated with pre-exercise hyperhydration in healthy individuals, and toxicity from excessive water intake is rare.[2] However, in some cases of hyponatremia in ultraendurance athletes, dilution of sodium by fluids ingested before, during, and perhaps after the exercise session is thought to be at least partly a cause.[1,77–80] Several studies by Zorbas and colleagues[81–86] of hyperhydration in endurance-trained athletes during restriction of their activities indicate that water loading attenuates plasma electrolyte and mineral changes, thereby minimizing the adverse effects of inactivity. For most of us (assuming normal health), water intoxication should not be a concern. Only in ultraendurance activities, during which large, excess volumes of water are intentionally consumed, might water intoxication pose a risk.

V. RECOMMENDATIONS

Maintaining hydration is one of the most important strategies for attaining peak performance during exercise and sports activities and for maintaining overall health. Many individuals are incognizant of what constitutes "enough" water to meet their needs. There are several ways to assess hydration status, and one or more of them must be adopted according to individual need.

At rest, or during short periods of light activity, one might rely on the sensation of thirst to promote rehydration. Although the perception of thirst lags considerably behind the need for rehydration,[1,8,35,87,88] most of the time it provides enough stimulus to replace fluids adequately. Thirst by itself is not a reliable indicator of the need to replenish fluids during exercise, however. As exercise increases in intensity or duration, the thirst sensation is blunted, further hampering our ability to know how much water is enough.[8,39]

The many popular books and magazines targeting active people, as well as nutrition and physiology textbooks, recommend that an individual monitor hydration by noting the frequency, amount, and color of the urine that is voided. The consensus is that infrequent voiding of small volumes of dark-colored urine is an indication of inadequate hydration. While an active person should not excrete less than 900 ml/day of urine,[89] a well-hydrated individual should be voiding 1000 to 1500 ml/day,[90] at intervals of 2 to 4 hr. The urine color should be no darker than pale yellow.[39] As a practical, expedient method in most situations, monitoring hydration status by noting urine color is effective.[91]

An alternative expedient method to monitor hydration status is to weigh oneself before exercise and then again at the end of an exercise session. Most of any weight lost will be water, and one should then drink about 1 l of water per kilogram of weight lost (or approximately 2 cups/lb).[39] Factors such as fluid composition (e.g., water, sports beverage, caffeinated beverage, etc.), drinking frequency and volume, the rate of gastric emptying, and fluid temperature all influence the effectiveness of rehydration.[92]

A. FLUID COMPOSITION

For most people, fluid replacement with plain water should suffice. For exercise sessions lasting longer than 30 min to 1 hr, especially if they are intense, and for endurance exercise, one must consider replacing carbohydrates and electrolytes. Fluid and electrolyte replacement is the subject of Chapter 9.

If an individual will be exercising for long periods or at great intensity, then carbohydrate-containing fluid replacement beverages might be indicated.[72] The aim would be to benefit performance by providing fluid for rehydration[1,18,25,75,93] as well as fuel for energy production.[1,94–97] If the carbohydrate content of a replacement beverage is great enough to slow gastric emptying time or to inhibit water absorption from the small intestine, then there is little to recommend that beverage for rehydration purposes (as carbohydrate content of a beverage increases, so does its osmolality, which reduces gastric emptying time).[8] One must also remember that if the object of an exercise program is to lose weight or to maintain a desirable weight, the various sports beverages, fruit juices, and sugar-sweetened carbonated beverages all provide energy (i.e., "contain calories"), whereas a 240-ml (1-cup) serving of water has no energy value. Most of the sports drinks available over the counter contain various sugars (e.g., glucose, sucrose, fructose, maltodextrins) in varying concentrations (from about 4 to 8%), with energy contributions of 40 to 68 kcal/237 ml (8 oz).[8]

Some athletes and exercise enthusiasts swear by caffeinated or alcohol-containing beverages, believing that they gain a competitive advantage by drinking these before, during, or after an exercise session. The evidence to indicate that caffeine has an ergogenic effect for endurance or high-intensity exercisers has been controversial.[98–107] However, the International Olympic Committee regards a urine caffeine concentration of ≥ 12 mg/ml as grounds to deny an athlete's participation in competition because of the stimulatory effects of the compound.[8] Caffeine is also a diuretic compound. This fact is often used in recommendations that active people avoid caffeine-containing substances, but some investigators have found that when caffeine is used in a carbohydrate–electrolyte beverage during moderate endurance exercise, body hydration status is not compromised.[108]

Alcohol (ethanol) may be perceived by some as an ergogenic compound, improving self-confidence and alertness, reducing inhibitions and anxiety, and alleviating aches, pains, and muscle tremors.[109] In fact, alcohol provides substantial energy (7 kcal/g) at the expense of the metabolism of other nutrients,[110] acts as a depressant on the central nervous system, acts as a diuretic, and can cause hypothermia in the cold by initiating peripheral vasodilation.[109] Some studies report little or no adverse effects of alcohol on thermoregulation or rehydration,[111,112] but the American College of Sports Medicine strongly advises against the use of alcohol by those who exercise or engage in sports.[113]

B. DRINKING FREQUENCY, VOLUME, AND TEMPERATURE

As mentioned above, it is possible to hyperhydrate by increasing fluid intake before exercise or competition. Cold water is preferable to warm water, because it attenuates changes in core temperature and peripheral blood flow, decreases sweat rate,[114] and speeds up gastric emptying time. Water is sufficient for rehydration for exercise lasting less than 1 hr, taken at the rate of 100 to 150 ml every 10 to 15 min and at a temperature of 4 to 10°C[6] (the American College of Sports Medicine[72] recommends 15 to 22°C). For those exercising for periods of more than 1 hr, Hultman et al.[36] make the following recommendations: if large quantities of fluids

($\geq$600 ml) are consumed at once, gastric emptying rate increases and may cause discomfort. Therefore, the amount of fluid consumed should be only about 100 to 200 ml every 10 to 15 min, which may be increased to 400 to 500 ml 10 to 15 min before commencing exercise. If the fluid is plain water, it will be difficult to hyperhydrate, because the kidneys will increase the rate of diuresis. Instead, those who will be engaging in exercise sessions of more than 1 hr may wish to drink fluids containing 50 to 100 g/l carbohydrate and 10 to 30 mM/l NaCl. Finally, cold fluids (temperature 6 to 12°C) facilitate gastric emptying and help to reduce body core temperature.

VI. SUMMARY

Water is one of the most important nutrients for anyone who exercises or participates in sports, and it assumes even greater importance during the exercise/sport session. Exercise performance is impaired if normal body weight decreases by as little as 2 to 3% as lost water, and greater losses lead to serious physiological changes and death.

Thirst usually prompts us to drink enough water to meet our daily needs. When exercising, however, water losses are greater than normal and the sensation of thirst is blunted, so that we must deliberately rehydrate by following a water replacement regimen. Each of us must decide, by trial and error, the best rehydration beverage for our needs (e.g., plain water, sports drink, diluted sports drink). If exercise sessions are intense or will last longer than 1 hr, then it may be advantageous to rehydrate by using fluids which contain carbohydrates and electrolytes. Despite the essential nature of water, there is a range of optimum intake which if exceeded can result in water toxicity. Fortunately, water intoxication, which is usually associated with deliberate overconsumption by ultraendurance athletes, is rare and is usually quickly resolved.

REFERENCES

1. Wilmore, J.H. and Costill, D.L., *Physiology of Sport and Exercise,* Human Kinetics, Champaign, IL, 1994, chap. 15.
2. National Research Council, Water and electrolytes, in *Recommended Dietary Allowances,* 10th ed., National Academy of Sciences, Washington, D.C., 1989, chap. 11.
3. Szlyk-Modrow, P.C., Francesconi, R.P., and Hubbard, R.W., Integrated control of body fluid balance during exercise, in *Body Fluid Balance. Exercise and Sport,* Buskirk, E.R. and Puhl, S.M., Eds., CRC Press, Boca Raton, FL, 1996, chap. 6.
4. Sawka, M.N., Montain, S.J., and Latzka, W.A., Body fluid balance during exercise–heat exposure, in *Body Fluid Balance. Exercise and Sport,* Buskirk, E.R. and Puhl, S.M., Eds., CRC Press, Boca Raton, FL, 1996, chap. 7.
5. Guyton, A.C. and Hall, J.E., *Human Physiology and Mechanisms of Disease,* 6th ed., W.B. Saunders, Philadelphia, 1997, chap. 20.
6. Pivarnik, J.M., Water and electrolytes during exercise, in *Nutrition in Exercise and Sport,* Hickson, J.F. and Wolinsky, I., Eds., CRC Press, Boca Raton, FL, 1989, chap. 8.

7. Christian, J.L. and Greger, J.L., *Nutrition for Living*, 4th ed., Benjamin/Cummings, Redwood City, CA, 1994, chap. 4.
8. Frye, S.L., Fluids, hydration, and performance concerns of all recreational athletes, in *Nutrition for the Recreational Athlete*, Jackson, C.G.R., Ed., CRC Press, Boca Raton, FL, 1995, chap. 8.
9. Oh, M.S., Water, electrolyte and acid–base balance, in *Modern Nutrition in Health and Disease*, 8th ed., Shils, M.E., Olson, J.A., and Shike, M., Eds., Lea & Febiger, Philadelphia, 1994, chap. 6.
10. Guyton, A.C. and Hall, J.E., *Human Physiology and Mechanisms of Disease*, 6th ed., W.B. Saunders, Philadelphia, 1997, chap. 6.
11. McArdle, W.D., Katch, F.I., and Katch, V.L., *Exercise Physiology. Energy, Nutrition, and Human Performance*, 3rd ed., Lea & Febiger, Philadelphia, 1991, chap. 18.
12. Wilmore, J.H. and Costill, D.L., *Physiology of Sport and Exercise*, Human Kinetics, Champaign, IL, 1994, chap. 2.
13. Guyton, A.C. and Hall, J.E., *Human Physiology and Mechanisms of Disease*, 6th ed., W.B. Saunders, Philadelphia, 1997, chap. 47.
14. Noakes, T.D., Adams, B.A., Myburgh, K.H., Greef, C., Lotz, T., and Nathan, M., The danger of an inadequate water intake during prolonged exercise, *Eur. J. Appl. Physiol.*, 57, 210, 1988.
15. Maughan, R.J., Shirreffs, S.M., Galloway, D.R., and Leiper, J.B., Dehydration and fluid replacement in sport and exercise, *Sports Exercise Inj.*, 1, 148, 1995.
16. Rothstein, A., Adolf, E.F., and Wills, J.H., Voluntary dehydration, in *Physiology of Man in the Desert*, Adolf, E.F. and Associates, Interscience, New York, 1947, chap. 16.
17. Adolf, E.F. and Associates, *Physiology of Man in the Desert*, Interscience, New York, 1947.
18. Szlyk, P.C., Francesconi, R.P., Rose, M.S., Sils, I.V., Mahnke, R.B., Jr., Matthew, W.T., and Whang, R., Incidence of hypohydration when consuming carbohydrate–electrolyte solutions during field training, *Mil. Med.*, 156, 399, 1991.
19. Burstein, R., Seidman, D.S., Alter, J., Moram, D., Shpilberg, O., Shemer, J., Wiener, M., and Epstein, Y., Glucose polymer ingestion — effect on fluid balance and glycemic state during a 4-d march, *Med. Sci. Sports Exercise*, 26, 360, 1994.
20. Singh, A.P., Majumdar, D., Bhatia, M.R., Srivastava, K.K., and Selvamurthy, W., Environmental impact on crew of armoured vehicles: effects of 24 h combat exercise in a hot desert, *Int. J. Biometeorol.*, 39, 64, 1995.
21. Mudambo, K.S., Leese, G.P., and Rennie, M.J., Dehydration in soldiers during walking/running exercise in heat and the effects of fluid ingestion during and after exercise, *Eur. J. Appl. Physiol.*, 76, 517, 1997.
22. Cheung, S.S. and McLellan, T.M., Influence of hydration status and fluid replacement on heat tolerance while wearing NBC protective clothing, *Eur. J. Appl. Physiol.*, 77, 139, 1998.
23. Fortney, S.M., Mikhaylov, V., Lee, S.M., Kobzev, Y., Gonzalez, R.R., and Greenleaf, J.E., Body temperature and thermoregulation during submaximal exercise after 115-day spaceflight, *Aviat. Space Environ. Med.*, 69, 137, 1998.
24. Rehrer, N.J., The maintenance of fluid balance during exercise, *Int. J. Sports Med.*, 15, 122, 1994.
25. Terrados, N. and Maughan, R.J., Exercise in the heat: strategies to minimize the adverse effects on performance, *J. Sports Sci.*, 13, S55, 1995.
26. Bates, G., Gazey, C., and Cena, K., Factors affecting heat illness when working in conditions of thermal stress, *J. Hum. Ergol. (Tokyo)*, 25, 13, 1996.
27. Aoyagi, Y., McLellan, T.M., and Shephard, R.J., Interactions of physical training and heat acclimation. The thermophysiology of exercising in a hot climate, *Sports Med.*, 23, 173, 1997.
28. Armstrong, L.E., Maresh, C.M., Gabaree, C.V., Hoffman, J.R., Kavouras, S.A., Kenefick, R.W., Castellani, J.W., and Ahlquist, L.E., Thermal and circulatory responses during exercise: effects of hypohydration, dehydration, and water intake, *J. Appl. Physiol.*, 82, 2028, 1997.
29. Burke, L.M., Fluid balance during team sports, *J. Sports Sci.*, 15, 287, 1997.
30. Falk, B., Radom-Isaac, S., Hoffmann, J.R., Wang, Y., Yarom, Y., Magazanik, A., and Weinstein, Y., The effect of heat exposure on performance of and recovery from high-intensity, intermittent exercise, *Int. J. Sports Med.*, 19, 1, 1998.

31. Fink, W., Costill, D.L., Van Handel, P., and Getchell, L., Leg muscle metabolism during exercise in the heat and cold, *Eur. J. Appl. Physiol.*, 34, 183, 1975.

32. Melin, B., Jimenez, C., Savourey, G., Bittel, J., Cottet-Emard, J.M., Pequignot, J.M., Allevard, A.M., and Gharib, C., Effects of hydration state on hormonal and renal responses during moderate exercise in the heat, *Eur. J. Appl. Physiol.*, 76, 320, 1997.

33. Wilmore, J.H. and Costill, D.L., *Physiology of Sport and Exercise,* Human Kinetics, Champaign, IL, 1994, chap. 11.

34. Wyndham, C.H. and Strydom, N.B., The danger of an inadequate water intake during marathon running, *S. Afr. Med. J.*, 43, 893, 1969.

35. Nieman, D.C., *Fitness and Sports Medicine. An Introduction,* Bull Publishing, Palo Alto, CA, 1990, chap. 9.

36. Hultman, E., Harris, R.C., and Spriet, L.L., Work and exercise, in *Modern Nutrition in Health and Disease,* 8th ed., Shils, M.E., Olson, J.A., and Shike, M., Eds., Lea & Febiger, Philadelphia, 1994, chap. 42.

37. Noakes, T.D., Dehydration during exercise: what are the real dangers? *Clin. J. Sport Med.*, 5, 123, 1995.

38. Murray, R., Fluid needs in hot and cold environments, *Int. J. Sport Nutr.*, 5, S62, 1995.

39. Clark, N., *Nancy Clark's Sports Nutrition Guidebook,* 2nd ed., Human Kinetics, Champaign, IL, 1997, chap. 9.

40. Greiwe, J.S., Staffey, K.S., Melrose, D.R., Narve, M.D., and Knowlton, R.G., Effects of dehydration on isometric muscular strength and endurance, *Med. Sci. Sports Exercise*, 30, 284, 1998.

41. Mitchell, J.W., Nadel, E.R., and Stolwijk, J.A.J., Respiratory weight losses during exercise, *J. Appl. Physiol.*, 32, 474, 1972.

42. Starling, E.H., Physiological factors involved in the causation of dropsy, *Lancet,* 1, 1405, 1896.

43. Guyton, A.C. and Hall, J.E., *Human Physiology and Mechanisms of Disease,* 6th ed., W.B. Saunders, Philadelphia, 1997, chap. 13.

44. Wilmore, J.H. and Costill, D.L., *Physiology of Sport and Exercise,* Human Kinetics, Champaign, IL, 1994, chap. 8.

45. Hawley, J.A., Dennis, S.C., and Noakes, T.D., Carbohydrate, fluid and electrolyte requirements during prolonged exercise, in *Sports Nutrition. Minerals and Electrolytes,* Kies, C.V. and Driskell, J.A., Eds., CRC Press, Boca Raton, FL, 1995, chap. 19.

46. Harrison, M.H., Effects of thermal stress and exercise on blood volume in humans, *Physiol. Rev.,* 65, 149, 1985.

47. Sherman, W.M. and Lamb, D.R., Nutrition and prolonged exercise, in *Perspectives in Exercise Science and Sports Medicine,* Vol. 1, Lamb, D.R. and Murray, R., Eds., Benchmark Press, Indianapolis, 1988, chap. 6.

48. O'Brien, C., Freund, B.J., Sawka, M.N., McKay, J., Hesslink, R.L., and Jones, T.E., Hydration assessment during cold-weather military field training exercises, *Arct. Med. Res.,* 55, 20, 1996.

49. Freund, B.J. and Young, A.J., Environmental influences on body fluid balance during exercise: cold exposure, in *Body Fluid Balance. Exercise and Sport,* Buskirk, E.R. and Puhl, S.M., Eds., CRC Press, Boca Raton, FL, 1996, chap. 8.

50. Rintamaki, H., Makinen, T., Oksa, J., and Latvala, J., Water balance and physical performance in cold, *Arct. Med. Res.,* 54, 32, 1995.

51. Mirkin, G., Nutrition for sports, in *Women and Exercise. Physiology and Sports Medicine,* 2nd ed., Shangold, M. and Mirkin, G., Eds., F.A. Davis, Philadelphia, 1994, chap. 6.

52. Kondo, N., Nishiyasu, T., and Ikegami, H., The sweating responses of athletes trained on land and in water, *Jpn. J. Physiol.*, 45, 571, 1995.

53. Kondo, N., Nishiyasu, T., Nishiyasu, M., and Ikegami, H., Differences in regional sweating responses during exercise between athletes trained on land and in water, *Eur. J. Appl. Physiol.,* 74, 67, 1996.

54. Epstein, M., Renal, endocrine, and hemodynamic effects of water immersion in humans, in *Body Fluid Balance. Exercise and Sport,* Buskirk, E.R. and Puhl, S.M., Eds., CRC Press, Boca Raton, FL, 1996, chap. 10.

55. Wada, F., Sagawa, S., Miki, K., Nagaya, K., Nakamitsu, S., Shiraki, K., and Greenleaf, J.E., Mechanism of thirst attenuation during head-out water immersion in men, *Am. J. Physiol.,* 268, R583, 1995.

56. Boning, D., Mrugalla, M., Maassen, N., Busse, M., and Wagner, T.O., Exercise versus immersion: antagonistic effects on water and electrolyte metabolism during swimming, *Eur. J. Appl. Physiol.,* 57, 248, 1988.

57. Wilmore, J.H. and Costill, D.L., *Physiology of Sport and Exercise,* Human Kinetics, Champaign, IL, 1994, chap. 12.

58. Singh, M.V., Rawal, S.B., and Tyagi, A.K., Body fluid status on induction, reinduction and prolonged stay at high altitude of human volunteers, *Int. J. Biometeorol.,* 34, 93, 1990.

59. Anand, I.S., Chandrashekhar, Y., Rao, S.K., Malhotra, R.M., Ferrari, R., Chandana, J., Ramesh, B., Shetty, K.J., and Boparai, M.S., Body fluid compartments, renal blood flow, and hormones at 6,000 m in normal subjects, *J. Appl. Physiol.,* 74, 1234, 1993.

60. Kayser, B., Nutrition and energetics of exercise at altitude. Theory and possible practical implications, *Sports Med.,* 17, 309, 1994.

61. Hoyt, R.W. and Honig, A., Environmental influences on body fluid balance during exercise: altitude, in *Body Fluid Balance. Exercise and Sport,* Buskirk, E.R. and Puhl, S.M., Eds., CRC Press, Boca Raton, FL, 1996, chap. 9.

62. Zaccaria, M., Rocco, S., Noventa, D., Varnier, M., and Opocher, G., Sodium regulating hormones at high altitude: basal and post-exercise levels, *J. Clin. Endocrinol. Metab.,* 83, 570, 1998.

63. Gunga, H.C., Kirsch, K., Baartz, F., Steiner, H.J., Wittels, P., and Rocker, L., Fluid distribution and tissue thickness changes in 29 men during 1 week at moderate altitude (2,315 m), *Eur. J. Appl. Physiol.,* 70, 1, 1995.

64. Bärtsch, P., Pluger, N., Audetat, M., Shaw, S., Weidmann, P., Vock, P., Vetter, W., Rennie, D., and Oelz, O., Effects of slow ascent to 4559 m on fluid homeostasis, *Aviat. Space Environ. Med.,* 62, 105, 1991.

65. Koller, E.A., Buhrer, A., Felder, L., Schopen, M., and Valloton, M.B., Altitude diuresis: endocrine and renal responses to acute hypoxia of acclimatized and non-acclimatized subjects, *Eur. J. Appl. Physiol.,* 62, 228, 1991.

66. Maw, G.J., MacKenzie, I.L., Comer, D.A., and Taylor, N.A., Whole-body hyperhydration in endurance-trained males determined using radionuclide dilution, *Med. Sci. Sports Exercise,* 28, 1038, 1996.

67. Hildebrandt, W., Schutze, H., and Stegemann, J., Higher capillary filtration rate in the calves of endurance-trained subjects during orthostatic stress, *Aviat. Space Environ. Med.,* 64, 380, 1993.

68. McArdle, W.D., Katch, F.I., and Katch, V.L., *Exercise Physiology. Energy, Nutrition, and Human Performance,* 3rd ed., Lea & Febiger, Philadelphia, 1991, chap. 25.

69. Colgan, M., *Optimum Sports Nutrition. Your Competitive Edge,* Advanced Research Press, New York, 1993, chap. 3.

70. Johnson, H.L., The requirements for fluid replacement during heavy sweating and the benefits of carbohydrates and minerals, in *Sports Nutrition. Minerals and Electrolytes,* Kies, C.V. and Driskell, J.A., Eds., CRC Press, Boca Raton, FL, 1995, chap. 18.

71. Coleman, E. and Steen, S.N., *The Ultimate Sports Nutrition Handbook,* Bull Publishing, Palo Alto, CA, 1996, chap. 9.

72. Convertino, V.A., Armstrong, L.E., Coyle, E.F., Mack, G.W., Sawka, M.N., Senay, L.C., Jr., and Sherman, W.M., American College of Sports Medicine. Position stand on exercise and fluid replacement, *Med. Sci. Sports Exercise,* 28, i, 1996.

73. Koenigsberg, P.S., Martin, K.K., Hlava, H.R., and Riedesel, M.L., Sustained hyperhydration with glycerol ingestion, *Life Sci.,* 57, 645, 1995.

74. Lyons, T.P., Riedesel, M.L., Meuli, L.E., and Chick, T.W., Effects of glycerol-induced hyperhydration prior to exercise in the heat on sweating and core temperature, *Med. Sci. Sports Exercise,* 22, 477, 1990.

75. Meyer, L.G., Horrigan, D.J., Jr., and Lotz, W.G., Effects of three hydration beverages on exercise performance during 60 hours of heat exposure, *Aviat. Space Environ. Med.,* 66, 1052, 1995.

76. Latzka, W.A., Sawka, M.N., Montain, S.J., Skrinar, G.S., Fielding, R.A., Matott, R.P., and Pandolf, K.B., Hyperhydration: thermoregulatory effects during compensable exercise–heat stress, *J. Appl. Physiol.*, 83, 860, 1997.

77. Noakes, T.D., Goodwin, N., Rayner, B.L., Branken, T., and Taylor, R.K., Water intoxication: a possible complication during endurance exercise, *Med. Sci. Sports Exercise*, 17, 370, 1985.

78. Frizzell, R.T., Lang, G.H., Lowance, D.C., and Lathan, S.R., Hyponatremia and ultramarathon running, *J. Am. Med. Assoc.*, 255, 772, 1986.

79. Zambraski, E.J., The kidney and body fluid balance during exercise, in *Body Fluid Balance. Exercise and Sport,* Buskirk, E.R. and Puhl, S.M., Eds., CRC Press, Boca Raton, FL, 1996, chap. 4.

80. Knochel, J.P., Clinical complications of body fluid and electrolyte balance, in *Body Fluid Balance. Exercise and Sport,* Buskirk, E.R. and Puhl, S.M., Eds., CRC Press, Boca Raton, FL, 1996, chap. 15.

81. Zorbas, Y.G., Federenko, Y.F., and Naexu, K.A., Urinary excretion of microelements in endurance-trained volunteers during restriction of muscular activity and chronic rehydration, *Biol. Trace Elem. Res.*, 40, 189, 1994.

82. Zorbas, Y.G., Federenko, Y.F., and Naexu, K.A., Phosphate-loading test influences on endurance-trained volunteers during restriction of muscular activity and chronic hyperhydration, *Biol. Trace Elem. Res.*, 48, 51, 1995.

83. Zorbas, Y.G., Sokiguchi, M.A., Johanson, O.A., and Federenko, Y.F., Zinc metabolism in endurance-trained volunteers during prolonged restriction of muscular activity and chronic hyperhydration, *Biol. Trace Elem. Res.*, 48, 185, 1995.

84. Zorbas, Y.G., Federenko, Y.F., and Naexu, K.A., Effect of daily hyperhydration on fluid-electrolyte changes in endurance-trained volunteers during prolonged restriction of muscular activity, *Biol. Trace Elem. Res.*, 50, 57, 1995.

85. Zorbas, Y.G., Federenko, Y.F., and Naexu, K.A., Potassium changes in trained subjects after potassium loading and during restriction of muscular activity and chronic hyperhydration, *Biol. Trace Elem. Res.*, 53, 95, 1996.

86. Zorbas, Y.G., Federenko, Y.F., and Naexu, K.A., Fluid electrolyte changes in trained subjects after water loading and during restriction of muscular activity and chronic hyperhydration, *Biol. Trace Elem. Res.*, 54, 251, 1996.

87. Adolf, E.F., Heat exchanges, sweat formation, and water turnover, in *Physiology of Man in the Desert,* Adolf, E.F. and Associates, Interscience Publishers, New York, 1947, chap. 3.

88. Guyton, A.C. and Hall, J.E., *Human Physiology and Mechanisms of Disease,* 6th ed., W.B. Saunders, Philadelphia, 1997, chap. 22.

89. Food and Nutrition Board, National Research Council, Water deprivation and performance of athletes, *Nutr. Rev.*, 32, 314, 1974.

90. McArdle, W.D., Katch, F.I., and Katch, V.L., *Exercise Physiology. Energy, Nutrition, and Human Performance,* 3rd ed., Lea & Febiger, Philadelphia, 1991, chap. 2.

91. Armstrong, L.E., Maresh, C.M., Castellani, J.W., Bergeron, M.F., Kenefick, R.W., LaGasse, K.E., and Riebe, D., Urinary indices of hydration status, *Int. J. Sport Nutr.*, 4, 265, 1994.

92. Costill, D.L. and Saltin, B., Factors limiting gastric emptying during rest and exercise, *J. Appl. Physiol.*, 37, 679, 1974.

93. Maughan, R.J. and Leiper, J.B., Fluid replacement requirements in soccer, *J. Sports Sci.*, 12, S29, 1994.

94. Maughan, R.J., Leiper, J.B., and Shirreffs, S.M., Factors influencing the restoration of fluid and electrolyte balance after exercise in the heat, *Br. J. Sports Med.*, 31, 175, 1997.

95. Millard-Stafford, M., Rosskopf, L.B., Snow, T.K., and Hinson, B.T., Water versus carbohydrate–electrolyte ingestion before and during a 15-km run in the heat, *Int. J. Sport Nutr.*, 7, 26, 1997.

96. Roberges, R.A., McMinn, S.B., Mermier, C., Leadbetter, G., 3rd, Ruby, B., and Quinn, C., Blood glucose and glucoregulatory hormone responses to solid and liquid carbohydrate ingestion during exercise, *Int. J. Sport Nutr.*, 8, 70, 1998.

97. Wilk, B., Kriemler, S., Keller, H., and Bar-Or, O., Consistency in preventing voluntary dehydration in boys who drink a flavored carbohydrate–NaCl beverage during exercise in the heat, *Int. J. Sport Nutr.*, 8, 1, 1998.
98. Tarnopolsky, M.A., Atkinson, S.A., MacDougall, J.D., Sale, D.G., and Sutton, J.R., Physiological responses to caffeine during endurance running in habitual caffeine users, *Med. Sci. Sports Exercise*, 21, 418, 1989.
99. Tarnopolsky, M.A., Caffeine and endurance performance, *Sports Med.*, 18, 109, 1994.
100. Nehlig, A. and Debry, G., Caffeine and sports activity: a review, *Int. J. Sports Med.*, 15, 215, 1994.
101. Graham, T.E. and Spriet, L.L., Metabolic, catecholamine, and exercise performance responses to various doses of caffeine, *J. Appl. Physiol.*, 78, 867, 1995.
102. MacIntosh, B.R. and Wright, B.M., Caffeine ingestion and performance of a 1,500-metre swim, *Can. J. Appl. Physiol.*, 20, 168, 1995.
103. McCarty, M.F., Optimizing exercise for fat loss, *Med. Hypotheses*, 44, 325, 1995.
104. Pasman, W.J., van Baak, M.A., Jeukendrup, A.E., and de Haan, A., The effect of different dosages of caffeine on endurance performance time, *Int. J. Sports Med.*, 16, 225, 1995.
105. Spriet, L.L., Caffeine and performance, *Int. J. Sport Nutr.*, 5, S84, 1995.
106. Thein, L.A., Thein, J.M., and Landry, G.L., Ergogenic aids, *Phys. Ther.*, 75, 426, 1995.
107. Trice, I. and Haymes, E.M., Effects of caffeine ingestion on exercise-induced changes during high-intensity, intermittent exercise, *Int. J. Sport Nutr.*, 5, 37, 1995.
108. Wemple, R.D., Lamb, D.R., and McKeever, K.H., Caffeine vs caffeine-free sports drinks: effects on urine production at rest and during prolonged exercise, *Int. J. Sports Med.*, 18, 40, 1997.
109. Wilmore, J.H. and Costill, D.L., *Physiology of Sport and Exercise*, Human Kinetics, Champaign, IL, 1994, chap. 13.
110. Kendrick, Z.V., Affrime, M.B., and Lowenthal, D.T., Effects of caffeine or ethanol on treadmill performance and metabolic responses of well-trained men, *Int. J. Clin. Pharmacol. Ther.*, 32, 536, 1994.
111. Desruelle, A.V., Boisvert, P., and Candas, V., Alcohol and its variable effect on human thermoregulatory response to exercise in a warm environment, *Eur. J. Appl. Physiol.*, 74, 572, 1996.
112. Shirreffs, S.M. and Maughan, R.J., Restoration of fluid balance after exercise-induced dehydration: effects of alcohol consumption, *J. Appl. Physiol.*, 83, 1152, 1997.
113. American College of Sports Medicine Position Statement, The use of alcohol in sports, *Med. Sci. Sports Exercise*, 14, ix, 1982.
114. Wimer, G.S., Lamb, D.R., Sherman, W.M., and Swanson, S.C., Temperature of ingested water and thermoregulation during moderate-intensity exercise, *Can. J. Appl. Physiol.*, 22, 479, 1997.

Chapter 6

SODIUM IN
EXERCISE AND SPORT

Elsworth R. Buskirk
William B. Farquhar

CONTENTS

I. INTRODUCTION: PHYSIOLOGICAL IMPORTANCE

The constancy of the internal environment (*milieu interieur*) was brought to our attention by Claude Bernard in 1865.[1] He proposed that the extracellular fluid (ECF) provided the medium in which cells are bathed. The solutes contained therein were regarded as being closely regulated with respect to their concentration so that vital functioning could be sustained. Bernard realized that the extracellular compartment contained ≈0.9% sodium chloride. Bernard also coined the term "homeostasis" to characterize the constancy of the internal environment. Homeostasis as a concept was further expanded by Walter Cannon.[2] Homer Smith[3] pointed out the important role of the kidneys in regulating the concentration of solutes in both ECF and intracellular fluid within rather precise limits under most circumstances where excess sweating or pathology is not present. Pitts[4] has stated that under conditions where diarrhea and excess sweating do not occur, 98% or more of ingested sodium is excreted in the urine. In simple terms, regulation of the cation sodium and the anion chloride is responsible for the regulation of ECF. There is mutual interdependence of these ions, but attention here will be on sodium.

The control systems for sodium, although studied by many for several years, are inadequately defined. Adaptations occur in both sodium intake and excretion. Changes in the following have been documented: plasma renin activity, plasma angiotensin II concentration, aldosterone production, atrial natiuretic peptide concentration, nitric oxide, sympathetic tone, substances produced in the gut, and Na^+K^+–adenosine triphosphatase (ATPase) activity. Thus, a change in sodium intake may initiate adaptations that minimize effects on total body sodium and ECF. In view of these adaptations, Luft[5] has pointed out that "whatever goes in must come out," but the greater the sodium chloride intake, the greater the ECF, plasma volume, blood volume, and cardiac output within compromised limits. In connection with adaptation, Hollenberg[6] referred to a "homeostasis set point" or a concentration of sodium that is defended. Simpson[7] proposed a "basal level" for sodium. Thus, when body sodium is above basal, the extra sodium is excreted and vice versa. Hollenberg[6] further emphasized that as body sodium tends to return to basal, any decrement below basal is constantly replenished by additional intake. Luft[5] has indicated that healthy people can maintain sodium chloride homeostasis at <10 mmol/day, which by current perspectives is a low intake.

The control of sodium movement is brought about by Na^+K^+–activated ATP (Na^+K^+–ATPase or Na^+K^+ pump), the first transport system found to be enzymatic in nature. Expressed in all cells and utilizing the energy derived from adenosine triphosphate (ATP) hydrolysis, it affects active countertransport of Na^+ and K^+ across plasma membranes. Movement of Na^+ out of and K^+ into cells establishes an electrochemical gradient that generates electrical activity in excitable tissues for movement of other ions and nutrients. Na^+K^+–ATPase is especially important to the reabsorption of Na^+ in renal tubules and sweat gland ducts, but it also functions in what has been called its "housekeeping" mode, controlling cell volume and composition. Regulation of Na^+K^+–ATPase is complex, involving a network of receptor-mediated intracellular signals. The review by Bertorello and Katz[8] should be consulted for further information.

Another control factor, particularly for sodium excretion, is nitric oxide (NO). It has been suggested that NO plays a pivotal role in maintaining the constancy of the extracellular fluid volume. Its role in exercise is relatively unknown, but physical activation of endothelial cells by such stimuli as pulsatile flow and shear stress induces NO synthesis. At this juncture, it is important to realize that NO plays an important role in arterial pressure control by regulation of sodium and water excretion.[9] Undoubtedly, more information about NO-induced actions will be forthcoming in the near future.

In regard to control systems and our understanding of them, the following quotation is pertinent:

> The problem is that while we can imagine, reason or predict why the body needs to adjust its sodium balance, we still have no idea how the body's regulatory system assesses its sodium status, or where the assessment is made.[10]

One of us earlier reviewed sodium involvement in the adaptation of high environmental temperature, exercise, and athletics.[11] In addition, there are a number of excellent reviews and books that deal with either sodium, sodium chloride (salt), or sodium and potassium. The interested reader would be well served by perusing them. See, for example, the following: Meneely and Battarbee,[12] Fregly,[13] Luft,[5,14] Michell,[10] and Moses.[15] Similarly, reviews are available describing the role of sodium in relation to exercise, such as Luetkemeier et al.,[16] Pivarnik and Palmer,[17] Pivarnik,[18] Fellman,[19] and Noakes.[20] Reviews on hyponatremia have been prepared by Goldberg[21] as well as Noakes.[22]

II. SOURCES, INTAKE, AND REQUIREMENTS

Sodium intake is required in the healthy person to sustain growth and provide replacement of obligatory losses. The quantity needed to support growth is associated with the rate at which ECF is expanded. In the adult with a relatively constant volume of ECF, sodium balance can be maintained on what might be regarded by many as a very low intake of sodium. The Recommended Dietary Allowances of sodium in relation to age and weight are presented in Table 1, along with respective caveats.[23] Thus, the estimated minimal allowance for adults (independent of gender) who are either resting or engaged in light activity that does not involve sweating is no more than 300 mg of NaCl per day, which corresponds to 5 meq/day or 115 mg/day of sodium. As should be noted, physical activity, environmental exposure, wearing heavy clothing, ingesting warm beverages, or taking pharmaceuticals can stimulate sweating and increase the need for greater sodium intake.

TABLE 1   Estimated Sodium Minimum
Requirements of Healthy
Persons[a]

Age	Weight (kg)[a]	Sodium (mg)[a,b]
Months		
0–5	4.5	120
6–11	8.9	200
Years		
1	11.0	225
2–5	16.0	300
6–9	25.0	400
10–18	50.0	500
>18[c]	70.0	500

[a] No allowance included for large, prolonged losses from the skin through sweat.

[b] There is no evidence that higher intakes confer any health benefits.

[c] No allowance included for growth. Values for those below 18 years assume a growth rate at the 50th percentile by the National Center for Health Statistics and averaged for males and females.

Adapted from Reference 23.

In the U.S. and most developed countries where processed foods are consumed in relatively large quantities or in lesser developed countries where salt is used as a preservative, a problem relates to excessive salt intake. There is also a penchant for many people to use the salt shaker liberally. In 1989 a committee of the Food and Nutrition Board recommended that the daily intake of NaCl be limited to 6 g or 2.4 g of sodium.[23]

Fregly[13] reviewed sodium intake data from the perspective of nondiscretionary (that contained in food, beverages, and processing) and discretionary (that added in cooking and from all adjuncts) sources. Fregly reported results of an FDA survey, which appear in Table 2. The daily sodium intake for an estimated 3900-kcal/day diet was about 7 g/day sodium from all sources or 1.8 g/1000 kcal/day. Such an analysis would presumably reflect that of a physically active individual. Fregly[13] also reviewed sources of sodium intake not commonly considered, such as drinking water (natural or softened) and drugs. Both sources can contribute as much as 500 mg or 1 g to daily intake. In terms of food categories that provide nondiscretionary salt intake, perhaps 20 to 35% comes from baked goods, cereals, and other grain products; 15 to 25% from meat, fish, and poultry; and about 10 to 20% from milk and milk products. Other food and beverage sources provide the remainder. Suffice it to say there is normally no problem in securing an adequate amount of sodium in the food and beverages commonly available to us. This includes individuals with

TABLE 2 Sodium Content by Food Composite of
3900-kcal Daily Diet Collected in FDA
Selected Minerals in Food Survey

Food composite	1978[a] Sodium	
	mg	mg/1000 kcal
Nondiscretionary		
Dairy products	792	203
Meat, fish, poultry	921	236
Grain and cereal products	2002	513
Potatoes	82	21
Leafy vegetables	22	6
Legume vegetables	258	62
Root vegetables	17	4
Garden fruits	284	73
Fruits	75	19
Oils and fats	406	104
Beverages	24	7
Total nondiscretionary	4886	1252
Discretionary		
Sugar, salt, and adjuncts[b]	2042	524
Total intake	6928	1776

[a] Mean value of eight market basket collections.
[b] Includes the salt normally used in home food preparation and for seasoning at the table.

Adapted from Fregly.[13]

a physically active lifestyle as well as athletes. In view of the salt link to the development of hypertension in genetically susceptible individuals, current labeling of packaged food and beverages showing the amount of sodium has helped many reduce their sodium intake to what are regarded as more healthy levels (i.e., consume amounts of sodium in keeping with physiological need).

Comparisons have been made between sodium intake derived from analytic measurements of food consumed and that calculated from urinary excretion, food surveys, or dietary records. An example is the study of Holbrook et al.,[24] who found that differences occurred with analytical intake usually somewhat higher than calculated intake. In addition, sodium intake also differed between men and women, but not when compared per 1000 kcal of dietary intake. Their results appear in Table 3. Urinary excretion of sodium amounted to 85 to 90% and was related to intake with a correlation coefficient of $r = 0.76$.

In a study of sodium replacement following a volume deficit induced by thermal and/or exercise sweating, Takamato et al.[25] found that the palatability ratings to hypertonic NaCl solutions were increased after a delay of 3 hr or more of rehydration. When ECF Na^+ content and plasma sodium concentration ($[Na^+]$) were decreased, palatability of hypertonic NaCl was increased. Osmotically induced thirst

TABLE 3   Determinants of Sodium Nutriture by Gender as Ascertained by Analytical or Calculated Techniques[a]

	Mean[b]		Men		Women	
Analytical intake (g/day)	3.4	(0.1)	4.2	(0.1)	2.7	(0.6)
Calculated intake (g/day)	2.9	(0.1)	3.5	(0.1)	2.4	(0.1)
Nutrient density (g/1000 kcal)	1.8	(0.03)	1.8	(0.1)	1.8	(0.1)
Urinary Na$^+$ (g/day)	2.9	(0.1)	3.4	(0.1)	2.4	(0.1)
Urinary excretion of Na$^+$ (% of intake)	85.8	(1.6)	82.1	(2.9)	89.5	(2.3)
Fecal Na$^+$ (mg/day)	56	(5)	76	(9)	34	(4)
Apparent absorption[c] (%)	98.5	(0.1)	98.3	(0.2)	98.7	(0.1)
Balance (g/day)	+0.47	(0.06)	+0.73	(0.24)	+0.26	(0.12)
Energy (kcal)	1985	(53)	2448	(60)	1638	(47)

[a] Mean (SEM).
[b] Mean of four balance periods, 16 women and 12 men.
[c] (Intake − fecal)/intake × 100.

Adapted from Holbrook et al.[24]

and renal water retention preceded what was regarded as Na$^+$ appetite. Thus, ECF volume was brought back toward normal by both the Na$^+$ appetite and lesser renal tubular Na$^+$ reabsorption.

Michell[10] has summarized the role of plasma sodium as being the main stimulus to thirst and antidiuretic hormone (ADH) secretion. An increase in plasma sodium associated with raising the concentration of interstitial fluid impinging on osmoreceptors is primarily responsible for thirst. Receptors reside in the hypothalamus. Although water is not primarily transported across membranes, it does follow osmotic gradients. With sodium largely constrained to ECF, the sodium pump (Na$^+$K$^+$–ATPase enzyme system) treats sodium as the osmotic skeleton of ECF and thereby influences ECF volume. The thirst associated with hypovolemia is mediated by angiotensin brought about by restricted renal perfusion and the release of renin.

The question of differences in salt or sodium appetite in relation to age or gender has not been satisfactorily resolved. Tiidus et al.[26] found that middle-aged and older men and women did not appear to have compromised sodium appetite. In contrast, by stressing elderly subjects with hypohydration, Rolls and Phillips[27] found that thirst and presumably sodium appetite were lessened in elderly subjects (i.e., the elderly failed to feel thirsty despite physiological need).

An important early observation regarding sodium sparing emanated from the life raft studies of Gamble[28] in 1946–47. Gamble pointed out the sparing effect of glucose intake on sodium retention in fasted hypohydrated men. Provision of 50 or 100 g of glucose not only conserved sodium but reduced the loss of ECF about 50%.

One interesting aspect of the caffeine-consumption ergogenic-enhancement story is that caffeine ingestion before exercise stimulates Na$^+$K$^+$ pump activity in muscle and aids in the regulation of plasma and intracellular [Na⁺] and [K⁺]. Action may be through epinephrine with the maintenance of a higher [Na⁺] and lower plasma [K⁺] during exercise and perhaps higher intracellular [K⁺] and membrane potential in contracting muscle. Also possible is a direct stimulating effect of caffeine on Na⁺K⁺ pump activity.[29]

III. STORAGE AND EXCHANGE COMPARTMENTS

Analysis of where sodium resides in the body was clarified by Forbes and Lewis,[30] who analyzed the carcasses of two adult men. The first specimen died of a fractured skull and the second was found dead in a hotel room. Further analysis revealed that the first man was healthy whereas the second showed evidence of cardiovascular and pulmonary disease. Data on sodium content of the various tissues analyzed appear in Table 4. The largest reservoirs of sodium are in bone and muscle. As analysis of ECF was not possible, this repository of sodium is missed with carcass analysis. Sodium assessment *in vivo* is accomplished using either of

TABLE 4   Distribution of Sodium and Water Content in the Carcasses of Two Adult Men

	1951 Specimen[a]			1953 Specimen[b]		
Organ	Weight (g)	Water (g)	Na⁺ (meq)	Weight (g)	Water (g)	Na⁺ (meq)
Skin	3,372	1,812	232	4,731	2,451	298
Skeleton	9,223	2,468	1,554	9,746	3,083	1,289
Tibia				1,004	138	166
Muscle	20,857	14,078	968	28,926	19,724	1,391
Nerve	1,570	1,166	103	1,534	1,270	144
Liver	1,225	841	66.8	1,714	1,059	74.6
Heart	271	165	10.8	430	295	18.7
Lungs	1,734	1,338	126	1,587	1,181	126
Kidney	270	191	18.0[c]	312	220	22.4
GI tract	975	748	32.4	1,087	937	47.4
Adipose	5,963	1,561	142	15,585	2,859	332
Remainder	5,998	3,402	322	4,661	2,645	252
Weight loss on dissection	1,400	1,400		1,600	1,600	
Total composition		55.2%	67.6 meq/kg		51.4%	57.1 meq/kg
Fat-free body	43,280	67.4%	82.6 meq/kg	53,220	70.4%	78.2 meq/kg

[a] 46-year-old man, 168.5 cm tall.
[b] 60-year-old man, 172 cm tall.
[c] Composition assumed.

Adapted from Forbes and Lewis.[30]

**TABLE 5   Predominant Methods for the
Assessment of Sodium in
Biological Samples and the
Common Sites for Sampling**

Sodium assessment	Flame photometry
	Ion-specific electrodes
Sodium sampling sites	Blood, plasma, serum
	Cells
	Bone
	Enteric fluids
	Saliva
	Sweat
	Tears
	Urine
	Feces
	Cerebrospinal fluid

two methods as set forth in Table 5. A variety of sites for sodium sampling are possible, but by far the most common are plasma or serum, urine, and sweat. In order to ascertain sodium balance, sampling of other sites is necessary.

IV. ABSORPTION: GASTROINTESTINAL HANDLING

Sodium is efficiently absorbed in the gastrointestinal (GI) tract, and only small amounts remain in feces in the healthy person. The colon is responsible for reducing sodium output in feces to virtually zero when sodium intakes are extremely low and body sodium depletion is eminent. Aldosterone is responsible for the almost complete sodium absorption. Also, the proximal segments of the intestine transport large quantities of sodium and water when sodium intake is more than adequate. Moreover, there is cotransport of sodium with such solutes as glucose and amino acids. In the GI tract, sodium gradients supply the bases for water movement and cotransport of other solutes. A highly selective amiloride-sensitive sodium channel protein has been identified in the colon which provides a rate-limiting step for aldosterone-responsive sodium reabsorption.[10] Among the mechanisms facilitating sodium movement are passive carriers, selective permeable channels, and energy-utilizing pumps. The main sodium pump is Na^+K^+–ATPase, which responds to glucocorticoids in the intestine and aldosterone in the colon. Nevertheless, regulatory effects are also influenced by modulation of receptor binding, the transport pathway, and intracellular signals.[10]

For the athlete, the main concern with GI absorption and handling is that involving processes brought about by poor judgment regarding sodium and related intakes with respect to timing and competition as well as diarrhea brought about by inappropriate nutrition, excessive apprehension, or severe exercise demands.

In summarizing studies on sodium flux in relation to intestinal water absorption from selected carbohydrate solutions made isotonic with NaCl, Gisolfi et al.[31] concluded that the lower the sodium concentration [Na$^+$] in a solution, the lower the net Na$^+$ flux. Net Na$^+$ absorption occurred at a luminal [Na$^+$] as low as 50 mM in a given segment of the intestine. Others had found a much higher absorption threshold for intraluminal [Na$^+$] of about 80 to 90 mM.[32] With little or no absorption from the stomach, sodium crosses the brush border by electroneutral and electrogenic processes. Coupled exchange across the brush border involves luminal Na$^+$ for cellular H$^+$. Sodium transport coupled with electroneutral nutrients such as the hexoses is electrogenic. The hexose transporter is maintained by the basolateral membrane sodium pump, which utilizes ATP for energy through action of Na$^+$K$^+$–ATPase. Amino acids are absorbed in conjunction with specific sodium-coupled transporters, an electrogenic process separate from the hexose transporter. In addition to membrane transport, paracellular transport also moves sodium. Transmucosal electrical potentials are responsible for Na$^+$ movement, with electrogenic sodium absorption promoting lumen negativity. In addition, the basolateral membrane has channels for cations as well as anions, in other words an Na$^+$ channel.[33]

Controversy exists regarding the influence of sodium on glucose bioavailability during exercise (65% $\dot{V}O_2$max). Hargreaves et al.[34] found that concentrations of beverage sodium from 0 to 50 mmol/l had essentially no effect on glucose availability when 400 ml of a 10% glucose solution was administered just prior to exercise. This finding contrasts with resting studies[35] where the addition of sodium increased the glycemic response to oral glucose. Because the test period was relatively short in the Hargreaves et al.[34] experiments, further studies during exercise are warranted, particularly because palatability of ingested fluids is enhanced if the [Na$^+$] is <50 mmol/l.

In man, intense exercise or exercising under hot conditions may reduce splanchnic blood flow without measurably altering intestinal absorption. Although the evidence for this is mixed, Sjovall et al.,[36] using splanchnic nerve stimulation during exercise, found reduced blood flow to the muscularis and crypts of the intestinal wall whereas the blood flow to the villi was unaffected. Whether different concentrations of sodium in relation to glucose would change absorbability under exercise conditions remains to be determined.

V. REGULATORY MECHANISMS

A. RENAL HANDLING
The long-term regulation of total body salt and therefore ECF volume is accomplished by the kidney. If sodium balance is to occur, the kidney must adjust the amount of sodium excreted to coincide with dietary sodium intake. In nearly all circumstances, the kidney does a remarkable job of maintaining the constancy of the internal environment despite lifelong adjustments in sodium intake due to cul-

tural preferences or acute changes in sodium intake due to dietary whims. Brief periods of positive or negative sodium balance follow acute increases or decreases in sodium intake, as well as increases or decreases in body weight, respectively.[37] Urinary sodium excretion is a function of the sodium filtered minus the sodium reabsorbed. Because sodium is a low-molecular-weight molecule that is not bound to protein, it is freely filtered through the glomerular capillaries into Bowman's space. During most circumstances, ~99% of the sodium filtered is reabsorbed, approximately two-thirds of which occurs in the proximal tubule. The transport of sodium occurs in all tubular segments except the descending limb of the loop of Henle. In the basolateral membrane of the tubules, acute sodium reabsorption occurs by Na^+K^+–ATPase pumps. These pumps actively transport sodium out of the tubular cell and into the interstitial fluid, thereby increasing the sodium gradient between the tubular lumen and cell interior. Sodium transport on the luminal side is location dependent along the nephron. For example, in the proximal tubule, sodium is transported with glucose and amino acids and also countertransported with hydrogen ions. At the distal end of the nephron, in the cortical-collecting duct, sodium mainly diffuses through sodium channels.[38]

Sodium excretion is under precise physiological control. Changes in sodium reabsorption are quantitatively more important than changes in sodium filtered, especially in the distal portion of the nephron. A partial controller of sodium reabsorption in the cortical-collecting duct is aldosterone, a steroid hormone produced by the adrenal cortex; it was discovered in 1953 by Simpson and co-workers (see Funder[39]). When aldosterone concentration is high, essentially all of the sodium reaching the collecting ducts is reabsorbed. Conversely, when aldosterone is absent, ~2% of the filtered sodium is excreted. Zambraski[40] makes the point that although the short-term effects of aldosterone on urinary excretion of sodium and water are minimal and largely overstated (because aldosterone is only responsible for ~2% of renal tubular reabsorption), the long-term control exerted by aldosterone is important for sodium and body fluid balance. Aldosterone acts in the cortical-collecting duct by inducing the synthesis of proteins that function as sodium channels in the luminal membrane and Na^+K^+–ATPase pumps in the basolateral membrane.[39]

The control of aldosterone secretion is due to changes in angiotensin II concentrations, which are ultimately determined by circulating levels of renin (see Figure 1). In resting humans, abrupt deprivation of sodium causes a decrease in plasma volume because sodium is initially lost in the urine before the kidney can respond by increasing sodium reabsorption (i.e., a period of negative sodium balance) and possibly decreasing the amount of sodium filtered. This decrease in plasma volume is sensed by the juxtaglomerular (JG) cells, which are located in the walls of the afferent arterioles. The JG cells respond by secreting renin. The JG cells also respond to enhanced renal sympathetic nerve activity and to signals originating in the macula densa, which are located in the ascending limb of the loop of Henle and sense the sodium and/or chloride concentration in the tubular fluid. All of these inputs to the JG cells can enhance renin secretion. Additionally, renal

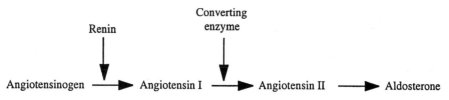

FIGURE 1   The control of aldosterone secretion. (Adapted from Vander et al.[38])

sympathetic nerves[41] and angiotensin II[42] act directly on the tubules to stimulate sodium reabsorption.

Physiological controls exist for inhibition of sodium reabsorption, such as atrial natriuretic factor or peptide (ANF or ANP). ANF is synthesized by cardiac atrial cells and responds to increases in plasma volume. ANF may also cause an increased glomerular filtration rate, which also increases sodium excretion.[38] The end result of this complex and somewhat redundant system of controls influencing renal sodium handling is, at least in normal individuals under resting conditions, increased sodium excretion in times of sodium excess and decreased sodium excretion during periods of sodium deficit.

During moderate to heavy acute exercise (>50% $\dot{V}O_2$max), the amount of sodium filtered decreases because the glomerular filtration rate declines. However, sodium excretion declines more than can be accounted for by a decrease in filtration rate alone; therefore, sodium reabsorption must be enhanced. Zambraski[40] has reviewed these data and points out that there are a number of factors that could potentially be responsible for the increase in renal tubular sodium reabsorption during acute exercise. These include increased renal sympathetic nerve activity, increased filtration fraction, increased plasma angiotensin II concentration, increased plasma aldosterone concentration, and increased plasma ADH concentration. The rapid time course of the response appears to support a neural (rather than hormonal) mechanism. Also, studies that have blocked angiotensin II show that renal sodium handling is not significantly altered,[43] further supporting a neural mechanism such as increased renal sympathetic nerve activity.

During light aerobic exercise, sodium excretion has been reported to be either unchanged or increased slightly. Possible reasons for a slight increase in sodium excretion during light exercise include an increase in ANF and an increase in renal perfusion pressure.[40]

B. SWEAT GLAND HANDLING

Sweat glands are innervated by sympathetic cholinergic nerve fibers and function by secreting hypotonic fluid that evaporates on the skin surface and aids in evaporative cooling. Like the kidney, the sweat gland actively reabsorbs sodium. In fact, the primary function of the sweat gland duct is the conservation of Na^+ and other electrolytes such as Cl^- and HCO_3.[44] In his review of water and elec-

TABLE 6   Comparative Average Electrolyte Concentrations in Sweat, Plasma, and Skeletal Muscle

Variable	[Na$^+$] (meq/l)	[Cl$^-$] (meq/l)	K$^+$ (meq/l)	Osmolarity (mosmol/l)
Sweat	40–60	30–50	1–5	80–150
Plasma	140	101	5	290
Muscle	9	6	162	290

Adapted from Pivarnik.[18]

trolytes during exercise, Pivarnik[18] illustrated the fact that sweat is composed largely of water but also contains significant quantities of electrolytes, particularly sodium and chloride. Due to active reabsorption, sodium concentration in sweat is considerably lower than other body fluids and cellular components. Average amounts are presented in Table 6. The importance of sodium reabsorption is clearly illustrated in patients with cystic fibrosis (discussed in Section XI), who sweat freely but are not able to conserve salt because of an inability to reabsorb NaCl. Some of these patients may be heat intolerant and may need additional salt to prevent dehydration.[45]

According to Sato,[44] Na$^+$ passively enters the two-layered (i.e., the luminal cell and the basal ductal cell) sweat gland ductal cell from the lumen through amiloride-sensitive Na$^+$ channels found at the luminal membrane. Na$^+$ is then actively pumped across the basal membrane via the Na$^+$K$^+$–ATPase pump. These two layers (or cell types) appear to be electrically coupled and act in concert with each other. The duct consists of the proximal coiled segment, a distal straight segment, and an intraepidermal sweat duct unit. The proximal portion of the sweat gland duct appears to contain greater Na$^+$K$^+$–ATPase activity, suggesting more reabsorption of NaCl. Aldosterone is known to cause greater sodium reabsorption;[46] however, overall pharmacological regulation of absorption is still poorly understood.[44]

Physical training in general enhances sweat production, electrolyte conservation, and redistribution of sweat gland activity. Thus potential adaptation to exercise in the heat can be achieved through regular physical exercise. Taylor[47] reviewed studies supporting these views and commented specifically on ion concentrations. For example, elevated sweat gland flow increases sodium content perhaps because of reduced reabsorption in sweat gland ducts at higher flow rates. In contrast, modified reabsorption that conserves sodium may be mediated by increased aldosterone secretion. Nadel et al.[48] have hypothesized that elevated peripheral sensitivity to temperature affects the sweat glands as a likely outcome of physical training. Sato and Sato[49] have associated heightened peripheral sensitivity with heightened cholinergic sensitivity and glandular hypertrophy.

The amount of sodium in the sweat of children tends to be lower than that of adults.[50] No significant gender differences were observed by maturational group. The authors concluded that children are at a lower risk than adults for development of hyponatremia and that the need for sodium replacement is lower under adverse conditions such as heat stress.

VI. EXERCISE EFFECTS

A variety of studies have described specific observations arising from exposure to different types, intensities, and durations of exercise. Examples of such studies are cited to provide a broad view of our knowledge concerning the movement of sodium and the reasons for such movement.

Edwards and Harrison[51] clearly demonstrated that moving from a sitting to a standing position prior to exercise always produced a decrease in blood volume and an increase in plasma [Na$^+$] and osmolality. Further [Na$^+$] increases were observed when exercise was performed. The exercise experiments varied from running 60 min at 62% of $\dot{V}O_2$max to 90 min at a similar intensity. Heating and cooling the body surface during running had little effect on [Na$^+$]. Thus, postural hemoconcentration is real and is comparable to the rapid hemoconcentration that occurs during the first few minutes of cycle ergometer exercise. Sitting down after running reverses hemoconcentration, and a rapid hemodilution occurs which is somewhat unrelated to the preceding exercise. Edwards and Harrison[51] concluded that the same before and after exercise posture as that during any upright exercise should be utilized to ascertain true exercise effects.

Such postural changes can have measurable effects on baseline values for experiments involving walking, running, or any other activity that involves upright exercise. Gore et al.[52] studied both running and cycling in ten men and found that the initial reduction in plasma volume during running involved no change in plasma [Na$^+$] (i.e., an isosmotic shift occurred). With cycling, a significant increase in plasma [Na$^+$] only occurred toward the end of exercise. The authors concluded that with similar plasma volume reductions ($\approx$6.5%) in both events, losses of Na$^+$ were approximately equivalent.

Another study designed to ascertain the effects of body posture during exercise on plasma volume and electrolyte shifts was conducted by Greenleaf et al.[53] Cycle ergometry to peak $\dot{V}O_2$max was undertaken in the sitting and supine positions. Serum [Na$^+$] increased only slightly in each position with peak exercise whereas plasma volume decreased about 16%. Slight differential time responses postexercise were observed, with [Na$^+$] returning to normal at a slower rate following the supine exercise. Sodium content in plasma was reduced about 16% with both types of exercise. It was concluded that the different hydrostatic pressure profiles induced by each type of exercise did not have an important effect on fluid shift.

Senay et al.[54] raised the question of differences in vascular volume changes with treadmill exercise and cycle ergometry. With treadmill exercise, [Na$^+$] increased about 3 meq/l at $\dot{V}O_2$max. In contrast, cycling produced practically no change in [Na$^+$]. The authors concluded that the differences could not be ascribed to any one cause but cited different contracting muscle masses, patterns of blood flow, lactate concentrations, cardiac output, etc. as possible factors associated with the differences in the [Na$^+$] response. They also noted that protein exited the vascular space during cycling but not during treadmill exercise. Considerable interindividual differences occurred in the [Na$^+$] response to both types of exercise.

Intense cycling exercise (e.g., 105% of peak $\dot{V}O_2$ for 3 min) produced a 17% reduction in plasma volume as well as an increase in plasma [Na$^+$] from 142.6 to 148.1 meq/l.[55] Osmolality increased from 283 to 299 mosmol/kg and plasma colloid osmotic pressure from 25.1 to 30.6 mmHg. Thus, the reduction of plasma volume was moderated during this intense exercise.

In studying marathoners during a race, Myhre et al.[56] found that the most significant changes in serum osmolality and [Na$^+$], about a 5% increase, occurred during the first 16 km of the race. Little change was evident thereafter or until the 42-km race was completed. In contrast, plasma volume at 16 km was reduced in the five runners from 2 to 21%, with expansion of plasma volume in only one subject during the remainder of the race. Any voluntary rehydration that occurred was with water.

In a study of marathon runners, Cade et al.[57] offered either water, 1:1 diluted Gatorade® (1/2 GE), or full-strength Gatorade® (GE) during the run. Plasma volume decreased somewhat more with 1/2 GE (≈10%) than GE (≈8%) and both were less than water (−12.3%). The cumulative loss of sodium was roughly equivalent (i.e., about 400 mmol), but plasma sodium concentration increased with GE from 144 to 146 mmol/l and with 1/2 GE from 143.5 to 145.4 mmol/l. Consumption of water produced only a marginal increase in serum [Na$^+$]. Considerable interindividual variation occurred with each treatment. Cade et al.[57] concluded that when the replacement solution contains sodium, a larger proportion of ingested water remains in the ECF and the vascular volume was better maintained. Thus, a marked fall in blood pressure was avoided because of the better maintenance of vascular volume.

When cycling exercise (84% $\dot{V}O_2$max) to exhaustion was performed with or without saline infusion (0.9% NaCl, mean volume 1280 ml), plasma volume decreased less with the infusion (−5.3% versus −13.7% control). This improved plasma volume retention was associated with a lower core temperature and heart rate and slightly improved thermoregulation, but no change was observed in endurance (time on cycle ergometer).[58]

Convertino et al.[59] investigated plasma volume, electrolyte, osmolality, arginine vasopressin (AVP), and plasma renin activity (PRA) during graded cycle ergometry exercise. Significant correlation coefficients were found between Δ [Na$^+$] and Δ osmolality ($r = 0.96$), Δ [Na$^+$] and AVP ($r = 0.88$), and Δ [Na$^+$] and Δ PRA ($r = 0.49$). In evaluating the data, they concluded that AVP may well be the primary hormone responsible for fluid and electrolyte balance restoration following exercise as well as the hyperosmolality associated with the net hypotonic plasma efflux during exercise. An exercise intensity exceeding 40% $\dot{V}O_2$max was required to increase plasma osmolality and [Na$^+$] to trigger AVP release. They concluded that graded exercise stimulates sympathetic nervous activity and thereby the renin–angiotensin system as part of a general stress response.

Walsh et al.[60] found impaired high-intensity cycle ergometer performance with slight hypohydration. The six trained subjects rode for 60 min at 70% $\dot{V}O_2$peak and then to exhaustion at 90% $\dot{V}O_2$peak. In one trial the subjects ingested 400 ml of 20 mmol/l NaCl followed by 120 ml every 10 min during the first 50 min of exercise. No fluid was ingested in the other trial. Environmental conditions were ambient temperature 0°C and relative humidity 60%. Plasma volume loss was about 18% in both trials. Total sodium losses were 115 mmol in the no fluid trial and 123 mmol in the NaCl fluid replacement trial. Fluid ingestion reduced the perceived exertion rating and ADH but had no effect on aldosterone. None of the measured variables accounted for the enhanced performance or the reduced perceived exertion rating with fluid ingestion.

Montain and Coyle[61] studied eight endurance-trained cyclists who exercised at 62 to 67% $\dot{V}O_2$max for 2 hr in a warm environment (33°C dry bulb, 50% relative humidity). On four separate occasions they were rehydrated at 0, 20, 48, or 81% of their sweat losses. Esophageal temperature (T_{es}) was highly correlated with both the increase in serum osmolality ($r \approx 0.90$) and sodium concentration ($r \approx 0.93$). Of the variables measured (i.e., blood volume, plasma volume, serum osmolality, [K^+], and [Na^+]), the increase in serum [Na^+] was the single variable that best predicted elevation in T_{es}. Serum [Na^+] with no fluid replacement increased from about 144 to 150 mmol/l. The fluid replacement solution was the carbohydrate–electrolyte beverage Gatorade®.

Several days of regular exercise in the heat produced an increase in renal sodium reabsorption. In addition, consumption of 180 to 250 meq Na^+ per day induced not only a positive sodium balance but plasma volume and extracellular fluid expansion. In an attempt to clarify the roles of PRA and aldosterone in these responses, Costill et al.[62] exercised a group of men at 60% $\dot{V}O_2$max for 1 hr. Urine sodium and volume were reduced postexercise for up to 48 hr. PRA and aldosterone were elevated during and immediately following exercise but returned to preexercise values by 6 to 12 hr. Thus the relatively short-lived effect of aldosterone on renal sodium conservation could not explain continued sodium conservation beyond the 6- to 12-hr period.

Prolonged exercise in warm or hot environments in which body temperature and heart rate are elevated induces hypertonic hypovolemia and large increases in several circulating hormones including ANF or ANP, AVP, adrenocorticotropic hormone, and cortisol. Hydration, particularly with dilute saline solutions, moderates these hormonal increases and preserves plasma volume. The ANP observations appear contrary to other results where plasma volume expansion was associated with increased circulating ANP. Follenius et al.[63] concluded from these experiments that the complex interaction of the hormones involved remains to be resolved.

Another study of ANP during and following intense upright or supine exercise revealed substantial increases in plasma ANP that were somewhat higher with supine exercise. Serum [Na^+] was also elevated with both types of exercise.[64] These authors concluded that atrial distention is the probable stimulus for ANP release, but it can be postulated the ANP exerts modulatory influences on the fluid-regulating hormonal system during exercise.

With acute intense (30 sec to exhaustion) cycling exercise, there is some evidence that [Na^+] in muscle increases slightly and [K^+] decreases. Simultaneous increases in serum [Na^+] were associated with the reduction in plasma volume.[65]

In an interesting study of heavy muscular exercise during a 90-km cross-country ski race under adverse environmental conditions involving low temperature (0°C), snowfall, and adverse wind, Refsum et al.[66] found a small negative correlation coefficient between serum [Na^+] and body weight loss ($r = -0.40$, $p < 0.01$). The serum [Na^+] showed an increase of 1.2 meq/l in ten men with the greatest weight loss (−3.2 kg) and a decrease of 2.6 meq/l in ten men with the smallest weight loss (0.7 kg). Depending on the extent of consumption of replacement beverages during the race or use of glucose or salt tablets, remarkably small disturbances of fluid and electrolyte balance occurred.

When the body becomes hypohydrated by different methods (e.g., physical activity, sauna bath, use of diuretics, or a combination of all three), changes from baseline measurements are not always the same. Caldwell et al.[67] studied these three methods of rapid weight loss, all of which are commonly used by athletes, especially wrestlers. Their results appear in Table 7. Although the respective changes from baseline are not exceptionally large, the diuretic (furosemide) produced the greatest deficit in plasma volume and the sauna the largest increase in serum [Na^+].

Armstrong et al.[68] utilized furosemide (40 mg) to evaluate the effects of hypohydration on competitive running performance which was adversely affected, particularly in the 5000- and 10,000-m running events. In association with these performance decrements, total urinary sodium loss over 5 hr averaged 134.8 meq in 1562 ml of urine but represented only 4.7% of the body pool of sodium (estimated at 2870 meq Na^+). The authors concluded that this acute loss of sodium and a smaller quantity of potassium had significant detrimental effects on muscle contractility. Although it does not alter sweating, furosemide exerts its effect by blocking sodium reabsorption in the renal tubules, thereby facilitating diuresis.

TABLE 7 Mean Changes in Baseline Measurements with Three Different Methods for Inducing Hypohydration

Variable	Physical Activity (n = 16)	Sauna (n = 16)	Diuretic (n = 15)	Combined (n = 47)	Control (n = 15)
Weight (kg)	−2.3[a,b]	−3.5[a,b]	−3.1[a,b]	−3.0[a,b]	−0.8
Plasma volume (%)	−0.9	−10.3[b]	−14.1[b]	−8.3[b]	3.3
Serum Na^+ (mmol/l)	1.7[a,b]	3.5[a,b]	0.6	2.0[a,b]	−0.3

[a] $p < 0.001$ after hypohydration.
[b] $p < 0.001$ when compared to controls.

Adapted from Caldwell et al.[67]

Although men and women appear to respond equally with respect to fluid and electrolyte shifts with exercise and heat exposure, the question was asked whether the menstrual cycle would modify responses and whether estrogen replacement therapy (ERT) could be used to help clarify the situation. Middle-aged women (48 ± 2 years) were given ERT for 14 to 23 days and then performed semireclined exercise for 60 min at an intensity of 40% $\dot{V}O_2$max in a 36°C environment.[69] ERT produced an isotonic hemodilution and greater sweat sodium concentration despite an unaltered aldosterone. Since no clear interpretation could be given, others are encouraged to follow up on this preliminary study.

VII. NATREMIA

A. HYPONATREMIA

Hyponatremia (serum sodium <130 meq/l) in the athlete is most usually associated with excessive dilute fluid intakes resulting in reduced extracellular sodium concentration to yield what amounts to water intoxication. When it occurs, the athlete commonly complains of such symptoms as weakness, agitation, confusion, nausea, or vomiting. Noakes[22] summarized some data and reported hyponatremia in a variety of endurance events (e.g., two runners in a Western States 100-mi run, five competitors in a Canadian Ironman Triathlon, and a 13 to 27% incidence in competitors in the 226-km Hawaiian Ironman Triathlon). In addition, Armstrong et al.[70] have documented a case study of an individual who consumed and retained a large quantity of water during a 4-hr bout of exercise in the heat. Significant hyponatremia resulted from the exposure. Several possible causes of hyponatremia are listed in Table 8, but the overriding solution for most athletes engaged in endurance events that could cause hyponatremia is the provision of proportional salt and water replacement so as to avoid the problem.

Perhaps the experience of Noakes et al.[71] in evaluating hyponatremia in endurance athletes is useful in summarizing the prevalence of the condition. They suggest that symptomatic hyponatremia (serum $[Na^+]$ <130 mmol/l) occurs in less than 0.3% of competitors even when they ingest little sodium chloride. Among col-

TABLE 8 Possible Causes of Hyponatremia with Exercise

- Excessive losses of sodium due to heavy sweating
- Excessive ingestion of water or dilute fluids in relation to fluid needs
- Extended training under adverse environmental conditions along with dieting and restricted sodium intake
- Lack of heat acclimatization, which promotes high concentrations of sodium in sweat
- Compromised kidney function with poor sodium reabsorption in the renal tubules and limited urine volume
- Failure to move protein into the intravascular space
- Elevation of serum ADH
- Translocation of sodium and other solutes into the GI tract

lapsed runners, however, a 9% incidence was found. They concluded that a regulated contraction of the ECF explains why the majority of the runners maintain normal or near normal serum [Na⁺] in the face of a considerable sodium deficit.

When present, hyponatremia must be considered serious and treated so as to avoid complications such as grand mal seizures, respiratory arrest or acute respiratory distress, and coma with elevated intracranial pressure. Others have recorded pulmonary edema and hypotension. In marathon runners, Noakes et al.[71] have found serum [Na⁺] as low as 112 mmol/l.

B. HYPERNATREMIA

Noakes et al.[71] also summarized findings from ultramarathon runners and ultratriathletes which suggest that the normal response to such exercise is a hypertonic, hypo- or normovolemic hypernatremia resulting from loss of sweat hypotonic to plasma and the renal conservation of sodium. Such hypertonic hypernatremia exists among many who become hypohydrated and hypovolemic.

In an intense exercise study involving an all-out timed swim (freestyle or butterfly) of 100 m, serum [Na⁺] increased 7 meq/l and osmolality 14 mosmol/l. Serum [Na⁺] exceeded 150 meq/l in about 40% of the subjects as a result of their respective swims. The correlation coefficient between the increase in osmolality and [Na⁺] was $r = 0.71$ ($p < 0.001$). Thus, many of the swimmers reached hypernatremic concentrations, that is, >150 meq/l. Presumably the movement of fluid out of the vascular space accounted for the changes observed. Such changes were not observed with longer submaximal swims.[72]

VIII. TRAINING EFFECTS

Evidence has been produced that resting blood volume can be increased with training within 3 days and that about 40% of the increase is associated with aldosterone activity, with the remainder explained by augmentation of intravascular protein.[73] Cycle ergometry training was undertaken for three consecutive days. Cycling duration was 2 hr and the intensity was maintained at 65% V̇O₂max. Half of the subjects were given 25 mg of spironolactone to inhibit aldosterone activity. Resting plasma volume increased about 500 ml in the trained subjects but only about 160 ml in the drug-treated subjects. Serum [Na⁺] and osmolality increased less with drug treatment, but urine volume was greater and sodium excretion tended to be higher. In conclusion, the authors suggested that aldosterone plays a significant role in plasma volume expansion and the movements of electrolytes such as sodium. Gillen et al.[74] found that after eight 4-min bouts of exercise at 85% V̇O₂max, plasma volume was expanded at 24 hr of recovery by about 4.0 ml/kg body weight. This expansion was accounted for by an increase of plasma albumin. Thus, any plasma volume response to a training regimen appears to begin early and progress more moderately for several days before reaching a training-induced plateau. Gillen et al.[74] maintain that plasma [Na+] could only account for a 24-hr postexercise hypervolemia of 1.0 ml/kg body weight.

The progressive loss of hypotonic sweat by well-trained runners reduces body content of sodium, yet many runners manage to preserve serum [Na+] with no[75] or moderate elevations.[56] Thus, in cool or warm weather competition in such events as the marathon, the need for supplemental electrolyte replacement is questionable. Perhaps the trained individual has indeed adapted to such competition through an elevated plasma volume, and sodium conservation in sweating tends to preserve sodium homeostasis. Learning reasonable fluid replacement strategies no doubt contributes to the adaptation process.

Freund et al.[76] recognized that the trained condition is associated with elevated plasma and blood volumes in trained individuals, a lessened diuresis, and sodium excretion during head-out water immersion or after water ingestion. Yet their observation of trained and untrained subjects who performed maximal treadmill exercise for 8 to 13 min revealed no differences in resting plasma osmolality, [Na+], ADH, aldosterone, PRA, or ANF but significantly higher osmolality and [Na+] values immediately following maximal exercise in the untrained group. Plasma volume was reduced equally in both groups. Plasma volume during recovery expanded faster in the trained group. They concluded that similar ADH responses but lower osmolality in the trained subjects may point to an increased ADH sensitivity to osmotic stimulation. Thus, some evidence for fluid/electrolyte adaptation with training was found.

Plasma hypervolemia following 8 days of aerobic training (65% $\dot{V}O_2$max) was associated with a ninefold elevation in both PRA and AVP during exhaustive exercise that facilitated sodium and water retention.[77] An associated chronic increase in plasma albumin content was also noted, which facilitated water transfer into the vascular space. [Na+] and osmolality remained essentially unchanged before and after training, although the performance of exhausting exercise produced about a 2% increase on each testing occasion. The chronic exercise regimen appeared to stimulate compensatory mechanisms for the expansion of plasma volume (in these experiments, 427 ml on average) by enhancing water and solute conservation through elevation of PRA and AVP. Any such effects were short-lived during recovery and had diminished substantially within 24 hr. Because the mean resting plasma osmolality remained relatively constant throughout the 8-day training regimen, an isotonic increase in total solute content is implicated. This suggests that the renin–angiotensin system was stimulated and the AVP release with exercise enhanced fluid, electrolyte, and protein conservation.

Melin et al.[78] studied the effects of cycling to exhaustion among men classified according to the extent of their physical training. The results were somewhat ambiguous, but they concluded that although plasma volume was reduced substantially with the exhausting exercise, evidence for a better water shift from previously active muscle to plasma is more marked in the trained subjects. [Na+] immediately following exhaustive exercise was slightly but nonsignificantly higher in the trained subjects, as was plasma osmolality. Somewhat lesser elevations were found among the trained subjects for AVP, renin, aldosterone, and neurophysin. A lesser lowering of plasma volume and greater sweat loss were noted among the trained men, but the respective differences among groups were small. The authors conclude that the different volemias probably accounted for the hormonal changes and that 5 months of training by other subjects produced similar results.

IX. ACCLIMATIZATION EFFECTS

It has been known for some time that exercise/heat acclimatization produces a decline in sweat sodium concentration.[79,80] Using a passive hyperthermia technique, Allan and Wilson[81] stimulated various rates of sweating in men before and after they had been acclimatized to heat. A significant reduction in sweat sodium concentration with acclimatization was observed over a wide range of sweat rates. Sweating was augmented about 70% with heat acclimatization and the sweat sodium concentration was proportionally less at the higher sweat rates. It was postulated that with higher sweat outputs, the capacity for sodium reabsorption was increased after heat acclimatization possibly due to an effect of aldosterone. Collins and Weiner[82] had a similar view.

Controversial evidence in regard to the effect of aldosterone has been presented by Bonner et al.,[83] who concluded that the expansion of the intravascular volume and increase in the ratio of $[Na^+]/[K^+]$ with heat acclimatization should reduce rather than increase aldosterone secretion, and aldosterone concentrations were indeed lower in three of five subjects, although the mean reduction was insignificant. Their results were consistent with the hypothesis that the adrenal cortex is not overly important in maintaining heat acclimatization if any negative salt balance is resolved. Similarly, Davies et al.[84] concluded that the increased sodium conservation with acclimatization is probably a normal response to exercise and heat exposure even in the absence of a negative sodium balance. They had prevented the latter by administering 1% saline to prevent any salt deficit.

In a study of drinking and water balance during heat acclimation involving exercise, Greenleaf et al.[85] observed a progressive increase in plasma volume over an 8-day exercise period. With acclimation, plasma $[Na^+]$ and osmolality were negatively correlated with voluntary fluid intake; that is, the lower concentrations were associated with more drinking. They concluded that of the two postulated mechanisms for control of fluid intake during exercise/heat acclimation, the renin–angiotensin system along with reductions in body water and intravascular fluid appear more important than the sodium–osmotic–vasopressin pathway.

X. LOSS REPLACEMENT

There are extreme conditions during which sweat losses are great, as are the losses of sodium. Perhaps ultraendurance events such as the marathon or longer running events, triathlons, cross-country skiing tours exceeding 30 km, etc. epitomize such conditions. For such competition, additional sodium in the diet or electrolyte- (Na^+) containing beverages is warranted. Saline intake before exercise causes an expansion of plasma volume that can be maintained for some time, and saline intake during exercise at moderate levels can help relative sodium homeostasis. Greenleaf[86] has reviewed the effects of sodium ingestion and has made several pertinent observations. Osmotic pressure is raised in the ECF, producing a shift of water from cells to ECF. Volume-sensitive osmoreceptors in the hypothalamus stimulate release of ADH. Renal distal tubule cells are stimulated by ADH and fluid is retained. The hypothalamus also senses the increase in plasma osmolality, which can stimulate drinking. Retained fluid serves to dilute [Na^+] toward its original concentration, but a relative hypervolemia is retained. Repeated bouts of exercise with or without heat exposure induce sodium retention.[87]

As a result of these actions (i.e., sodium retention and hypervolemia), improvements in performance have been noted perhaps due to maintained cardiac output (stroke volume) during exercise and an enhanced capability for thermoregulation.[16]

XI. IMBALANCE PATHOLOGIES: TOXICITY

The amount of salt intake that can be regarded as lethal is not well established, but some information is available. On the basis of a case study of a 17-year-old (102-kg) girl who consumed an estimated 150 g of salt and experienced severe toxic symptoms, Schatz[88] stated that 3 g/kg should be regarded as lethal but that smaller amounts were likely to kill more susceptible subjects. Gosslin et al.[89] set the lethal dose between 0.5 and 5.0 g/kg, whereas Battarbee and Meneely[90] observed edema in healthy men on intakes of 35 to 40 g NaCl per day. They also called attention to the balance between sodium and potassium and the role greater intakes of potassium would have in ameliorating the adverse effects of sodium. Although Americans in general consume excess salt (i.e., 10 to 15 g/day), it is not clear that these intakes are incompatible with health among those who are not salt sensitive.[13] Clearer interpretation of excess salt intake and hypertension has only been exposed in susceptible animals and population studies. Fregly[13] also points out that no studies have reported mutagenic properties of NaCl.

It was discovered in 1953 by di Sant'Agnese et al.[91] that cystic fibrosis patients had abnormally high concentrations of Na^+ and Cl^- in their sweat, and they were regarded as being potentially heat intolerant. Orenstein et al.[92] determined that they secrete normal volumes of sweat but that they do indeed lose more sodium and chloride in their sweat. In a follow-up study to ascertain their tolerance of exercise and heat stress, Orenstein et al.[93] found that cystic fibrosis patients can acclimatize to heat, showing lower body temperature and heart rate responses, but that their sweat electrolytes were unaltered. Thus, they suffer greater electrolyte losses on a continuing basis as they acclimatize to heat. Despite these observations, the authors concluded that the cystic fibrosis patients responded well enough to the acclimatization process that there was no need for salt supplementation. More recent work has characterized the genetic components of the disease and describes the role of transmembrane conductance regulation in electrolyte channel regulation.[94]

A variety of conditions can affect sodium balance in the athlete. These include use of various drugs (diuretics), diarrhea, use of fluid-reducing techniques such as wearing water-vapor-impermeable suits, sauna or hot baths, and excessive water consumption. Other clinically related sodium imbalances and conditions such as hyperthermia, chronic renal disease, sweat gland dysfunctions, and endocrine disorders have been extensively treated by others (e.g., Michell,[10] Goldberg,[21] Moses,[15] and Fregly[13]).

XII. NEW ROLE: SODIUM CHANNEL

A new role has been postulated for the stimulating action of Ca^+ flux on heart muscle and perhaps skeletal muscle by opening of Na^+ channels to facilitate Ca^+ passage.[95] This so-called "slip-mode conductance" was estimated to account for 30% of Ca^+ flux, particularly when protein kinase A is activated. The investigators also indicate that phosphorylation of Na^+ is probably necessary for the Na^+ channel to facilitate Ca^+ transfer. Cardotonic steroids also were implicated as activators of "slip-mode conductance." They were said to bind to the Na^+ pump, possibly altering protein–protein interaction between Na^+K^+–ATPase and the Na^+ channel to initiate "slip-mode conductance." The authors conclude that "slip-mode conductance" is probably a general signaling pathway. Thus, the uniqueness of the Na^+ channel has further evolved into an important ion transfer mechanism with multiple functions.

XIII. SUMMARY

Investigations regarding the role of salt and in particular sodium on the body have a long history related primarily to studies of salt appetite, thirst, and body fluid regulation. The regulation of sodium movement within the body is only partially understood. That sodium is an essential element for healthy bodily function is now a given, but the fact that our culture consumes excess sodium has posed some problems, with hypertension in susceptible individuals perhaps of most consequence. Absorption and gastrointestinal handling of sodium is an efficient process, with very little sodium excreted in feces. Renal handling in normal kidneys is also efficient, with conservation of sodium by reabsorption generally proportional to physiological need. Important losses of sodium occur in sweat, but sweat gland handling is modified by both regular physical exercise that produces sweating and regular exposure to environmental heat and other conditions that activate the acclimatization process. Several hormones, enzymes such as Na^+K^+–ATPase, NO, and other factors modify sodium handling and movement within the GI tract, the kidney, sweat glands, and tissue to tissue and fluid to tissue or vice versa. Toxicity can exist with excessive intakes or defects in handling, but such situations are rare. That sodium has ubiquitous effects within the body is illustrated by the discovery of a new role for sodium channels in tissue membranes regarding the facilitation of calcium ion movement. Other roles for sodium may well appear as investigations continue.

REFERENCES

1. Bernard, C., *Les Phenomenes de la Vie,* Loudres, Baillière, Tindall and Cox, Paris, 1878.
2. Cannon, W.B., Organization for physiological homeostasis, in *Homeostasis: Origins of the Concept,* Langley, L.L., Ed., Dowden, Hutchinson, and Ross, Stroudsburg, PA, 1973, 250.
3. Smith, H.W., *From Fish to Philosopher: The Story of Our Internal Environment,* CBA Pharmaceutical Products, Summit, NY, 1959.
4. Pitts, R.F., *Physiology of the Kidney and Body Fluids,* Year Book Medical Publishers, Chicago, 1974.
5. Luft, F.C., Salt, water, and extracellular volume regulation, in *Present Knowledge in Nutrition,* Zeigler, E.E. and Filer L.J., Eds., International Life Sciences Institute Press, Washington, D.C., 1996, 265.
6. Hollenberg, N.K., Set point for sodium homeostasis: surfeit, deficit and their implications, *Kidney Int.,* 17, 423, 1980.
7. Simpson, F.O., Sodium intake, body sodium and sodium excretion, *Lancet,* 2, 25, 1988.
8. Bertorello, A.M. and Katz, A.I., Regulation of Na^+K^+ pump activity: pathways between receptors and effectors, *News Physiol. Sci.,* 10, 253, 1995.
9. Salazar, F.J. and Llinas, M.T., Role of nitric oxide in the control of sodium excretion, *News Physiol. Sci.,* 11, 62, 1996.
10. Michell, A.R., *The Clinical Biology of Sodium,* Elsevier, New York, 1995.
11. Buskirk, E.R., Sodium and adaptation to high environmental temperatures, work and athletics, in *Sodium in Medicine and Health — A Monograph,* Moses, C., Ed., Reese Press, Baltimore, 1980, 75.
12. Meneely, G.R. and Battarbee, H.D., Sodium and potassium, *Nutr. Rev.,* 34, 225, 1976.
13. Fregly, M.J., Sodium and potassium, *Annu. Rev. Nutr.,* 1, 69, 1981.
14. Luft, F.C., Sodium, chloride, and potassium, in *Present Knowledge in Nutrition,* Brown, M.L., Ed., International Life Sciences Institute–Nutrition Foundation, Washington, D.C., 1990, 233.
15. Moses, C., Ed., *Sodium in Medicine and Health — A Monograph,* Reese Press, Baltimore, 1980.
16. Luetkemeier, M.J., Coles, M.G., and Askew, E.W., Dietary sodium and plasma volume levels with exercise, *Sports Med.,* 23, 279, 1997.
17. Pivarnik, J.M. and Palmer, R.A., Water and electrolyte balance during rest and exercise, in *Nutrition in Exercise and Sport,* Wolinsky, I. and Hickson, J.F., Eds., CRC Press, Boca Raton, FL, 1994, 245.
18. Pivarnik, J.M., Water and electrolytes during exercise, in *Nutrition in Exercise and Sport,* Hickson, J.F. and Wolinsky, I., Eds., CRC Press, Boca Raton, FL, 1989, 185.
19. Fellmann, N., Hormonal and plasma volume alterations following endurance exercise — a brief review, *Sports Med.,* 13, 37, 1992.
20. Noakes, T.D., Fluid replacement during exercise, in *Exercise and Sport Sciences Review,* Holloszy, J.O., Ed., Williams and Wilkins, Baltimore, 1993, 297.
21. Goldberg, M., Hyponatremia, *Med. Clin. North Am.,* 65, 251, 1981.
22. Noakes, T.D., The hyponatremia of exercise, *Int. J. Sport Nutr.,* 2, 205, 1992.
23. National Research Council, *Recommended Dietary Allowances,* 10th ed., National Academy Press, Washington, D.C., 1989.

24. Holbrook, J.T., Patterson, K.Y., Bodner, J.E., Douglas, L.W., Veillon, C., Kelsay, J.L., Mertz, W., and Smith, J.C., Sodium and potassium intake and balance in adults consuming self-selected diets, *Am. J. Clin. Nutr.,* 40, 786, 1984.
25. Takamato, A., Mack, G.W., Gillen, C.M., and Nadel, E.R., Sodium appetite, thirst, and body fluid regulation in humans during rehydration without sodium replacement, *Am. J. Physiol. Regulatory Integrative Comp. Physiol.,* 266, R1493, 1994.
26. Tiidus, P., Shephard, R.J., and Montelpare, W., Overall intake of energy and key nutrients: data for middle-aged and older middle-class adults, *Can. J. Sport Sci.,* 14, 173, 1989.
27. Rolls, B.J. and Phillips, P.A., Age and disturbances of thirst and fluid balance, *Nutr. Rev.,* 48, 137, 1990.
28. Gamble, J.L., Physiological information gained from studies on the life raft ration (1947), *Nutr. Rev.,* 47, 247, 1989.
29. Lindinger, M.I., Graham, T.E., and Spriet, L.L., Caffeine attenuates the exercise-induced increase in plasma [K$^+$] in humans, *J. Appl. Physiol.,* 74, 1149, 1993.
30. Forbes, G.B. and Lewis, A.M., Total sodium, potassium and chloride in adult man, *J. Clin. Invest.,* 35, 596, 1956.
31. Gisolfi, C.V., Summers, R.W., Schedl, H.P., and Bleiler, T.L., Intestinal water absorption from select carbohydrate solutions in humans, *J. Appl. Physiol.,* 73, 2142, 1992.
32. Spiller, R.C., Jones, B.J.M., and Silk, D.B.A., Jejunal water and electrolyte absorption from two proprietary enteral feeds in man: importance of sodium content, *Gut,* 28, 681, 1987.
33. Schedl, H.P., Maughan, R.J., and Gisolfi, C.V., Intestinal absorption during rest and exercise: implications for formulating an oral rehydration solution (ORS), *Med. Sci. Sports Exercise,* 26, 267, 1994.
34. Hargreaves, M., Costill, D., Burke, L., Mcconell, G., and Febbraio, M., Influence of sodium on glucose bioavailability during exercise, *Med. Sci. Sports Exercise,* 26, 365, 1994.
35. Ferrannini, E., Barrett, E., Bevilacqua, S., Dupre, J., and DeFronzo, R.A., Sodium elevates the plasma glucose response to glucose ingestion in man, *J. Clin. Endocrinol. Metab.,* 54, 455, 1982.
36. Sjovall, H., Redfors, S., Hallback, D., Eklund, S., and Jodal, M., The effect of splanchnic nerve stimulation on blood flow distribution, villous tissue osmolality and fluid and electrolyte transport in the small intestine, *Acta Physiol. Scand.,* 117, 359, 1983.
37. Reineck, H.J., Stein, J.H., and Seldin, D.W., Integrated responses of the kidney to alterations in extracellular fluid volume, in *The Kidney: Physiology and Pathophysiology,* Seldin, D.W. and Giebisch, G., Eds., Raven Press, New York, 1985, 1137.
38. Vander, A., Sherman, J., and Luciano, D., Eds., *Human Physiology: The Mechanics of Body Function,* 7th ed., WCB McGraw-Hill, Boston, 1998, chap. 16.
39. Funder, J.W., Aldosterone action, *Annu. Rev. Physiol.,* 55, 115, 1993.
40. Zambraski, E.J., The kidney and body fluid balance during exercise, in *Body Fluid Balance: Exercise and Sport,* Buskirk, E.R. and Puhl, S.M., Eds., CRC Press, Boca Raton, FL, 1996, 75.
41. Slick, G.L., Aguilera, A.J., Zambraski, E.J., DiBona, G.F., and Kaloyanides, G.J., Renal neuroadrenergic transmission, *Am. J. Physiol.,* 229, 60, 1975.
42. Hall, J.E., Guyton, A.C., Smith, M.J., and Coleman, T.G., Chronic blockade of angiotensin II formation during sodium deprivation, *Am. J. Physiol.,* 237, F424, 1979.
43. Wade, C.E., Ramee, S.R., Hunt, M.M., and White, C.J., Hormonal and renal responses to converting enzyme inhibition during maximal exercise, *J. Appl. Physiol.,* 63, 1796, 1987.
44. Sato, K., The mechanism of eccrine sweat secretion, in *Perspectives in Exercise Science and Sports Medicine,* Gisolfi, C.V., Lamb, D.R., and Nadel, E.R., Eds., Brown and Benchmark, Dubuque, IA, 1993, 85.
45. Bar-Or, O., Blimkie, C.J.R., Hay, J.A., MacDougall, J.D., Ward, D.S., and Wilson, W.M., Voluntary dehydration and heat intolerance in cystic fibrosis, *Lancet,* 339, 696, 1992.
46. Sato, K. and Dobson, R.L., The effect of intracutaneous d-aldosterone and hydrocortisone on the human eccrine sweat gland function, *J. Invest. Dermatol.,* 54, 450, 1970.
47. Taylor, N.A.S., Eccrine sweat glands: adaptation to physical training and heat acclimation, *Sports Med.,* 3, 387, 1986.

48. Nadel, E.R., Pandolf, K.B., Roberts, M.F., and Stolwijk, J.A.J., Mechanisms of thermal acclimation to exercise in the heat, *J. Appl. Physiol.,* 37, 515, 1974.

49. Sato, K. and Sato, F., Individual variations in structure and function of human eccrine sweat glands, *Am. J. Physiol.,* 245, R203, 1983.

50. Meyer, F. and Bar-Or, O., Fluid and electrolyte loss during exercise: the paediatric angle, *Sports Med.,* 18, 4, 1994.

51. Edwards, R.J. and Harrison, M.H., Intravascular volume and protein responses to running exercise, *Med. Sci. Sports Exercise,* 16, 247, 1984.

52. Gore, C.J., Scroop, G.C., Marker, J.D., and Catcheside, P.G., Plasma volume, osmolarity, total protein and electrolytes during treadmill running and cycle exercise, *Eur. J. Appl. Physiol.,* 65, 302, 1992.

53. Greenleaf, J.E., Van Beaumont, W., Brock, P.J., Morse, J.T., and Mangseth, G.R., Plasma volume and electrolyte shifts with heavy exercise in sitting and supine positions, *Am. J. Physiol.,* 236, R206, 1979.

54. Senay, L.C., Jr., Rogers, G., and Jooste, P., Changes in blood plasma during progressive treadmill and cycle exercise, *J. Appl. Physiol. Respir. Environ. Exercise Physiol.,* 49, 59, 1980.

55. Mohsenin, V. and Gonzalez, R.R., Tissue pressure and plasma oncotic pressure during exercise, *J. Appl. Physiol. Respir. Environ. Exercise Physiol.,* 56, 102, 1984.

56. Myhre, L.G., Hartung, G.H., and Tucker, D.M., Plasma volume and blood metabolites in middle-aged runners during a warm-weather marathon, *Eur. J. Appl. Physiol.,* 48, 227, 1982.

57. Cade, R., Packer, D., Zauner, D., Kaufmann, D., Peterson, J., Mars, D., Privette, M., Hommen, N., Fregly, M.J., and Rogers, J., Marathon running: physiological and chemical changes accompanying late-race deterioration, *Eur. J. Appl. Physiol.,* 65, 485, 1992.

58. Deschamps, A., Levy, R.D., Cosio, M.G., Marliss, E.B., and Magder, S., Effect of saline infusion on body temperature and endurance during heavy exercise, *J. Appl. Physiol.,* 66, 2799, 1989.

59. Convertino, V.A., Keil, L.C., Bernauer, E.M., and Greenleaf, J.E., Plasma volume, osmolality, vasopressin, and renin activity during graded exercise in man, *J. Appl. Physiol. Respir. Environ. Exercise Physiol.,* 50, 123, 1981.

60. Walsh, R.M., Noakes, T.D., Hawley, J.A., and Dennis, S.C., Impaired high intensity cycling performance time at low levels of dehydration, *Int. J. Sports Med.,* 15, 392, 1994.

61. Montain, S.J. and Coyle, E.F., Influence of graded dehydration on hyperthermia and cardiovascular drift during exercise, *J. Appl. Physiol.,* 73, 1340, 1992.

62. Costill, D.L., Branam, G., Fink, W., and Nelson, R., Exercise induced sodium conservation: changes in plasma renin and aldosterone, *Med. Sci. Sports Exercise,* 8, 209, 1976.

63. Follenius, M., Candas, V., Bothorel, B., and Brandenberger, G., Effect of rehydration on atrial natriuretic peptide release during exercise in the heat, *J. Appl. Physiol.,* 66, 2516, 1989.

64. Perrault, H., Cantin, M., Thibault, G., Brisson, G.R., Brisson, G., and Beland, M., Plasma atrial natriuretic peptide during brief upright and supine exercise in humans, *J. Appl. Physiol.,* 66, 2159, 1989.

65. Kowalchuk, J.M., Heigenhauser, G.J.F., Lindinger, M.I., Sutton, J.R., and Jones, N.L., Factors influencing hydrogen ion concentration in muscle after intense exercise, *J. Appl. Physiol.,* 65, 2080, 1988.

66. Refsum, H.E., Tveit, B., Meen, H.D., and Stromme, S.B., Serum electrolyte, fluid and acid–base balance after prolonged heavy exercise at low environmental temperature, *Scand. J. Clin. Lab. Invest.,* 32, 117, 1973.

67. Caldwell, J.E., Ahonen, E., and Nousiainen, U., Differential effects of sauna-, diuretic-, and exercise-induced hypohydration, *J. Appl. Physiol. Respir. Environ. Exercise Physiol.,* 57, 1018, 1984.

68. Armstrong, L.E., Costill, D.L., and Fink, W.J., Influence of diuretic-induced dehydration on competitive running performance, *Med. Sci. Sports Exercise,* 17, 456, 1985.

69. Tankersley, C.G., Nicholas, W.C., Deaver, D.R., Mikita, D., and Kenney, W.L., Estrogen replacement in middle-aged women: thermoregulatory responses to exercise in the heat, *J. Appl. Physiol.,* 73, 1238, 1992.

70. Armstrong, L.E., Curtis, W.C., Hubbard, R.W., Francesconi, R.P., Moore, R., and Askew, E.W., Symptomatic hyponatremia during prolonged exercise in heat, *Med. Sci. Sports Exercise*, 25, 543, 1993.

71. Noakes, T.D., Norman, R.J., Buck, R.H., Godlonton, J., Stevenson, K., and Pittaway, D., The incidence of hyponatremia during prolonged ultraendurance exercise, *Med. Sci. Sports Exercise*, 22, 165, 1990.

72. Felig, P., Johnson, C., Levitt, M., Cunningham, J., Keefe, F., and Boglioli, B., Hypernatremia induced by maximal exercise, *J. Am. Med. Assoc.*, 248, 1209, 1982.

73. Luetkemeier, M.J., Flowers, K.M., and Lamb, D.R., Spironolactone administration and training-induced hypervolemia, *Int. J. Sports Med.*, 15, 295, 1994.

74. Gillen, C.M., Lee, R., Mack, G.W., Tomaselli, C.M., Nishiyasu, T., and Nadel, E.R., Plasma volume expansion in humans after a single intense exercise protocol, *J. Appl. Physiol.*, 71, 1914, 1991.

75. Maron, M.B., Horvath, S.M., and Wilkerson, J.E., Acute blood biochemical alterations in response to marathon running, *Eur. J. Appl. Physiol.*, 34, 173, 1975.

76. Freund, B.J., Claybaugh, J.R., Dice, M.S., and Hashiro, G.M., Hormonal and vascular fluid responses to maximal exercise in trained and untrained males, *J. Appl. Physiol.*, 63, 669, 1987.

77. Convertino, V.A., Brock, P.J., Keil, L.C., Bernauer, E.M., and Greenleaf, J.E., Exercise training-induced hypervolemia: role of plasma albumin, renin, and vasopressin, *J. Appl. Physiol. Respir. Environ. Exercise Physiol.*, 48, 665, 1980.

78. Melin, B., Eclache, J.P., Geelen, G., Annat, G., Allevard, A.M., Jarsaillon, E., Zebidi, A., Legros, J.J., and Gharib, C., Plasma AVP, neurophysin, renin activity, and aldosterone during submaximal exercise performed until exhaustion in trained and untrained men, *Eur. J. Appl. Physiol.*, 44, 141, 1980.

79. Bass, D.E., Kleeman, C.R., Quinn, M., Henschel, A., and Hegnauer, A.H., Methods of acclimatization to heat in man, *Medicine*, 34, 323, 1955.

80. Dill, D.B., Hall, F.G., and Edwards, H.T., Changes in composition of sweat during acclimatization to heat, *Am. J. Physiol.*, 123, 412, 1932.

81. Allan, J.R. and Wilson, C.G., Influence of acclimatization on sweat sodium concentration, *J. Appl. Physiol.*, 30, 708, 1971.

82. Collins, K.J. and Weiner, J.S., Endocrinological aspects of exposure to high environmental temperatures, *Physiol. Rev.*, 48, 785, 1968.

83. Bonner, R.M., Harrison, M.H., Hall, C.J., and Edwards, R.J., Effect of heat acclimatization on intravascular responses to acute heat stress in man, *J. Appl. Physiol.*, 41, 708, 1976.

84. Davies, J.A., Harrison, M.H., Cochrane, L.A., Edwards, R.J., and Gibson, T.M., Effect of saline loading during heat acclimatization on adrenocortical hormone levels, *J. Appl. Physiol. Respir. Environ. Exercise Physiol.*, 50, 605, 1981.

85. Greenleaf, J.E., Brock, P.J., Keil, L.C., and Morse, J.T., Drinking and water balance during exercise and heat acclimation, *J. Appl. Physiol.*, 54, 414, 1983.

86. Greenleaf, J.E., Problem: thirst, drinking behavior, and involuntary dehydration, *Med. Sci. Sports Exercise*, 24, 645, 1992.

87. Wenger, C.B., Human heat acclimatization, in *Human Performance Physiology and Environmental Medicine at Terrestrial Extremes*, Pandolf, K.B., Sawka, M.N., and Gonzalez, R.R., Eds., Cooper Publishing Group, Carmel, IN, 1988, 153.

88. Schatz, W.J., Treatment based on physical principles followed by recovery in sodium chloride poisoning, *Med. Rec.*, 145, 487, 1937.

89. Gosslin, R.E., Hodge, H.E., Smith, R.P., and Gleason, M.N., *Clinical Toxicology of Commercial Products, Acute Poisoning*, Williams and Wilkins, Baltimore, 1976, 87.

90. Battarbee, H.D. and Meneely, G.R., The toxicity of salt, *CRC Crit. Rev. Toxicol.*, 5, 355, 1977.

91. di Sant'Agnese, P.A., Darling, R.C., Perera, G.A., and Shea, E., Abnormal electrolyte composition of sweat in cystic fibrosis of pancreas, *Pediatrics*, 12, 549, 1953.

92. Orenstein, D.M., Henke, K.G., Costill, D.L., Doershuk, C.F., Lemon, P.J., and Stern, R.C., Exercise and heat stress in cystic fibrosis patients, *Pediatr. Res.*, 17, 267, 1983.

93. Orenstein, D.M., Henke, K.G., and Green, C.G., Heat acclimation in cystic fibrosis, *J. Appl. Physiol. Respir. Environ. Exercise Physiol.*, 57, 408, 1984.
94. Frizzell, R.A., The molecular physiology of cystic fibrosis, *News Physiol. Sci.*, 8, 117, 1993.
95. Santana, L.F., Gomez, A.M., and Lederer, W.J., Ca^{2+} flux through promiscuous cardiac Na^+ channels: slip mode conductance, *Science,* 279, 1027, 1998.

Chapter 7

CHLORIDE IN
EXERCISE AND SPORT

Carmen R. Roman-Shriver
L. Mallory Boylan

CONTENTS

I. INTRODUCTION

Throughout history and different cultures, salt has taken on a variety of symbolic and religious meanings that have been perpetuated by verbal and artistic expressions, traditions, and rituals.[1] Today, salt has a lesser value in our society, and it is often implicated in a more negative context in our lives. Regardless of the perceived negative association, the components of salt (particularly sodium and chloride) are considered vital to life. Sodium and chloride are considered dietary essentials and are abundantly present in food sources. Until recently, the importance of chloride was often overshadowed by its close association with elements like sodium and hydrogen in compounds such as table salt and hydrochloric acid secretions in the stomach. Chloride gained status of importance when metabolic alkalosis and death were documented in infants receiving formulas deficient in the mineral.[2]

Chloride is the major negatively charged ion of the extracellular compartment. Approximately 88% of the total chloride in the body is found outside the cell, where along with sodium it passively maintains fluid, osmotic, and electrochemical balance. Shifts in chloride tend to be proportional to changes in sodium. Despite the small amounts contained within the intracellular compartment (12% of the total), chloride plays a major role in acid–base balance, at times shifting from the extracellular into the intracellular compartment in coordination with bicarbonate ions.[3] Changes in body chloride are usually inversely related to those of bicarbonate. Chloride also plays a role as a passive anion that can easily shift its cellular distribution to maintain electrochemical gradients vital in the conduction of nerve transmission and muscle contraction.[3] The approximate distribution of chloride in the body as reported by various sources is summarized in Table 1.[3–7]

II. PHYSIOLOGIC AND METABOLIC ROLES OF CHLORIDE

A. GASTRIC ACID SECRETION

Along with hydrogen ions, chloride is needed in the parietal cells of the gastric mucosa for the synthesis of hydrochloric acid (HCl). The passage of chloride from the plasma into the parietal cell, and ultimately into the lumen of the stomach, involves the exchange of several electrolytes including bicarbonate, sodium, and hydrogen. The flux of these electrolytes occurs in a series of cotransport mechanisms that facilitate the movement of chloride into the cell against concentration gradients.[8] Upon stimulation, strong acid is released into the lumen of the stomach, where it activates pepsinogen into pepsin. This activation is essential in the initia-

TABLE 1 Chloride Content in the Body

	meq/l[a]
Plasma/serum/interstitial fluid	96–111
Intracellular fluid	2–4
Muscle	6
Spinal fluid	124
Gastric juices	120–169
Intestinal juices	69–127
Fecal	traces–45
Glomerular filtrate	108
Urine	138[b]
Sweat	traces–110

[a] Ranges and values adapted from References 3 to 7.
[b] Highly variable with dietary intake.

tion of protein digestion. The low pH in the stomach contributed by HCl is also vital for the absorption of vitamin B_{12}, the conversion of ferric to ferrous iron, and the prevention of bacterial overgrowth. All these make important nutritional and functional contributions to the body under all physiologic conditions, including physical activity.

B. FLUID AND OSMOTIC BALANCE

Chloride shares with sodium a role in the maintenance of fluid and osmotic balance, which is vital for proper homeostatic adaptations during physical activity. As fluid losses occur during physical exertion, converging regulatory mechanisms are initiated to evade drastic hemoconcentration and to reestablish plasma fluid balance. Regulatory mechanisms for chloride are indirectly exerted by mechanisms involved in the control of sodium, including neural, hormonal, and renal mechanisms.[9] Bicarbonate is also involved in chloride balance as part of the acid–base equilibrium maintained in the body.[10]

C. ACID–BASE BALANCE

Chloride maintains the negative electrochemical environment as changes in bicarbonate become necessary to adjust for alterations in pH. The renal proximal tubules[10] and the red blood cells[5] are major sites for the anionic exchange which maintains acid–base balance. The type of renal exchange between bicarbonate and chloride is favored by the acid–base environment prevalent in the body. As the renal retention of bicarbonate increases, such as in metabolic alkalosis, the excretion of chloride is enhanced, with a concurrent decrease in plasma levels. Conversely, loss of bicarbonate by the kidneys results in a retention of chloride to maintain electrochemical balance of the negative ions. This is typical of metabolic acidosis.[10] Therefore, the causes for alterations in plasma chloride levels must be ascertained and corrected by treating the underlying problem rather than merely improving the chloride status. The erythrocytes play an important role in supporting the carbon dioxide–bicarbonate equilibrium. This chemical reaction is essential in disposing of the CO_2 produced during energy metabolism, including that generated during physical activity. As CO_2 generated by the tissue is transported in circulation, a portion is dissolved, while another portion reacts to form carbamino compounds, and yet another portion reacts with water to form carbonic acid and ultimately bicarbonate, in the presence of the enzyme carbonic anhydrase. It is this bicarbonate, as it is formed in the red blood cells, that diffuses out of the cells in exchange for chloride ions. This chloride shift results in a higher content of chloride in venous red blood cells than in the arterial red blood cells, particularly during exercise.[11] As bicarbonate is removed in the pulmonary capillary bed (by shifting back into carbonic acid, which then dissociates into CO_2 and water), the chloride shifts back into the plasma from the red blood cells.[11]

III. POTENTIAL CAUSES OF CHLORIDE DEFICIENCY

Hypochloremia or a below normal serum chloride level is associated with many diseases and conditions. In some cases it reflects a deficit of chloride in the body, but it may also be influenced by acid–base or fluid balance abnormalities. A reference range for serum chloride is 96 to 111 meq/l or mmol.[10] Table 2 presents some diseases or conditions under which hypochloremia has been noted.[5,10–13]

Dietary deficiency of chloride as a cause for hypochloremia is extremely rare, and a high loss of chloride from the body is only slightly more common as a cause of hypochloremia. In many cases the hypochloremia is present in conjunction with other electrolyte abnormalities, which makes pinpointing the exact role of hy-

**TABLE 2   Conditions Associated with
            Hypochloremia**

- Overhydration
- Congestive heart failure
- Syndrome of inappropriate antidiuretic hormone secretion
- Vomiting or gastric suctioning
- Chronic respiratory acidosis
- Salt-losing nephritis
- Addison's disease
- Severe burns or trauma
- Metabolic alkalosis
- Diuretic use
- Hypokalemia
- Diarrhea
- Excessive sweating
- Cystic fibrosis
- Dietary chloride deficiency

pochloremia in the symptomatology or pathology associated with the disease or condition very difficult.

A. EXCESS LOSS
1. Vomiting

Vomiting or removal of the gastric secretions by chronic gastric suctioning can lead to a high loss of chloride from the body. Gastric fluid contains 1.5 to 3 times more chloride than sodium due to the high content of hydrochloric acid in normal gastric secretions.[10,13] Any chronic condition resulting in frequent vomiting, such as congenital hypertrophic pyloric stenosis or self-induced vomiting in bulimia or purging anorexia nervosa, can result in hypokalemic, hypochloremic alkalosis.

Kassirer and Schwartz[12] studied the effect of repeated gastric drainage on five young healthy male volunteers to characterize the effects of depletion of hydrochloric acid on the body. The gastric aspirates were analyzed and subjects were refed the amount of sodium and potassium (as the chloride) in the aspirate the next day. Subjects developed alkalosis (elevation of blood pH and plasma bicarbonate); plasma and urine chloride values decreased; and as urinary potassium excretion rose, plasma potassium levels fell. The absence of chloride from the urine is a consistent finding in hypochloremia resulting from vomiting.[13] When chloride is lacking, bicarbonate is substituted for it in the glomerular filtrate. To conserve sodium and prevent its loss in the urine along with the bicarbonate, which would result in sodium depletion and contraction of extracellular fluid, the kidney resorbs the sodium without chloride, which accelerates sodium–cation exchange, resulting in alkalosis and potassium depletion.[14]

2. Diarrhea

Diarrhea can lead to dehydration and loss of sodium, chloride, potassium, and in some cases bicarbonate in the stool. Severe diarrhea generally causes metabolic acidosis if not managed adequately by intravenous or oral rehydration. Oral rehydration solutions for children usually contain 35 to 65 meq chloride per liter in addition to sodium (20 to 25 meq/l) and potassium (45 to 75 meq/l).

A few cases of an unusual form of diarrhea associated with metabolic alkalosis due to congenital chloridorrhea have been reported in children.[15] These individuals lose excessive quantities of chloride in their stool due to a defect in the electrogenic chloride pump in the ileum. This reversal of the chloride–bicarbonate pump also causes bicarbonate resorption as well as the chloride secretion, resulting in acidic stools. This disorder leads to hypovolemia, secondary aldosteronism, and severe hypokalemic alkalosis

3. Cystic Fibrosis and Sweat Loss

Cystic fibrosis is a hereditary disorder characterized by dysfunction of the exocrine glands.[16] One characteristic of the disorder is elevated levels of sodium and chloride in the sweat due to a chloride channel defect in the sweat glands. A sweat chloride content of 40 to 60 meq/l is suggestive of and a value greater than 60 meq/l is diagnostic for cystic fibrosis. Especially under conditions which increase sweating such as heat, exercise, or fever, individuals with cystic fibrosis are vulnerable to hyponatremia, hypochloremia, hypovolemia, aldosteronism, and possibly hypokalemic alkalosis. Hypochloremic, hypokalemic metabolic alkalosis has been reported in infants with cystic fibrosis during their first year.[17] Even in individuals who are not hyponatremic and do not have hypokalemic alkalosis, hyperreninemia and aldosteronism are common.[13]

4. Diuretic Use and Urinary Loss

Loop diuretics such as furosemide (Lasix®) inhibit chloride uptake at the loop of Henle, and thiazide diuretics inhibit chloride reuptake at the distal nephron.[10] As sodium is also lost, hypochloremia and contraction alkalosis may develop during diuretic usage. Urine chloride can vary widely depending on dietary intake.[10] Urine values of 0 to 10 meq/l are often found in metabolic alkalosis. Urinary excretions of sodium and chloride generally parallel each other, but excretion of large amounts of other cations (e.g., potassium, [K+], ammonium [NH_4^+], calcium [Ca^{++}], or hydrogen [H^+]) can induce a disproportionately high excretion of chloride. Elevated urine chloride excretion without elevated urine sodium is indicative of metabolic acidosis and the renal elimination of excessive acid as ammonium chloride. The urinary ion gap, which is

$$(U_{Na} + U_K) - U_{Cl}$$

can be used to determine if acidosis is from an alkali loss from a cause such as diarrhea versus renal tubular acidosis. Generally, in renal tubular acidosis the patient has hypokalemia, a urinary pH above 5.3, and the urinary ion gap is positive.

In diarrhea, excretion of urinary hydrogen ions usually causes the urine to be acidic, but hypokalemia can enhance ammonia synthesis by the proximal renal tubules.[10] Even with acidemia, excess urine ammonia accepts a hydrogen ion, producing ammonium, which can increase the urine pH in some cases of diarrhea. The ammonium ion in turn accepts chloride ions, promoting chloride excretion in the urine and causing a negative urine ion gap.

5. Bartter's Syndrome

Bartter's syndrome was first described in 1962 by Bartter and co-workers[18] and is characterized by hypochloremic, hypokalemic metabolic alkalosis, primary aldosteronism, hyperreninemia, and excessive production of prostaglandin E_2 by the kidney.[13,18] Hyperplasia and hypertrophy of the juxtaglomerular complex in the kidney and a chloride reabsorption defect in the loop of Henle that is prostaglandin independent are noted in individuals with Bartter's syndrome.[13,18,19] Subjects with Bartter's syndrome are found to have slow growth, tetany, polydipsia, anorexia, salt craving, weakness, fatigue, vomiting, abdominal pain, are normotensive, and generally are mentally retarded or have memory defects.[18,20]

B. PRIMARY CHLORIDE DEFICIENCY

Dietary chloride deficiency syndrome was identified by Grossman et al.[2] in infants fed either Neo-Mull-Soy or Cho-Free infant formulas which were deficient in chloride. This is the only report of humans developing chloride deficiency alone from dietary lack of chloride. The signs and symptoms reported in these infants are listed in Table 3. The plasma chloride levels in the 12 infants evaluated ranged from 61 to 93 meq/l, and the urine chloride values were 0 to 7 meq/l. Most of the subjects were fed the formulas for 3 to 5 months before loss of appetite, failure to thrive, and weakness were noted. Following supplementation with potassium or sodium chloride, laboratory values improved and signs and symptoms reverted toward normal. The authors concluded that chloride deficiency resulted in a decrease in extracellular volume with substitution of ions which are poorly reabsorbed for chloride. Thus, these infants developed negative hydrogen and potassium balances, which promoted the development of hypokalemic metabolic alkalosis.

C. SIGNS AND SYMPTOMS OF CHLORIDE DEFICIENCY

Chloride deficiency caused by lack of dietary chloride intake is exceedingly rare and is only referred to in the literature by Grossman and co-workers[2] in regard to infants fed chloride-deficient infant formulas. The signs and symptoms of chloride deficiency as described in these infants are presented in Table 3. Symptoms and signs are similar in individuals with primary chloride deficiency and those exhibiting chloride depletion due to conditions resulting in excessive chloride loss from the body.

TABLE 3   Signs and Symptoms of Chloride Deficiency[a]

- Anorexia
- Failure to thrive/weight loss
- Muscular weakness
- Hypokalemia
- Metabolic alkalosis
- Lethargy
- Erythrocyturia

[a] As reported by Grossman et al.[2] in infants fed chloride-deficient formula.

IV. POTENTIAL CAUSES OF HYPERCHLOREMIA

A. CONDITIONS ASSOCIATED WITH HYPERCHLOREMIA

Hyperchloremia is defined as a serum chloride value exceeding the normal range (96 to 111 meq/l or mmol/l).[10] Often, a high serum chloride value is associated with abnormalities of fluid and acid–base balance and may not be indicative of excessive levels of chloride in the body. Conditions associated with hyperchloremia are presented in Table 4.[3,5,8] There is currently some evidence that high dietary intakes of chloride may induce hypertension in some animal models as well as in some humans.[21–23] The hypertensive effect of chloride seemed more pronounced when the chloride was given in the form of sodium chloride.[24] Similarly, in some instances hypertension occurred only when sodium was given in the form of sodium chloride.[23]

Kaup et al.[22] studied the effects of feeding different types and levels of chloride salts on blood pressure in normal Sprague–Dawley rats. As compared to the rats fed a moderate chloride level in the diet, hypertension was found in all rats fed high levels of chloride in conjunction with sodium, potassium, or lysine with or without calcium and magnesium. Kidneys of the animals fed a high level of chloride were found to be hypertrophied, but creatinine clearance and fluid regulation were not altered. The kidneys were found to have elevated levels of potassium. The authors concluded that changes in renal function appeared to induce the high blood pressure in these rats.[21,25]

In Dahl salt-sensitive rats, rats given angiotensin II intraperitoneally,[24] and deoxycorticosterone acetate–salt-fed rats,[26,27] sodium and chloride together appear necessary to cause a rise in blood pressure. High dietary chloride does appear to

TABLE 4   Conditions Associated with Hyperchloremia

- Dehydration
- Brain stem injury
- Cardiac decompensation
- High reabsorption of chloride secondary to ureterointestinal anastomoses
- Diabetes insipidus
- Parenteral nutrition solutions containing a chloride:sodium ratio greater than one
- Renal conditions in which the kidneys cannot conserve bicarbonate, such as obstruction, pyelonephritis, and renal tubular acidosis
- Cushing's syndrome
- Eclampsia
- Multiple myeloma
- Metabolic acidosis
- Hyperventilation
- Gastrointestinal loss of bicarbonate such as in ileal obstruction or small intestine fistulas
- Use of medications including acetazolamide, corticosteroids, guanethidine, nonsteroidal anti-inflammatory drugs, androgens, estrogens, chlorothiazide, ammonium chloride, and methyldopa

cause a decrease in renal blood flow in placebo- and angiotensin-II-treated rats even though blood pressure was not elevated.[24] Whitescarver and co-workers[25] also reported no blood pressure alteration in Dahl or renin-dependent, one-kidney, one-clip Sprague–Dawley rats subjected to dietary chloride loading alone.

Kotchen and Kotchen[21] include calcium or potassium deficiency and a high simple carbohydrate intake as factors which may potentiate hypertension in those sensitive to sodium chloride. In rats give deoxycorticosterone and sodium chloride, Kurtz and Morris[27] reported hypercalciuria. More research is needed to elucidate the role of chloride in blood pressure regulation and renal functioning.

B. SIGNS AND SYMPTOMS

Signs and symptoms specific to hyperchloremia are difficult to distinguish from those caused by other factors related to the conditions which induced the hyperchloremia.[3,10] In conjunction with parallel shifts in sodium levels, lethargy, weakness, and deep breathing may occur. In cases where acidosis is present, signs and symptoms may include headache, drowsiness, tachypnea, bradycardia, hyperkalemia, stupor, coma, and convulsions, but it is not clear to what extent hyperchloremia contributes to these problem associated with acidosis. Sodium bicarbonate can be used to help manage cases of acute toxicity of chloride.

V. CHLORIDE IN EXERCISE AND SPORTS

A. ATHLETIC PERFORMANCE

Because chloride actions and activities in the body are tightly related to sodium and other electrolytes, most studies deal with the impact of multiple electrolytes on athletic performance or endurance or the effect of exercise on electrolyte content in the body. Alterations in total body electrolytes, although significant under some environmental conditions and strenuous physical activities, do not appear to significantly impact performance or endurance in well-trained, properly hydrated athletes. Training has been associated with an enhanced ionic regulation during intense exercise.[28] Powers et al.[29] found no significant performance benefits or significant differences in laboratory values, including plasma chloride, with the use of beverages supplemented with electrolytes among nine trained cyclists.

B. EFFECTS OF EXERCISE ON CHLORIDE STATUS

Studies suggest that profuse and prolonged sweating may result in significant losses of sodium and chloride. Despite these losses, the sweat remains hypotonic when compared to the blood. Electrolyte losses, including chloride, must be evaluated within the context of fluid losses and the implications of these imbalances. Even if losses of total body chloride are significant, a proportional loss of fluid results in an apparent normal concentration in plasma. Therefore, caution must be exercised in interpreting laboratory data after strenuous physical activity. Overall increases in blood osmolality may be more significant than the loss of total body water in regard to the development of thermoregulatory complications.[4,7,30]

Reports of changes in the serum chloride during exercise are variable in different studies, ranging from significant increases[31] to relatively constant concentrations.[32] It is important to note that even when significant increases are noted from pre- to postevent performance, the serum concentrations are within normal physiologic values. These findings imply a very tight control by the body in maintaining chloride balance. Some studies suggest that during distance running, the losses of chloride, as well as sodium, are highly correlated with the losses of fluid. Decreases in the total circulating plasma chloride value in a group of well-trained and experienced marathon runners paralleled the loss of plasma volume.[32,33] Costill et al.[31] noted a significant decrease in total circulating plasma chloride values after different levels of dehydration in men exercising in the heat. Again, while total chloride value was lower, the serum concentration was higher after dehydration. Muscle chloride content also remained unchanged with dehydration. These alterations in water and electrolytes were not found to cause significant changes in muscle cell membrane excitability. Therefore, replenishment of chloride after intense exercise should not exceed the usual amounts found in common foods and beverages. The use of salt replacements or beverages with high electrolyte content is not warranted because the plasma concentration of chloride is maintained within normal levels or is slightly increased even when very strenuous activities are performed.[32]

C. CHLORIDE NEEDS
1. Estimated Minimum Requirements
The Committee on the Recommended Dietary Allowances (RDAs) from the Food and Nutrition Board of the National Research Council[34] suggests 750 mg of chloride per day as a minimum requirement for healthy individuals. Additional allowances need to be included for losses associated with profuse and sustained sweating, but no health benefits have been linked to intakes higher than the minimum.

2. Dietary Sources
The major contributor of chloride in the diet is sodium chloride, from table salt and processed foods and to a lesser extent potassium chloride. Natural sources include foods (eggs, meats, seafoods) and water.[3]

D. SUPPLEMENTATION DURING EXERCISE AND SPORT
1. Nutritional/Sports Beverages
While some support exists for the use of athletic beverages containing additional electrolytes and salt tablets, their benefits have not been fully sup-

ported in the literature.[4,11,29,32,35,36] As a major negative ion, chloride plays an essential role in maintaining fluid, osmotic, and electrochemical balance during athletic performance and endurance, but no advantage has been associated with a large electrolyte supplementation of any type. Hyperosmolar solutions contributed by electrolyte replacement beverages can be counterproductive, as the usual problem during and following physical performance varies between hypertonic and isotonic dehydration.

Heat cramps may be present as a complication of heat exhaustion after profuse losses of electrolytes in sweat.[7] While heat cramps are a rare problem, prolonged exercise in a hot environment, if the individual is poorly acclimated and practices improper fluid replacement (lacking electrolytes), may result in painful muscle cramps. Treatment involves the use of an oral or parenteral solution of sodium chloride.[7]

2. Toxicity Risks

According to the Committee on the RDAs,[34] the only dietary link with excessive chloride levels in the blood is secondary to water-deficiency dehydration. Excessive intake of chloride salt has also been associated with hypertension, as previously discussed.

VI. SUMMARY/RECOMMENDATIONS

As the public interest in exercise and sports increases, a wider range of people with different physiologic and metabolic makeup will become involved in physical activities. As a result, the chances that individuals with genetic aberrations, chronic conditions, and eating disorders that are associated with electrolyte imbalances will become involved in physical activities also increase. Therefore, it is important to recognize rare and less conspicuous medical problems that can create altered balances in electrolytes, such as chloride.

REFERENCES

1. De Santo, N.G., Bisaccia, C., De Santo, R.M., De Santo, L.S., Petrelli, L., Gallo, L., Cirrillo, M., and Capasso, G., Salt: a sacred substance, *Kidney Int.,* 52, S111, 1997.
2. Grossman, H., Duggan, E., McCamman, S., Welchert, E., and Hellerstein, S., The dietary chloride deficiency syndrome, *Pediatrics,* 66, 366, 1980.
3. Groff, J.L., Gropper, S.S., and Hunt, S.M., *Advanced Nutrition and Human Metabolism,* West Publishing, St. Paul, MN, 1995, 346.
4. Wolinsky, I., *Nutrition in Exercise and Sport,* 3rd ed., CRC Press, Boca Raton, FL, 1998, chap. 11, 12.
5. Berdanier, C.D., Macrominerals, in *Advanced Nutrition: Micronutrients,* CRC Press, Boca Raton, FL, 1998, 157.
6. Harper, H.A., Rodwell, V.W., and Mayes, P.A., *Review of Physiological Chemistry,* 16th ed., Lange Medical Publications, Los Altos, CA.

7. Fike, S., Kanter, M., and Markley, E., Fluid and electrolyte requirements of exercise, in *Sports Nutrition,* 2nd ed., Benardot, D., Ed., The American Dietetic Association, Chicago, 1992, 38.

8. Berne, R.M. and Levy, R.N., *Physiology,* C.V. Mosby, St. Louis, 1983, 777.

9. Luft, F.C., Sodium, chloride and potassium, in *Present Knowledge in Nutrition,* Brown, M.L., Ed., International Life Sciences Institute, Washington, D.C., 1990, 233.

10. Traub, S.L., *Basic Skills in Interpreting Laboratory Data,* American Society of Health-System Pharmacists, Bethesda, MD, 1996, 104.

11. McArdle, W.D., Katch, F.I., and Katch, V.L., *Exercise Physiology: Energy, Nutrition and Human Performance,* Lea and Febiger, Philadelphia, 1991.

12. Kassirer, J.P. and Schwartz, W.B., The response of normal man to selective depletion of hydrochloric acid, *Am. J. Med.,* 40, 10, 1966.

13. Simpoulos, A.P. and Bartter, F.C., The metabolic consequences of chloride deficiency, *Nutr. Rev.,* 38, 201, 1980.

14. Schwartz, W.B., van Ypersele de Strihou, C., and Kassirer, J.P., Role of anions in metabolic alkalosis and potassium deficiency, *N. Engl. J. Med.,* 279, 630, 1968.

15. Turnberg, L.A., Abnormalities in intestinal electrolyte transport in congenital chloridorrhoea, *Gut,* 12, 544, 1971.

16. Hunt, M., Cystic fibrosis, in *Pediatric Nutrition in Chronic Diseases and Developmental Disorders,* Ekvall, S., Ed., Oxford University Press, New York, 1993, 387.

17. Beckerman, R.C. and Taussig, L.M., Hypoelectrolytemia and metabolic alkalosis in infants with cystic fibrosis, *Pediatrics,* 63, 580, 1979.

18. Bartter, F.C., Pronove, P., Gill, J.R., and MacCardle, R.C., Hyperplasia of the juxtaglomerular complex with hyperaldosteronism and hypokalemic alkalosis, *Am. J. Med.,* 33, 811, 1962.

19. Gill, J.R. and Bartter, F.C., Evidence for a prostaglandin-independent defect in chloride reabsorption in the loop of Henle as a proximal cause of Bartter's syndrome, *Am. J. Med.,* 65, 766, 1978.

20. Simpoulos, A.P. and Bartter, F.C., Growth characteristics and factors influencing growth in Bartter's syndrome, *J. Pediatr.,* 81, 56, 1972.

21. Kotchen, T.A. and Kotchen J.M., Dietary sodium and blood pressure: interactions with other nutrients, *Am. J. Clin. Nutr.,* 65, 706S, 1997.

22. Kaup, S.M., Greger, J.L., Marcus, M.S.K., and Lewis, N.M., Blood pressure, fluid compartments and utilization of chloride in rats fed various chloride diets, *J. Nutr.,* 121, 330, 1991.

23. Kurtz, T.W., Al-Bander, H.A., and Morris, R.C., "Salt-sensitive" essential hypertension in men, *N. Engl. J. Med.,* 317, 1043, 1987.

24. Passmore, J.C. and Jimenez, A.E., Effect of chloride on renal blood flow in angiotensin II induced hypertension, *Can. J. Physiol. Pharmacol.,* 69, 507, 1991.

25. Whitescarver, S.A., Holtzclaw, B.J., Downs, J.H., Ott, C.E., Sowers, J.R., and Kotchen, T.A., Effect of dietary chloride on salt-sensitive and renin-dependent hypertension, *Hypertension,* 8, 56, 1986.

26. Passmore, J.C., Whitescarver, S.A., Ott, C.E., and Kotchen, T.A., Importance of chloride for deoxycorticosterone acetate–salt hypertension in the rat, *Hypertension,* 7, 1115, 1985.

27. Kurtz, T.W. and Morris, R.C., Dietary chloride as a determinant of disordered calcium metabolism in salt-dependent hypertension, *Life Sci.,* 26, 921, 1985.

28. McKenna, M.J., Heigenhauser, G.J., McKelvie, R.S., MacDougall, J.D., and Jones, N.L., Sprint training enhances ionic regulation during intense exercise in men, *J. Physiol.,* 501, 687, 1997.

29. Powers, S.K., Lawler, J., Dodd, S., Tulley, R., Landry, G., and Wheeler, K., Fluid replacement drinks during high intensity exercise: effects on minimizing exercise-induced disturbance homeostasis, *Eur. J. Appl. Physiol.,* 60, 54, 1990.

30. Sawka, M.N., Francesconi, R.P., Young, A.J., and Pandolf, K.B., Influence of hydration level and body fluids on exercise performance in the heat, *J. Am. Med. Assoc.,* 252, 1165, 1984.

31. Costill, D.L., Cote, R., and Fink, W., Muscle, water and electrolytes following varied levels of dehydration in man, *J. Appl. Physiol.,* 40, 6, 1976.

32. Cohen, I. and Zimmerman, A.L., Changes in serum electrolyte levels during marathon running, *S. Afr. Med. J.,* 53, 449, 1978.

33. Riley, W.J., Pyke, F.S., Roberts, A.D., and England, J.F., The effect of long-distance running on some biochemical variables, *Clin. Chim. Acta,* 65, 83, 1975.

34. National Research Council, *Recommended Dietary Allowances,* 10th ed., National Academy Press, Washington, D.C., 1989.

35. Lamb, D.R. and Brodowicz, G.R., Optimal use of fluids of varying formulations to minimize exercise-induced disturbances in homeostasis, *Sports Med.,* 3, 247, 1986.

36. Wells, C.L., Schrader, T.A., Stern, J.R., and Krahenbuhl, G.S. Physiological response to a 20-mile run under three fluid replacement treatments, *Med. Sci. Sports Exercise,* 17, 364, 1985.

Chapter **8**

POTASSIUM IN EXERCISE AND SPORT

———————————————————————— Leo C. Senay, Jr.

CONTENTS

I. INTRODUCTION

Exercise, whether anaerobic or aerobic, demands the contraction of skeletal muscle. To bring about the interaction of actin and myosin necessary for tension development, calcium (Ca^{++}) must be released from the sarcoplasmic reticulum, and to do this, an action potential must be initiated on and within the sarcolemma.[1,2] To adequately respond to an action-potential-provoking stimulus, the sarcolemma must possess a proper resting membrane potential, and this, in turn, is largely determined by the distribution of potassium ions across the sarcolemma.[2] Such basic facts have stimulated exercise physiologists to investigate the effect of exercise on both the body content and distribution of potassium and to consider the physiologic consequences of perturbations in both. Before describing the dynamics of potassium in exercise, certain basic information related to potassium metabolism should be understood.

II. DISTRIBUTION OF POTASSIUM AMONG BODY FLUID COMPARTMENTS

The distribution of K^+ among the fluid compartments of humans has been addressed in numerous publications, and those referenced here are a representative rather than an exhaustive group.[3-5] In general, the total amount of K^+ in an adult human is between 3000 and 4000 meq.[4,5] Approximately 92% of the total K^+ is readily exchangeable. As noted elsewhere, "readily exchangeable" indicates that the ion under discussion rapidly equilibrates with the radioactive ion of the same species.[3] Of the total amount of K^+, 50 to 70 meq is in the extracellular fluid (plasma and interstitial fluid), with the remainder residing within cells.[3-5] Whereas the concentration of K^+ in extracellular fluids usually lies between 4 and 5 meq/l, the concentration within cells such as nerve and muscle is said to be 140 to 150 meq/l of cell water. This state of affairs is dependent upon the ability of the ionic pump resident within the cell membrane to move K^+ into while moving sodium (Na^+) out of the cell.[6] The membrane-resident carrier complex has been dubbed Na^+–K^+–ATPase. Using energy supplied by oxidative metabolism in the form of adenosine triphosphate (ATP), the membrane carrier moves three Na^+ out of the cell while moving two K^+ into the cell. In both instances, the movement of the ion is against a concentration gradient.[3] As a result of the activity of Na^+–K^+–ATPase, the water content of the cells is controlled, and, most importantly for excitable tissue, the cell membrane carries a charge much like a capacitor. The resting membrane potential is due to the distribution of K^+ across the cell membrane, with the inside of the membrane negative to the outside.[2,7] This state of affairs mainly exists because K^+ leaks out of the cell down its concentration gradient and the exiting K^+ separates from intracellular negative charges across the cell membrane.[7]

Skeletal muscle makes up approximately 40% of a person's body weight; if one considers the standard 70-kg man, then 28 kg of his body mass is skeletal muscle which is, in turn, 75% water and contains an approximate total of 3150 meq of potassium.[3] It would seem of interest to gather information as to how alterations in potassium distribution would affect muscle function.

In conclusion, the distribution of K^+ between extra- and intracellular compartments is the result of an active process. As will be seen below, a number of events can modify K^+ distribution.

III. CONTROL OF BODY POTASSIUM CONTENT

A. DIETARY INTAKE

The amount of potassium ingested in most diets in the U.S. ranges from 60 to 115 meq for each 1000 cal (1 kg cal or 4186 J) of dietary intake.[8] For example, the K^+ content of orange or grapefruit juice is 40 to 50 meq/l, while vegetables in particular are rich sources of K^+.[8] In fact, most dietary items are rich in potassium and sodium poor.[8]

1. Mechanisms Buffering a Rise in Blood Potassium

Most of the K^+ ingested is absorbed, although at a somewhat slower rate than Na^+.[9] Monitoring blood plasma K^+ concentrations after a meal has shown that plasma K^+ increases are insignificant in healthy subjects.[10] Simple calculations emphasize that buffering of absorbed K^+ has occurred. Suppose a 1000-cal meal with a K^+ content of 70 meq is ingested and all the K^+ has been absorbed. Assuming an extracellular volume of 14 l, and if no other process has interfered, the extracellular $[K^+]$ would rise some 5 meq/l. The absorbed K^+ is first taken up into the cells of the body and the excess is eventually eliminated via the kidney some 6 to 8 hr later.[7,10,11]

As noted above, in order for K^+ to enter most cells of the body, it must do so against a concentration gradient. This eliminates passive diffusion and leaves us with the activity of Na^+–K^+–ATPase. Before the absorption of the K^+ in the meal, the K^+ in the cells was in equilibrium with the K^+ outside the cells. Clearly, the uptake of K^+ by cells must involve an increase in the activity of the Na^+–K^+–ATPase. Several agents have been shown to so act. One of these is insulin. Separate from its effect on glucose movement across the cell membrane, insulin increases the activity of ATPase, thus increasing cell uptake of K^+.[12]

Blocking the activity of insulin with somatostatin has been shown to reduce K^+ uptake.[13] K^+ uptake has also been shown to be influenced by catecholamines.[14,15] Stimulation of the beta-2 receptors present in a variety of tissues has been shown to accelerate K^+ movement into cells. Beta blockers (propranolol) decrease cell uptake of K^+. Interestingly, alpha receptor blockade appears to assist in the lowering of extracellular K^+ by decreasing the rate of K^+ escape from the cell.[16] It appears that norepinephrine (alpha receptors) guards against hypokalemia, while epinephrine (beta receptors) assists in preventing hyperkalemia.[16] The applicability of these two catecholamine functions to events in exercise will be addressed below. If the action of insulin and catecholamines is prevented concomitantly with an increase in extracellular [K⁺], the uptake of K⁺ is not abolished because the rise in K⁺ concentration stimulates Na⁺–K⁺–ATPase.[17]

Na⁺–K⁺–ATPase is also stimulated by an increase in the concentration of intracellular [Na⁺] and, while not of great importance at rest, becomes significant with exercise.[18,19]

Two other events change the resting [K⁺] within the extracellular fluid. When changing from a supine to an upright position, the concentration of K⁺ in plasma increases.[20] An increase in the activity of postural muscles probably accounts for the increase. Lastly, the concentration of K⁺ in extracellular fluid undergoes a diurnal variation.[21] The kidney does not appear to be involved because excretion of K⁺ does not accompany the decrease in plasma K⁺. The investigators concluded that the decrease was due to cell uptake of K⁺.[21]

B. KIDNEY EXCRETION

The amount of K⁺ excreted in the urine of normal subjects depends upon the dietary intake. Given a K⁺-deficient diet such that the plasma [K⁺] is reduced from 4 to 3 meq/l, the excretion of K⁺ can be as low as 1% of that contained in the glomerular filtrate.[22] At the other extreme, a gradual increase in the daily K⁺ intake from 80 to 100 meq/day to 500 meq/day is met by a more rapid excretion in the urine.[23] Thus, through kidney adaptation, the ingestion of a K⁺ load that normally would be fatal is nullified. In real life, subjects on a mixed diet excrete 5 to 10% of the filtered K⁺.[24] If the 24-hr volume of glomerular filtrate is 180 l with a [K⁺] of 4 meq/l, the 24-hr urine volume would contain from 36 to 72 meq of K⁺. If the amount excreted matches the amount ingested, potassium balance is attained.

1. The Interrelationship of Sodium, Potassium, Aldosterone, and the Kidney

In the preceding paragraph, the amount of K⁺ excreted was expressed in relationship to the amount filtered. For the uninitiated to renal vocabulary, this would seem to imply that 5 to 10% of the filtered K⁺ zips right through the tubules and out through the collecting duct. This is not true. In a normal subject on a mixed diet, virtually all the K⁺ that is filtered is reabsorbed before the filtrate reaches the late distal tubule.[7,22] The K⁺ that appears in the urine had been added in the late distal tubule and the collecting duct through the activity of the principal cells.[25] These cells are responsible for secreting K⁺ into the duct lumen. Also present in the same portions of the kidney tubule are the intercalated cells which apparently reabsorb K⁺ when plasma [K⁺] decreases. How, then, is the secretion of K⁺ controlled in the distal tubule and collecting duct?

How much K^+ is excreted into the urine depends upon three items: (1) the concentration gradient for K^+ between the cells lining the tubular lumen and the lumen contents, (2) the rate at which fluid is flowing within the tubular lumen, and (3) the electrical potential that exists across the luminal-facing cell membrane.[22] The concentration gradient is important because the so-called secretion of K^+ in the distal tubule and collecting duct is mainly a passive process. K^+ is moved into the tubule cells via Na^+–K–ATPase resident in the basolateral membranes of the cell. K^+ then moves out of the cell through the apical portion of the cell membrane which faces the tubular lumen. Clearly, the K^+ gradient across the luminal cell wall is a function of the fluid flow rate within the tubule. The slower the flow, the greater the concentration of K^+ within the tubule, thus diminishing the K^+ concentration gradient from inside to outside the luminal-facing cell. Also assisting in maintaining the proper direction of K^+ movement into the tubular lumen is the electrical potential that exists across the cell membrane. The magnitude of this potential appears to depend upon the passive movement of Na^+ into the principal cells followed by chloride (Cl^-) movement. Na^+ is then moved out of the cell via the usual pump, and at the same time, K^+ is transported into the cell. Prevention of Na^+ movement into luminal cells reduces K^+ excretion, while an increase in Na^+ movement into these cells is accompanied by an increase in K^+ excretion.[7,22]

Superimposed upon these basic items that influence K^+ excretion are the activities of several entities, chief of which is aldosterone. The secretion of aldosterone mainly depends upon two factors: one is the $[K^+]$ in the blood and the other is the presence of angiotensin II.[25] For a full explanation of the production of angiotensin II, textbooks concerned with renal physiology should be consulted. Angiotensin II has a number of actions, and most of these are aimed at maintaining systemic blood pressure.[22] One of the ways to maintain or increase systemic blood pressure is to conserve or increase the amount of Na^+ in the extracellular space. Angiotensin II does so indirectly by stimulating the secretion of aldosterone. Aldosterone acts upon cytosolic receptors within the cells lining the connecting segment of the distal tubule and collecting duct which in turn produce proteins that act to increase Na^+ and K^+ channels in the apical cell membrane and to increase the number of Na^+–K^+–ATPase units.[22,26] The end result of aldosterone action would be to increase Na^+ reabsorption and K^+ excretion.

Finally, the acid–base status of arterial blood will also affect K^+ excretion.[24] Alkalosis increases K^+ excretion, while acidosis decreases K^+ excretion. As in most instances of dealing with acid–base balance, a variety of scenarios can be constructed wherein these general statements are not operative.

C. POTASSIUM IN SWEAT

Aerobic exercise, when conducted with appropriate intensity and duration, precipitates sweating. Stimulation of eccrine sweat glands by cholinergic sympathetic nerves stimulates the glands to secrete a fluid similar to that of blood plasma but lacking protein.[25,27] As the fluid flows to the skin surface through the sweat ducts, ions, particularly Na^+ and Cl^-, are reabsorbed.[25-28] The sweat that reaches the surface is a hypotonic fluid. The Na^+ content is considerably reduced, but the $[K^+]$ is equal to or slightly greater than that in blood plasma.[25,26] Aldosterone also acts on sweat glands to increase the reabsorption of Na^+.[25] However, K^+ secretion is not affected. The consequences of sweating in regard to body fluids have been addressed elsewhere.[3] The question as to whether or not sweat secretion is a significant avenue of K^+ loss can be answered with simple calculations. If an individual sweats 2 l/hr, this would be considered a high sweat rate. Allow the subject to sweat thus for 4 hr, and total K^+ loss would probably range between 32 and 48 meq. Clearly, this loss is readily replaced in the diet (see above).

IV. ROLE OF POTASSIUM IN MUSCLE FUNCTION

During rhythmic exercise, the blood level of K^+ increases.[29,30] In general, the level depends upon the intensity of the exercise.[31] The basis for this occurrence can be found in the processes leading to the activation of the contractile mechanism. As noted above, the distribution of K^+ across the sarcolemma is responsible for the resting membrane potential of some 70 to 90 mV, inside negative to the outside.[2] When nerve impulses arrive at motor end plates on each muscle fiber, the relative impermeability of the sarcolemma to Na^+ is lost, and because of the chemical and electrical gradient that exists for Na^+, Na^+ rapidly diffuses into the cell and is responsible for the rising phase of the action potential.[2] Once underway, the action potential sweeps to the end of the sarcolemma and into the T-tubules, leading to the release of Ca^{++} from the sarcoplasmic reticulum and the eventual joining of actin and myosin.[1] It is important to remember that the initiation of the action potential depends upon the presence of an adequate resting membrane potential.[7] If the resting membrane potential is reduced (hypopolarization) or increased (hyperpolarization) sufficiently, an action potential cannot be initiated. This can occur if the interstitial $[K^+]$ is increased or lowered, respectively.[7] For heuristic purposes, consider chronic renal failure: here, K^+ excretion is reduced, leading to an increased extracellular fluid concentration of K^+. Included in the symptoms of this disease are muscular weakness and abnormal conduction of the cardiac electrical impulse.[5,7]

With the initiation of the action potential, Na^+ conductance increases, and Na^+ rushes into the muscle fiber. As the Na^+ impermeability of the sarcolemma is reestablished, the K^+ conductance increases and K^+ moves out of the muscle fiber, thus balancing the electrical charges carried into the fiber by the Na^+ ions.[25] Therefore, in one stimulation of a muscle fiber, there is an increase in internal $[Na^+]$ and a decrease in internal $[K^+]$.[2,32] Taken as an isolated act, these events act to stimulate the activity of Na^+–K^+–ATPase and the distribution of K^+ and Na^+ across the sarcolemma will be reestablished. However, what happens when stimulation of skeletal muscle fibers is rapidly repetitive and involves a large number of fibers?

V. POTASSIUM DYNAMICS DURING EXERCISE

The concentration of K^+ that appears in the blood during rhythmic exercise is subject to several determining factors. The intensity of the exercise, size and contents of interstitial space, the osmotic movement of water out of the systemic circulation into active skeletal muscle, the amount of blood flowing through the stimulated muscle, the activity of Na^+–K^+–ATPase, inactive tissue uptake of K^+, the acid–base status of the contracting muscle, the duration of exercise, and the training status of the individual all play a role in determining the net increase in $[K^+]$ during exercise.[7,31,33–37]

Of this group, the main determinants of plasma $[K^+]$ appear to be exercise intensity, training status, Na^+–K^+–ATPase activity, and inactive tissue uptake of K^+.

A. EXERCISE INTENSITY

In terms of percent of maximum oxygen consumption ($\dot{V}O_2$max), exercise levels below 60% max cause a net increase in plasma $[K^+]$ in the range of 1 meq/l for the duration of the exercise. Below this exercise intensity, the increases in plasma $[K^+]$ are measured in fractions of a milliequivalent.[31,38–40] In studies incorporating progressive increases in exercise intensity, plasma $[K^+]$ also increased progressively.[41] When exercise intensities were set at 85, 90, 100, and 200% of $\dot{V}O_2$max in separate studies, the higher the intensity, the greater the increase in plasma $[K^+]$.[38,42–44] At 200% $\dot{V}O_2$max, the increase was above 4 meq/l. As noted by Lindinger, at the highest exercise intensities, the plasma $[K^+]$ rose progressively and peaked at exhaustion.[31]

In prolonged exercise, such as standard marathons, contestants usually suffer an increase in plasma $[K^+]$.[45] The increase over the course of the race is the net result of fluid deficits, muscular exercise, K^+ reabsorption by active and inactive tissue, and sweat gland activity. The increase seldom surpasses 1 meq/l.

B. NA^+–K^+–ATPASE

For the duration of a bout of rhythmic exercise, the number of muscle action potentials is proportional to the exercise. As noted above, with each action potential, Na^+ enters and K^+ leaves the muscle cell interior.[1,2] Clearly, if this situation continued without modification, the resting membrane potential would become more positive (for example, moving from −90 to −70 mV), and such hypopolarization could render the muscle cell membrane refractory to the initiation of an action potential by the end plate potential.[1,2,7,25] Thus, repetitive muscle contractions depend upon the ratio of intracellular to extracellular $[K^+]$. As noted above, the ionic movements that occur during and following the action potential stimulate the activity of Na^+–K^+–ATPase.[19] Upon onset of exercise, there is a lag of 6 to 8 sec before an increase in $[K^+]$ is detected in the blood; the delay is due to accumulation of K^+ within the muscle interstitial space.[31] During this interval, activity of Na^+–K^+–ATPase is stimulated and, in supramaximal exercise, reaches a maximum within 30 sec from onset of exercise.[46] The amount of K^+ diffusing into the venous blood must equal the total amount moving out of the sarcolemma minus lymph content and the amount returned to the cell interior by Na^+–K^+–ATPase. In the case of Na^+–K^+–ATPase, the amount of K^+ returned to the muscle cell is proportional to the number of Na^+–K^+–ATPase sites within the muscle cell membrane. In trained subjects, the maximal *in vivo* rate of uptake has been found to be 5.5 meq/kg wet weight per minute, while untrained subjects have a rate some 15 to 20% less (see below).[48] In human subjects performing leg extension exercise at 100% $\dot{V}O_2$max, each contraction was calculated to release 17 µeq of K^+ per kilogram of muscle wet weight, an amount considerably less than that calculated for Na^+–K^+–ATPase activity.[38,47] To exceed the transport capacity of Na^+–K^+–ATPase, the exercise intensity must be three to four times that recorded at 100% $\dot{V}O_2$max.[42,44] Clearly, this exercise is of short duration.

If the exercise intensity results in a K^+ release below that of the transport maximum for K^+, why does $[K^+]$ increase in the plasma? First, the K^+ diffuses away from the cell membrane where the Na^+–K^+–ATPase resides, and second, the activity of the carrier may not be maximally stimulated. In other words, not only is K^+ release proportional to the intensity of the exercise, but the activity of the Na^+–K^+–ATPase system may also be.

During sprint or endurance exercises, activation of the sympathetic nervous system results in increased circulating amounts of epinephrine and norepinephrine.[49] Epinephrine attaches to the beta-2 receptors on the muscle fiber and stimulates increased activity of Na^+–K^+–ATPase.[49] Evidence obtained from rat muscle experiments indicates that physiologic increases in epinephrine double the activity of Na^+–K^+–ATPase in resting muscle.[50]

The effectiveness of Na^+–K^+–ATPase activity during exercise is best appreciated by following the plasma $[K^+]$ after a bout of vigorous (>80% $\dot{V}O_2$max) exercise. Immediately upon exercise cessation, the plasma $[K^+]$ begins to fall in a rapid and exponential fashion, reaching control levels within 2 to 3 min.[41,44] Medbo and Sejersted noted that, regardless of the intensity of exercise and peak $[K^+]$, the half-times for all exponential curves were virtually the same, thus indicating that the higher the $[K^+]$ at end of exercise, the greater the Na^+–K^+–ATPase activation.[44] The exponential character of the curve also indicates that even as K^+ is being removed from the extracellular fluid, the activity of Na^+–K^+–ATPase is decreasing. However, the activity of Na^+–K^+–ATPase does not appear to immediately return to baseline activity, for the $[K^+]$ continues to fall below pre-exercise levels.[31,41,44] The resulting hypokalemia (levels of $[K^+]$ some 1 to 2 meq/l below control), if sustained, could have physiologic consequences.[31] However, $[K^+]$ does return to control levels usually within 15 min of end of exercise.[41,44] The reduction in activity of Na^+–K^+–ATPase involves the reduction in intracellular Na^+ and extracellular K^+ and a decrease in epinephrine secretion.

1. Possible Physiologic Consequences of Hyperkalemia and Hypokalemia

In exercising subjects, the plasma [K$^+$] can be doubled, and in postexercise, it can be reduced some 25 to 40% below normal levels.[31,41,44] Do such shifts cause cardiac events in persons who exercise? While laboratory evidence obtained from animal studies supports possible cardiac electrical problems, there is little hard evidence that either hyperkalemia or hypokalemia that occurs in exercising individuals is life-threatening.[31]

C. CHANGES IN POTASSIUM DYNAMICS DUE TO TRAINING

There are a number of changes that take place in skeletal muscle during training, and among them are changes in [K$^+$] dynamics.[37,51] Both sprint and endurance training lower the amount of K$^+$ appearing in the blood during the performance of a given submaximal absolute work load (see Lindinger[31] and McKenna et al.[52] for summary). When subjects are endurance trained and tested at the same absolute work load, venous [K$^+$] decreases some 25 to 50% depending upon the level of exercise.[48,54] The plasma [K$^+$] of sprint-trained subjects performing supermaximal exercise to fatigue did not differ from pretrained levels. However, the work output was increased, and when expressed as changes in [K$^+$] per unit of work, the trained subjects had a 10 to 15% decrease in venous K$^+$.[53] The same studies have also shown that the decrease in [K$^+$] depends to some degree on the experimental protocol used (i.e., intermittent maximal exercise, exercise to fatigue, etc.).[37,53]

Depending on the experimental format, the [K$^+$]work^{-1} generally decreases from 12 to 30% after sprint and endurance training. In one study based upon 8 weeks of knee extension training, K$^+$ release was lowered some 50%.[54]

The decrease in K$^+$ release coupled with a decrease in muscle blood flow at similar absolute work loads results in a decrease in venous and arterial [K$^+$] after training. Training also increases blood volume, thus increasing the total volume for K$^+$ distribution.[3,55] Depending on the exercise and the subject, there is a reduction in plasma volume during exercise because of the increase in osmotically effective substances within skeletal muscle.[55,56] This decrease contributes to but only partially accounts for the increase in plasma [K$^+$].

1. Training and Na$^+$–K$^+$–ATPase

The K$^+$ leaving active muscle fibers faces two prospects: the K$^+$ can diffuse away from the membrane into the interstitial space or the K$^+$ can be reabsorbed by the membrane-resident Na$^+$–K$^+$–ATPase. How much K$^+$ can be reabsorbed depends directly upon the number of carrier molecules within the muscle membrane and their maximal rates of Na$^+$ and K$^+$ transfer. Both sprint and endurance training increase the number of ATPase sites some 14 to 16%.[48,57,58] Interestingly, in a study on elderly men, those who had trained for 12 to 17 years had 30 to 40% more Na$^+$–K$^+$–ATPase sites than did nontrained control subjects.[59] Although Na$^+$–K$^+$–ATPase sites are increased after training, it is not clear that this is the cause of the decrease in plasma [K$^+$] per work load.[37]

One other possibility exists that could account for a reduction in K$^+$ appearance in the systemic circulation: an increased activation of Na$^+$–K$^+$–ATPase. Endurance training either reduced or did not change the catecholamine levels at a given work load, and at the same time, the plasma [K$^+$] was reduced.[37] Sprint training (see above) did lessen the increase in [K$^+$]/work load in supramaximal exercise, and there is suggestive evidence that there are subtle differences in the K$^+$ dynamics of sprint- and endurance-trained subjects.[44]

D. INACTIVE TISSUE UPTAKE OF K$^+$

Earlier, the buffering of dietary loads of K$^+$ was discussed, and it appears that inactive (noncontracting) tissue removes K$^+$ from the extracellular fluid.[7] There is no reason to believe that such uptake does not exist during and following exercise. Exercise-induced increases in extracellular K$^+$ and catecholamines certainly will serve to increase the activity of Na$^+$–K$^+$–ATPase regardless of the cell membrane in which it is situated (see above). However, the evidence to support this belief is sparse.[31] The role of erythrocytes in K$^+$ uptake in exercise has been the one exception to this statement. K$^+$ uptake by erythrocytes has been shown to occur in high-intensity exercise but not in moderate-intensity exercise.[46,60–62]

E. INFLUENCE OF [K$^+$] ON RESPIRATION AND CIRCULATION

Increased interstitial [K$^+$] has been related to increases in minute volume of respiration. The source for this response is said to be stimulation of certain C nerve fiber endings by the increase in [K$^+$] in active tissue.[63–66] Small increases in heart rate have also been related to C-fiber stimulation.[67] Finally, increased plasma [K$^+$] has been shown to play a role in the vasodilatation that accompanies muscle contraction.[68] Infusion of K$^+$ into the brachial artery raised brachial vein [K$^+$] 1 meq/l and was accompanied by a 25 to 30% decrease in forearm vascular resistance.[68] With forearm exercise, forearm vascular resistance fell 83%, although plasma [K$^+$] only increased 0.5 meq/l.[68] Recent experiments indicate that K$^+$-induced vasodilation involves the activation of ATP-sensitive K$^+$ channels in smooth muscle in resistance blood vessels.[69] When activated, these channels lead to hyperpolarization of the smooth muscle membrane and subsequent vasodilation.[69]

F. K$^+$ AND SKELETAL MUSCLE FATIGUE

As noted in the introduction and discussed in Section IV, both increases and decreases of interstitial [K$^+$] can cause the muscle cell membrane to become refractory to nervous stimulation. In those levels of exercise that cause continuous or marked acute alterations in internal and external [K^+], the resting membrane potential has been calculated as reaching levels of hypopolarization that could cause muscle to become nonresponsive.[38,44,70]

Using the concept of "strong ion differences" developed by Stewart,[71] Lindinger and Heigenhauser[72] have linked the exit of K^+ from the muscle cells to the increase in [H^+] as a factor in fatigue.

VI. POTASSIUM IN REPLACEMENT BEVERAGES

Fluid loss and fluid replacement during and after exercise have been thoroughly discussed elsewhere.[3] To be addressed is whether or not K^+ needs to be added to beverages used for fluid replacement after exercises in which fluid deficits occur. The manufacturers of such beverages seem to believe that it is necessary to add K^+ to their products. When reading the content labels of these fluids, one readily notices the different concentrations of K^+ included. The author's casual survey of the drinks available in local markets has found [K^+] ranging from 2.1 to 5.3 meq/l, a difference of 152%! Compared to the Na^+ contents of such beverages, there seems to be a bit of uncertainty as to just how much K^+ is needed. The intake of K^+ and its loss were discussed in Section III. Given reasonable training regimens even in warm weather, dietary replacement of K^+ seems likely. As noted elsewhere, this does not seem to be the case for Na^+.[3] Is K^+ at the concentrations listed above deleterious? Referring to Section III.B, the answer is no! Between cell uptake of K^+ and kidney excretion, the chance of such levels of intake causing cardiac arrhythmias is remote. In fact, the replacement of K^+ is not addressed in the latest position stand of the American College of Sports Medicine on exercise and fluid replacement.[73]

VII. SUMMARY AND CONCLUSIONS

Exercise requires that skeletal muscles contract.[1] They do so after electrical changes occur on the muscle cell membrane.[1,2] This event causes Na^+ to move into the muscle cell and K^+ to move out of the cell. Such movement stimulates the activity of cell-membrane-bound Na^+–K^+–ATPase, and reuptake of K^+ is accelerated.[31] However, in proportion to the exercise intensity, K^+ also diffuses out of muscle interstitial space into the blood, where it is distributed throughout the tissues of the body.[41–46] Both inactive tissue and skeletal muscle Na^+–K^+–ATPase are stimulated by a number of agents, chief of which are [K^+], catecholamines, insulin, and for active skeletal muscle intracellular Na^+.[7,14,19,42,58] Cessation of exercise often results in short-term hypokalemia.[31,44] However, neither the hyperkalemia nor hypokalemia of exercise has been shown to be physiologically harmful. For a given absolute work load, training reduces the amount of K^+ that escapes from skeletal muscle, and this is mainly due to an increase in the number and/or catecholamine sensitivity of Na^+–K^+–ATPase carriers in the muscle cell membrane.[14,19,37,57,58]

Increase in interstitial [K^+] has been implicated in local vasodilatation as well as increases in heart rate and minute volume of respiration.[64–69] Loss of K^+ from skeletal muscle has been implicated in fatigue.[38,70–72] Although K^+ dynamics in exercise are dramatic and K^+ is lost in sweat, a person on an adequate diet need not increase K^+ intake because K^+ intake usually exceeds K^+ loss.

REFERENCES

1. Huxley, A.F., Muscular contraction, *Annu. Rev. Physiol.*, 50, 1, 1988.
2. Katz, B., *Nerve, Muscle, and Synapse,* McGraw-Hill, New York, 1968.
3. Senay, L.C., Jr., Water and electrolytes during physical activity, in *Nutrition in Exercise and Sport,* Wolinsky, I., Ed., CRC Press, Boca Raton, FL, 1997, chap. 11.
4. Bland, J.H., Basic considerations of body water and electrolytes, in *Clinical Metabolism of Body Water and Electrolytes,* Bland, J.H., Ed., W.B. Saunders, Philadelphia, 1963, chap. 2.
5. Pitts, R.F., *Physiology of the Kidney and Body Fluids,* 3rd ed., Year Book Medical Publishers, Chicago, 1974, chap. 2, 15.
6. Sweadner, K.J. and Goldin, S.M., Active transport of sodium and potassium ions: mechanism, function, and regulation, *N. Engl. J. Med.*, 302, 777, 1980.
7. Rose, B.D., *Clinical Physiology of Acid–Base and Electrolyte Disorders,* McGraw-Hill, New York, 1989, chap. 7, 14, 28, 30.
8. Scientific tables, in *Documenta Geigy,* 6th ed., Diem, K., Ed., Geigy Pharmaceuticals, Ardsley, NY, 1962.
9. Gisolfi, C.V., Summers, R.W., and Schedl, H.P., Intestinal absorption of fluids during rest and exercise, in *Fluid Homeostasis During Exercise,* Gisolfi, C.V. and Lamb, D.R., Eds., Cooper, Carmel, IN, 1990, chap. 4.
10. Sterns, R.H., Cox, M., Feig, P.U., and Singer, I., Internal potassium balance and the control of the plasma potassium concentration, *Medicine,* 69, 339, 1981.
11. Brown, R.S., Extrarenal potassium homeostasis, *Kidney Int.,* 30, 116, 1986.
12. Clausen, T. and Flatman, J.A., Effect of insulin and epinephrine on Na^+–K^+–ATPase and glucose transport in soleus muscle, *Am. J. Physiol.,* 252, E492, 1987.
13. DeFronzo, R.A., Felig, P., Ferrannini, E., and Wahren, J., Effect of graded doses of insulin on splanchnic and peripheral potassium metabolism in man, *Am. J. Physiol.,* 238, 421, 1980.
14. D'Silva, J., The action of adrenaline on serum potassium, *J. Physiol.,* 86, 219, 1935.
15. De Fronzo, R.A., Bia, M., and Birkhead, G., Epinephrine and potassium homeostasis, *Kidney Int.,* 20, 83, 1981.
16. Williams, M.E., Gervino, E.V., Tosa, R.M., Landsber, L., Young, J.B., Silva, P., and Epstein, F.H., Catecholamine modulation of rapid potassium shifts during exercise, *N. Engl. J. Med.,* 312, 823, 1985.
17. De Fronzo, R.A., Lee, R., Jones, A., and Bia, M., Effect of insulinopenia and adrenal hormone deficiency on acute potassium tolerance, *Kidney Int.,* 17, 586, 1980.
18. Everts, M. and Clausen, T., Excitation-induced activation of the Na^+–K^+ pump in rat skeletal muscle, *Am. J. Physiol.,* 266, C925, 1994.
19. Clausen, T., Regulation of active Na^+–K^+ transport in skeletal muscle, *Physiol. Rev.,* 66, 542, 1986.
20. Sonkodi, S., Nicholls, M.G., Cumming, A.M., and Robertson, J.I., Effects of change in body posture on plasma and serum electrolytes in normal subjects and in primary aldosteronism, *Clin. Endocrinol.,* 14, 63, 1981.

21. Solomon, R., Weinberg, M.S., and Dubey, A., The diurnal rhythm of plasma potassium: relationship to diuretic therapy, *J. Cardiovasc. Pharm.*, 17, 854, 1991.
22. Valtin, H. and Shafer, J.A., *Renal Function*, 3rd ed., Little, Brown, Boston, 1995, chap. 7, 11.
23. Hayslett, J.P. and Binder, H.J., Mechanism of potassium adaptation, *Am. J. Physiol.*, 243, F103, 1982.
24. Pitts, R.F., *Physiology of the Kidney and Body Fluids*, 3rd ed., Year Book Medical Publishers, Chicago, 1974, chap. 7.
25. Guyton, A.C., *Textbook of Medical Physiology*, 8th ed., W.B. Saunders, Philadelphia, 1991, chap. 7, 29, 73.
26. Garg, L.C., Knepper, M.A., and Burg, M.B., Mineralocorticoid effects on Na–K–ATPase in individual nephron segments, *Am. J. Physiol.*, 240, F536, 1981.
27. Sato, K., The mechanism of eccrine sweat secretion, in *Perspectives in Exercise Science and Sports Medicine*, Vol. 6, Gisolfi, C., Lamb, D.L., and Nadel, E.R., Eds., Brown and Benchmark, Dubuque, IA, 1993, chap. 3.
28. Costill, D.L., Sweating: its composition and effects on body fluids, in *The Marathon: Physiological, Medical, Epidemiological, and Psychological Studies*, Vol. 301, Milvey, P., Ed., New York Academy of Sciences, New York, 1977, 160.
29. Laurell, H. and Pernow, B., Effect of exercise on plasma potassium in man, *Acta Physiol. Scand.*, 66, 241, 1966.
30. Kilburn, K.H., Muscular origin of elevated plasma potassium during exercise, *J. Appl. Physiol.*, 21, 675, 1966.
31. Lindinger, M.I., Potassium regulation during exercise and recovery in humans: implications for skeletal and cardiac muscle, *J. Mol. Cell. Cardiol.*, 26, 1011, 1995.
32. Hodgkin, A.L., The ionic basis of electrical activity in nerve and muscle, *Biol. Rev.*, 26, 339, 1951.
33. Vyskocil, F., Hnik, P., Vejsada, R.M., and Ujec, E., The measurement of K+e concentration changes in human muscles during volitional contractions, *Pflugers Arch.*, 399, 235, 1983.
34. Sjogaard, G., Adams, R.P., and Saltin, B., Water and ion shifts in skeletal muscle of humans with intense dynamic knee extension, *Am. J. Physiol.*, 248, R190, 1985.
35. Vollestad, N.K., Hallen, J., and Sejersted, O.M., Effect of exercise intensity on potassium balance in muscle and blood of man, *J. Physiol.*, 475, 359, 1994.
36. Hermansen, L. and Osnes, J., Blood and muscle pH after maximal exercise in man, *J. Appl. Physiol.*, 32, 304, 1972.
37. McKenna, M.J., Effects of training on potassium homeostasis during exercise, *J. Mol. Cardiol.*, 27, 241, 1995.
38. Sjogaard, G., Water and electrolyte fluxes during exercise and their relation to muscle fatigue, *Acta Physiol. Scand.*, 140 (Suppl. 583), 1, 1990.
39. Wilkerson, J.E., Horvath, S.M., Gutin, B., Molnar, S., and Diaz, F.J., Plasma electrolyte content and concentration during treadmill exercise in humans, *J. Appl. Physiol.*, 53, 1529, 1982.
40. Sessard, J., Vincent, M., Annat, G., and Bizollon, C.A., A kinetic study of plasma renin and aldosterone during changes of posture in man, *J. Clin. Endocrinol. Metab.*, 42, 20, 1976.
41. Marcos, E. and Ribas, J., Kinetics of plasma potassium concentrations during exhausting exercise in trained and untrained men, *Eur. J. Appl. Physiol.*, 71, 207, 1995.
42. Lindinger, M.I., Spriet, L.L., Hultman, E., Putman, T., McKelvie, R.S., Lands, L.C., Jones, N.L., and Heigenhauser, G.J.F., Plasma volume and ion regulation during exercise after low- and high-carbohydrate diets, *Am. J. Physiol.*, 266, R1896, 1994.
43. Vollestad, N.K., Hallen, J., and Sejersted, O.M., Effect of exercise intensity on potassium balance in muscle and blood of man, *J. Physiol.*, 475, 359, 1994.
44. Medbo, J.K. and Sejersted, O.M., Plasma potassium changes with high intensity exercise, *J. Physiol.*, 421, 105, 1990.
45. Rocker, K., Kirsch, K.A., Heyduck, B., and Altenkirch, H.-U., Influence of prolonged physical exercise on plasma volume, plasma proteins, electrolytes and fluid-regulating hormones, *Int. J. Sports Med.*, 10, 270, 1989.

46. Lindinger, M.I., Heigenhauser, G.J.F., McKelvie, R.S., and Jones, N.L., Blood ion regulation during repeated maximal exercise and recovery in humans, *Am. J. Physiol.,* 262, R126, 1992.

47. Kjeldsen, K., Muscle Na, K pump dysfunction may expose the heart to dangerous K levels during exercise, *Can. J. Sport Sci.,* 16, 33, 1991.

48. Green, H.J., Chin, E.R., Ball-Burnet, M., and Ranney, D., Increases in human skeletal muscle Na$^+$–K$^+$-ATPase concentration with short term training, *Am. J. Physiol.,* 264, C1538, 1993.

49. Williams, M.E., Gervino, E.V., Rosa, R.M., Landsberg, L., Young, J.B., Silva, P., and Epstein, F.H., Catecholamine modulation of rapid potassium shifts during exercise, *N. Engl. J. Med.,* 312, 823, 1985.

50. Clausen, R. and Flatman, J.A., The effect of catecholamines on Na–K transport and membrane potential in rat soleus muscle, *J. Physiol.,* 270, 383, 1977.

51. Rogers, M.A. and Evans, W.J., Changes in skeletal muscle with aging: effects of exercise training, in *Exercise and Sports Sciences Reviews,* Vol. 21, Holloszy, J.O., Ed., Williams and Wilkins, Baltimore, 1993, chap. 3.

52. McKenna, M.J., Harmer, A.R., Fraser, S.F., and Li, J.L., Effects of training on potassium, calcium, and hydrogen ion regulation in skeletal muscle and blood during exercise, *Acta Physiol. Scand.,* 156, 335, 1996.

53. McKenna, M.J., Heigenhauser, G.J., McKelvie, R.S., MacDougall, J.S., and Jones, N.L., Sprint training enhances ionic regulation during intense exercise in men, *J. Physiol.,* 501, 687, 1997.

54. Kiens, B. and Saltin, B., Endurance training of man decreases muscle potassium loss during exercise, *Acta Physiol. Scand.,* 126, P5, 1986.

55. Convertino, V., Blood volume: its adaptation to endurance training, *Med. Sci. Sports Exercise,* 23, 1338, 1991.

56. Senay, L.C., Jr. and Pivarnik, J.M., Fluid shifts during exercise, in *Exercise and Sport Sciences Reviews,* Vol. 13, Terjung, R.L., Ed., MacMillan, New York, 1985.

57. McKenna, M.J., Schmidt, T.H., Hargreaves, M., Cameron, L., Skinner, S.L., and Kjeldsen, K., Sprint training increases human skeletal muscle Na$^+$–K$^+$–ATPase concentration and improves potassium regulation, *J. Appl. Physiol.,* 75, 173, 1993.

58. Madsen, K., French, J., and Claussen, T., Effects of intensified endurance training on the concentration of Na, K–ATPase and Ca–ATPase in human skeletal muscle, *Acta Physiol. Scand.,* 150, 251, 1994.

59. Klitgaard, H. and Clausen, T., Increased total concentration of Na–K pumps in vastus lateralis muscle of old trained human subjects, *J. Appl. Physiol.,* 67, 2491, 1989.

60. McKelvie, R.S., Lindinger, M.I., Heigenhauser, G.J.F., and Jones, J.L., Contribution of erythrocytes to the control of electrolyte changes of exercise, *Can. J. Physiol. Pharmacol.,* 69, 984, 1991.

61. Vollestad, N., Hallen, J., and Sejersted, O.M., Effect of exercise intensity on potassium balance in muscle and blood of man, *J. Physiol.,* 475, 359, 1994.

62. Boning, D., Tibes, U., and Schweigart, U., Red cell hemoglobin, hydrogen ion and electrolyte concentrations during exercise in trained and untrained subjects, *Eur. J. Appl. Physiol.,* 25, 243, 1976.

63. Liu, C.T., Huggins, R.A., and Hoff, H.E., Mechanisms of intraarterial potassium induced cardiovascular and respiratory responses, *Am. J. Physiol.,* 217, 969, 1969.

64. Hnik, P., Kriz, N., Vyskocil, F., Smusko, V., Mejsnar, J., Ujec, E., and Holas, M., Work-induced potassium changes in muscle venous effluent blood measured by ion-specific electrodes, *Pflugers Arch.,* 338, 177, 1973.

65. Newstead, C.G., Donaldson, G.C., and Sneyd, J.R., Potassium as a respiratory signal in humans, *J. Appl. Physiol.,* 69, 1799, 1990.

66. Linton, R.A.F., Lim, M., Wolff, C.B., Wilmhurst, P., and Band, D.M., Arterial potassium measured continuously during exercise in man, *Clin. Sci.,* 67, 427, 1984.

67. Mitchell, J.H., Reardon, W.C., and McCloskey, D.I., Reflex effects on circulation and respiration from contracting skeletal muscle, *Am. J. Physiol.,* 233, H374, 1977.

68. Wilson, J.R., Kapoor, S.C., and Krishna, G.G., Contribution of potassium to exercise-induced vasodilation in humans, *J. Appl. Physiol.,* 77, 2552, 1994.

69. Bonitt, P.F., Smits, P., Williams, S.B., Ganz, P., and Creager, M.A., Activation of ATP-sensitive channels contributes to reactive hyperemia in humans, *Am. J. Physiol.,* 271, H1594, 1996.

70. Fitts, R.H., Cellular mechanisms of muscle fatigue, *Physiol. Rev.,* 74, 49, 1994.

71. Stewart, P.A., *How to Understand Acid–Base: A Quantitative Acid–Base Primer for Biology and Medicine,* Elsevier, New York, 1981.

72. Lindinger, M.I. and Heigenhauser, G.J.F., The roles of ion fluxes in skeletal muscle fatigue, *Can. J. Physiol. Pharmacol.,* 69, 246, 1991.

73. American College of Sports Medicine, Position stand on exercise and fluid replacement, *Med. Sci. Sports Exercise,* 28, i, 1996.

Chapter 9

FLUID AND ELECTROLYTE REPLACEMENT

Christopher T. Minson
John R. Halliwill

CONTENTS

I. INTRODUCTION

To fully understand the regulation of body fluid balance and the importance of fluid and electrolyte replacement during and after exercise, an understanding of the fluid compartments and forces that affect the movement between these compartments is necessary. Although a complete discussion of the physiological regulation is beyond the scope of this chapter and is covered in numerous textbooks,[1,2] a review of the basic concepts is warranted. For the purpose of this chapter, the review focuses on the factors that maintain fluid within the separate compartments of the body and how physiologic changes during heat stress and exercise alter these compartments. We hope this will allow the educated layman and undergraduate student to gain a general understanding of the principles that govern fluid homeostasis, providing the basic concepts necessary to decipher information from the volumes of research papers on fluid replacement.

To maintain homeostasis, the total amount of body fluid and solutes must be relatively constant. In order to maintain this constancy, despite extreme variances in fluid and solute intake and loss, there must be continuous exchange of fluid and solutes with the external environment and within the internal compartments of the body. As such, during rest and exercise, water is continuously exchanged between fluid compartments. The regulation and maintenance of fluid and electrolytes are so imperative that derangements of fluid and electrolyte balance (or maintenance) are among the most common medical disturbances of the athlete.[3] Indeed, even a small amount of dehydration (1% of body weight) can increase cardiovascular strain, as evidenced by a disproportionate elevation of heart rate and by a limited ability of the body to dissipate heat.[4] This alteration in physiological function will result in a greater rate of heat storage, leading to further detriments to exercise performance.

II. DISTRIBUTION OF FLUID WITHIN THE BODY

Water is the largest component of the body, representing approximately 50% of body weight for the adult female and 60% of body weight for the adult male. Total body fluid is distributed among two major compartments: the extracellular fluid compartment and the intracellular compartment (Figure 1). The extracellular fluid is comprised of all the fluid that is outside the cells and is further divided into the interstitial fluid and the noncellular part of the blood called the plasma (or intravascular fluid). A separate compartment of fluid called transcellular fluid also exists, composed of fluid in the synovial joints, intracellular spaces, peritoneal and pericardial spaces, and cerebrospinal fluid. The transcellular fluid only comprises about 2% of total body fluid and will not be specifically addressed in this chapter.

The water content of lean body mass is fairly constant at approximately 71 to 72 ml/100 g of tissue. Therefore, water normally comprises about 72% of lean body mass for both adult men and women.[5] Body fat, on the other hand, is

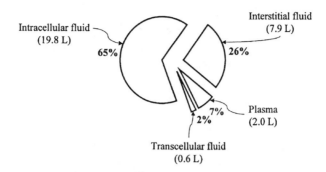

FIGURE 1 Distribution of total body water. Total body water can be divided into intracellular, transcellular, and interstitial fluids and plasma. Intracellular fluid accounts for two-thirds whereas extracellular fluid (transcellular, interstitial, and plasma) accounts for one-third of total body water.

relatively free of water at approximately 10 ml/100 g of tissue. Differences in total body water and the ratio of body water to body weight (expressed as milliliters per kilogram body weight) with gender, age, and degree of obesity can be explained almost entirely on the basis of alterations in percent body fat.[6] Figure 2 displays approximate values of body fluid contained in the various compartments for an "average" 55-kg female with 25% body fat and an "average" 70-kg male with 15% body fat.

Using the female as an example, we can estimate the volumes of the separate fluid compartments. Of the approximately 30 l of fluid in the female body, about 20 l is inside the cells to sustain cell integrity and function. The total extracellular fluid is approximately 10.3 l, of which 7.9 l is in the interstitial space and 2.4 l is plasma. The hematocrit (or packed red cell volume) is the percent of blood composed of red blood cells and will vary depending on gender and age, affecting the plasma volume in the blood. Typical hematocrit values are ~37% for young females and 42% for young males. Therefore, the total blood volume for this female is approximately 3.9 l. The blood is often considered its own compartment, as it is contained within the vascular system. In addition to the extracellular fluid (plasma) contained in the blood, water is also contained in the red blood cells (intracellular fluid).

Returning to the earlier example regarding body water loss and performance, we can estimate that the 1% of body weight loss during exercise sufficient to alter physiological function during exercise translates to only 0.55 l of water loss in the 55-kg female described above. During exercise in a warm environment, fluid loss due to sweating can easily exceed 1 l/hr in an average trained individual. In this case, the "average" female can lose this volume of fluid in 40 min or less.

This example highlights the importance of understanding proper hydration techniques prior to and during exercise to minimize the effects of hypohydration. As will be discussed later in this chapter, many contributing factors must be considered when determining appropriate hydration techniques.

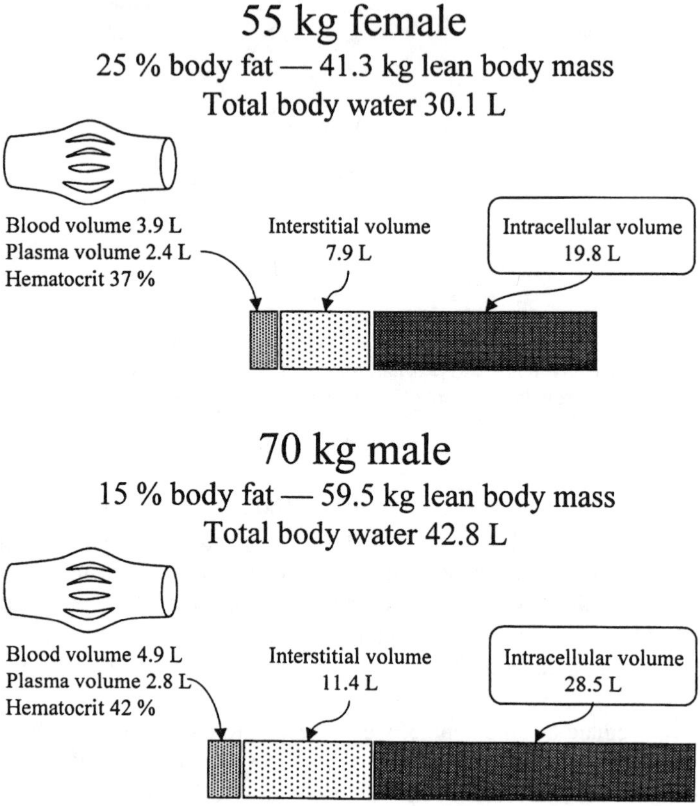

55 kg female
25 % body fat — 41.3 kg lean body mass
Total body water 30.1 L

Blood volume 3.9 L
Plasma volume 2.4 L
Hematocrit 37 %

Interstitial volume
7.9 L

Intracellular volume
19.8 L

70 kg male
15 % body fat — 59.5 kg lean body mass
Total body water 42.8 L

Blood volume 4.9 L
Plasma volume 2.8 L
Hematocrit 42 %

Interstitial volume
11.4 L

Intracellular volume
28.5 L

FIGURE 2 Fluid volumes for average female and male. Typical values for plasma, interstitial, and intracellular fluid volumes are represented for a 55-kg female and 70-kg male.

III. FLUID MOVEMENT BETWEEN COMPARTMENTS

As stated above, water is the primary component of plasma and is essential to maintain blood volume. If blood volume is compromised, circulatory function will be altered and performance diminished. In this context, it is important to note that the compartments are not static volumes, but represent a dynamic fluid exchange with numerous factors affecting turnover rates between compartments. As will be discussed, the fluid exchange helps to maintain circulatory function by transferring water from the intracellular fluid space to minimize the effects of fluid loss on blood volume. The type of exercise, body posture in which the exercise is performed, and other contributing factors such as the amount of heat stress will modify the volumes and turnover rates of water between the fluid compartments. This concept is central to understanding body fluid balance and how dehydration and fluid replacement before or during exercise will impact performance.

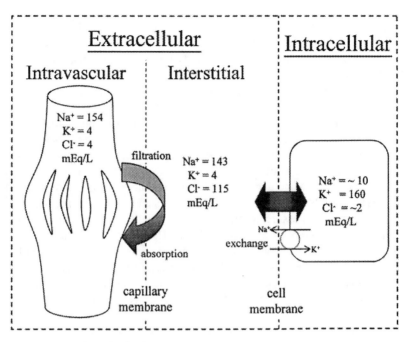

FIGURE 3 Major solutes by fluid compartment.

A. INTRAVASCULAR AND INTERSTITIAL COMPARTMENTS

The primary electrolytes are covered in Chapters 6 to 8. Therefore, they will only be covered briefly here, with particular attention to how fluid movement and balance are affected by changes in electrolyte concentration as a whole. The volume of each compartment is fixed by the total amount of solute within it. As displayed in Figure 3, the extracellular fluid contains large amounts of sodium and chloride ions and only small amounts of potassium. The similarity in composition between these two compartments is striking and is explained by the fact that these two compartments are separated by a semipermeable membrane, the capillary endothelium, which allows free diffusion of solutes of low molecular weight. Fluid exchange between the intravascular and interstitial space also occurs at the capillary, so that the ionic composition between the intravascular and interstitial spaces is similar. The main difference between plasma and interstitial fluid is in the concentration of proteins, which are largely excluded from the interstitial compartment by the capillary endothelium. These proteins have a net negative charge and tend to bind positively charged ions such as sodium and potassium, keeping these values slightly higher in the plasma. Hence, a difference of about 5% in the concentrations of diffusible ions exists between the two compartments. In other words, the concentration of cations is slightly greater in plasma than in the interstitial fluid, and the concentrations of diffusible anions are slightly smaller in plasma than in the interstitial fluid. Thus, the differences in composition between plasma and interstitial fluid can be accounted for almost entirely by the unequal distribution of proteins. The osmotic pressure caused by the plasma proteins is called the plasma oncotic pressure (also termed the colloid osmotic pressure). Some of these proteins "leak" through the capillary membrane, pulling water with them. This, in turn, is termed the tissue oncotic pressure (or tissue colloid osmotic pressure).

The movement of water between the two compartments is governed not solely by osmotic differences but by a balance of all pressures (i.e., of the oncotic and hydrostatic pressures in both compartments). The importance of these forces in determining fluid exchange across the capillary endothelium was first outlined by Ernest Starling in 1896, in what he termed the *milieu interieur*, or internal environment. A hydrostatic pressure results from the weight of water and is therefore proportional to the height of the water column. The steady size of the plasma and the interstitial compartments at rest is therefore determined by the balance of these Starling forces: the intercapillary hydrostatic pressure and the interstitial oncotic pressure favoring fluid movement out of the capillary, and plasma oncotic pressure and interstitial hydrostatic pressure favoring movement of fluid in the opposite direction.

The major force promoting filtration of fluid out of the capillary into the interstitium is the hydrostatic pressure within the capillaries. This pressure declines along the course of the capillary, and a small amount of protein leaks out of the capillaries. Although most of this protein is returned to the systemic circulation via the lymph channels, some remains, giving rise to a small interstitial oncotic pressure of approximately 5 mmHg, which also promotes filtration out of the capillary. These two forces are opposed by the plasma oncotic pressure and a small amount of pressure that is due to the fluid pressure within the interstitium. The balance of these forces is such that there is a net filtration of fluid out of the capillary along slightly more than one-half of the length of the capillary and a net reabsorption of fluid into the capillary as it approaches the venule. The slight excess of fluid that is filtered into the interstitium is returned to the systemic plasma by the lymph channels, so that in the steady state the volumes of the two compartments remain constant.

Vasoconstriction and vasodilation of the precapillary sphincters will greatly affect fluid movement through the capillary and are the primary mechanisms responsible for changes in fluid compartments during posture changes and the initiation of exercise. When these relax, the resulting increase in capillary hydrostatic pressure is sufficient to promote net filtration; when they constrict, hydrostatic pressure may be so low that only reabsorption of fluid into the capillary can occur.

The rate of fluid flow across the capillary endothelium is also a function not only of the Starling forces but also of the filtration coefficient, K_f. These relationships are expressed in the formula

$$q = K_f \left[(P_c - P_i) - (\pi_p - \pi_i) \right]$$

where q = the rate of fluid movement across the capillary wall, K_f = the filtration coefficient, P_c = the capillary hydrostatic pressure, P_i = the interstitial hydrostatic pressure, π_p = the plasma oncotic pressure, and π_i = the interstitial oncotic pressure.

The filtration coefficient is proportional to the total surface area of capillaries, as well as to capillary permeability per unit of surface area. Therefore, when precapillary sphincters contract, many capillaries are actually shut off from the arterial circulation. An example of this is during postural maneuvers such as standing. The constriction of the precapillary sphincters reduces total capillary surface area. Thus, activity of the precapillary sphincters governs fluid flow across the capillary endothelium by its effect on both the intracapillary hydrostatic pressure and the filtration coefficient. In general, the balance between vasodilation and vasoconstriction throughout the body is such that the net return of fluid to the plasma equals its net filtration from this compartment, and the return via the lymphatic circulation makes only a minor contribution at rest. During exercise, the pumping action of the muscles will greatly increase the amount of lymph flow, increasing the total amount of protein in the plasma.[7] This serves the purpose of increasing the plasma oncotic pressure, thereby minimizing fluid loss to the interstitium during exercise.

Mean arterial pressure is the primary factor modulating changes in capillary pressure. During maximal exercise, mean arterial pressure is typically increased about 10 to 20 mmHg, leading to an increase in capillary pressure.[8] Miles et al.[9] have shown that the magnitude of plasma volume loss was directly proportional to the increase in mean arterial pressure. Subjects performed either arm or leg cycle ergometry at a given oxygen consumption. Arm exercise resulted in a greater hemoconcentration than leg ergometry. Because the rise in mean arterial pressure was greater during arm ergometry, the investigators controlled the increase in mean arterial pressure in a second trial to match the mean arterial pressure during cycle exercise. The decreases in plasma volume were similar, indicating that pressure and not the type of exercise is most important in hydrostatic fluid shifts.

As pointed out earlier, the change in pre- and postcapillary resistance can greatly alter the amount of filtration, particularly if the vascular beds have relatively large surface areas and permeabilities. In addition, vasoactive hormones that are increased in response to exercise and heat stress (vasopressin, aldosterone, epinephrine, norepinephrine, etc.) alter the pre- and postcapillary sphincters, influencing fluid movement between the intravascular and extravascular spaces. Most of the effects of these hormones act through the influence of changes in blood pressure. However, evidence suggests that catecholamines and vasopressin may also inhibit the efflux of proteins from the vasculature by affecting factors which mediate capillary permeability.[10]

During rest, the interstitial hydrostatic pressure is near zero. During exercise, the interstitial hydrostatic pressure can greatly increase due to muscle contractions and may equal the capillary hydrostatic.[11] This increase in interstitial hydrostatic pressure will oppose the increase in capillary pressure, serving to limit the amount of filtration and maintain plasma volume and circulatory function.

The rate of albumin escape from the capillaries is increased during exercise and is also dependent upon the increase in blood pressure[12] and the exercise intensity.[13] However, during exercise, an increase in plasma oncotic pressure can occur despite the movement of proteins into the interstitial space, due in part to an increase in plasma protein concentration from the lymphatic circulation and the greater interstitial pressure resulting from fluid efflux from plasma.[7,14]

B. INTERSTITIAL AND INTRACELLULAR COMPARTMENTS

The intracellular compartment is separated from the interstitial fluid by the cell membrane, which, unlike the capillary endothelium, has selective permeabilities not only for proteins but also for certain other ions. In addition, the membranes of most cells have pumps that remove sodium from the cells and move potassium into them. The primary pump is the sodium–potassium ATPase pump. This process requires energy, and when the cells are deprived of energy, such as occurs during extreme cold or hypoxia, they gain sodium and chloride and with these solutes water. More than one-third of the metabolic energy of most cells is expended in transporting sodium, thereby maintaining cellular volume. Active pumping of sodium out of cells offsets the oncotic pressure of nondiffusible organic phosphates and proteins and thereby ordinarily prevents swelling and bursting of cells. Therefore, movement of water between the interstitial and intracellular compartments is dependent entirely on osmotic gradients.[15]

The intracellular and interstitial compartments have the greatest electrolyte concentration difference because they are separated by this cell membrane (Figure 3). Thus, the striking differences in composition between the intracellular and extracellular fluids result from the combined effects of selective permeabilities, metabolic pumps, and ion binding. It is important to note that the osmolality (a function of the number of discrete particles in solution) of the intracellular compartment is the same as the interstitial osmolality, mainly because sodium is actively removed from cells.

In 1947, Adolf[16] reported that water lost during dehydration during desert walks was not drawn equally from all body compartments. He reported that the volume lost from the plasma volume was disproportionately higher than the decrease in total body water. However, as pointed out by Senay,[17,18] comparing the ratio of body water losses to plasma volume losses is inappropriate because the plasma is approximately 90% water compared to 60% water for the remainder of the body. Therefore, more direct measurement of the changes in fluid compartments is necessary.

During dehydration, plasma osmolality increases in proportion to the decrease in body weight due to the loss of hypotonic sweat.[16,19] This increase in plasma osmolality will promote movement of water from the intracellular space to the interstitium and plasma. However, fluid loss from the various compartments is influenced by the type of dehydration and amount of solute loss. Nose and co-workers[20] have shown that sweat sodium concentration determines the volume of fluid mobilized from the intracellular fluid compartment. Subjects performed 2 hr of cycle exercise in the heat to induce dehydration followed by 1 hr of recovery without fluid intake. Plasma volume was reduced by 9.4% immediately following exercise, but this deficit was restored to –5.6% after 30 min of recovery and to –5.0% after 60 min of recovery. The partial restoration of plasma volume came at the expense of the interstitial and intracellular fluid spaces. The increase in plasma osmolality during dehydration was primarily a function of free water clearance, and the decrease in the intracellular compartment was closely related to the increased plasma osmolality. Therefore, water distribution from the intracellular to extracellular fluid compartments follows the osmotic gradient. Thus, a more dilute sweat, as observed with heat acclimation, allows a greater conservation of plasma volume during dehydration primarily due to the greater influx of water from the intracellular fluid compartment.

Kozlowski and Saltin[21] compared fluid loss from the various compartments during different dehydration procedures. Subjects performed three separate experimental trials designed to result in similar losses of total body water: (1) dehydration by exposure to 80°C for 2.5 hr, (2) dehydration by light exercise in a hot environment (38°C) for 3 hr, and (3) dehydration by heavy exercise in a cool environment (18°C) for 3 hr. The results from these experiments are shown in Figure 4. Plasma water loss accounted for 22.7% of total body water loss during heat stress alone, 11.4% during light exercise in the heat, and only 2.8% during heavy exercise. Almost all of the water lost during heavy exercise was from the intracellular space but only accounted for 50 to 60% in the two heated conditions. This may reflect the influence of a high skin blood flow on plasma volume loss. Harrison[22] proposed that fluid leaves the intravascular space as a result of increased perfusion of cutaneous capillaries. Skin blood flow is greatly elevated during passive heating[23] and cannot attain similar values during exercise in the heat[24] due to restraint of active vasodilation.[25] Therefore, the greater loss of plasma volume during passive heating or exercise in the heat may reflect primarily transient shifts between the compartments due to the high skin blood flow.

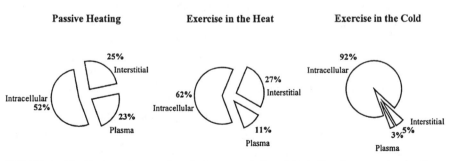

FIGURE 4 Distribution of water loss that occurs during dehydration from passive heating, exercise in the heat, and exercise in the cold. (Data adapted from Kozlowski and Saltin.[21])

IV. MECHANISMS OF FLUID SHIFTS AND LOSS

Body posture, type of exercise, or intensity can alter plasma volume and solute concentration even before any body fluid loss from sweating or ventilation has occurred. Upon assumption of the upright posture, a translocation of fluid to the dependent veins of the lower legs causes an increase in tissue hydrostatic pressure. After prolonged standing, this can cause a 10 to 12% reduction in plasma volume.[26] In order to maintain sufficient blood pressure and cerebral perfusion, precapillary vasoconstriction occurs, which, as described previously, normally favors net absorption from the interstitium across the capillary. However, during standing, either no or little venoconstriction occurs, so there is a rapid initial loss of fluid into the interstitium. During prolonged standing, the venous valves are forced open, causing a greater backpressure on the capillary to be exerted from the resulting hydrostatic column of blood. This shift in capillary pressure in the dependent limbs immediately causes a decrease in plasma volume, which continues until a new equilibrium between the Starling forces is obtained. The majority of the fluid shifts take approximately 30 to 40 min. However, it may take more than 60 minutes to reach a new equilibrium or "steady state."[26]

A. TREADMILL RUNNING

These posture-induced changes in plasma volume are important when evaluating studies on changes in fluid compartments during exercise and are often overlooked. For example, if a pre-exercise blood sample is obtained in a supine or seated posture, the exercise-induced hemoconcentration during treadmill running from rest to exercise is similar in magnitude to that expected for the posture change alone.[27] The lack of control for these posture changes has led to many controversial findings in the literature regarding a potential hemoconcentration during treadmill running. These considerations have been reviewed by Harrison[27] and Harrison et al.[28] and are discussed here only briefly. When the hemoconcentration associated with posture change is accounted for during treadmill exercise by having the subject stand for 20 to 30 min, no hemoconcentration is observed. Most investigators have shown that this observation is not affected by exercise intensity.[14,29,30] Senay and colleagues[29] found no relationship between exercise intensity ($\dot{V}O_2$) and vascular volume fluid shifts in subjects while walking on a treadmill at 6 km/hr at grades that increased 3% every 3 min. Furthermore, returning to the initial posture will reverse the hemoconcentration and a rapid hemodilution occurs, due in part to the increased osmolality of the plasma.

Other considerations that must be addressed when evaluating studies of treadmill exercise and plasma volume include the environment in which the exercise is performed and the level of hydration prior to exercise. For example, when treadmill exercise is combined with heat stress, hemodilution is commonly observed.[14,31,32] Sawka and colleagues[31] measured plasma volume changes in 12 male and female subjects under euhydrated (normally hydrated) and hypohydrated (5% decline from baseline body weight) conditions during thermoneutral rest and light-intensity treadmill exercise in a hot environment. The subjects walked at approximately 30% of $\dot{V}O_2$max for two 25-min periods separated by a 10-min rest period. The authors measured plasma volume during standing rest and at minute 20 of each exercise bout. During rest, hypohydration elicited a 5% decrease in plasma volume. During exercise, plasma volume decreased an additional 4% from rest in the hypohydrated condition; however, plasma volume increased 4% in the euhydrated condition. They concluded that hydration level alters exercise-induced vascular fluid shifts in the heat. The authors speculated that this hemodilution during treadmill running in the euhydrated state is oncotically mediated, due to the muscle action increasing lymph turnover, thereby increasing protein in the intra-vascular space. This increase in plasma protein could exert an oncotic pressure and cause a proportionate (as discussed above) increase in fluid movement from the interstitium to the plasma.

It is important to note that a 5% level of hypohydration results in a 38% reduction in interstitial fluid,[33] most likely resulting in a reduction in the amount of fluid entering the lymph duct for a given amount of protein. This smaller volume of more viscous lymph could result in reduced flow during exercise for a given amount of skeletal muscle pump activity. This would effectively return less protein to the circulatory system and further have the effect of increasing vascular fluid efflux by the increased interstitial colloid oncotic pressure.

B. CYCLE EXERCISE

Evidence suggests that cycle exercise, on the other hand, tends to result in hemoconcentration, although this response is heavily dependent on the intensity of exercise. This hemoconcentration can be divided into two distinct phases. The initial hemoconcentration will occur during the first 5 to 10 min of exercise, most likely mediated via an increase in hydrostatic capillary filtration. Miles et al.[9] reported that the amount of plasma volume reduction was related to the increase in mean arterial pressure during cycle exercise with the arms or legs. The increase in mean arterial pressure probably reflected capillary hydrostatic pressures, favoring net filtration into the interstitium. This initial hemoconcentration has been reported despite an increase in plasma protein gain.[34] The secondary hemoconcentration occurs more slowly, most likely due to a gradual reduction in plasma protein loss related to an increase in skin blood flow.[28]

Exercise posture will also affect the plasma volume shifts during cycling exercise. Diaz and colleagues[35] measured plasma volume shifts during rest and exercise in the upright, low-sit, and supine posture in a hot environment. They found that the reduction in plasma volume from rest to exercise was 11% in the supine posture, 7.1% in the low-sit posture, and 2.7% in the upright posture. Interestingly, these authors also reported that some fluid was being lost from the red blood cells (intracellular compartment).

C. SWEAT FLUID LOSS

The increase in whole body metabolism during endurance exercise can exceed resting metabolism by 15-fold. However, approximately 80% of the increase in metabolism with exercise is converted to heat and needs to be dissipated to minimize an increase in core temperature. Heat can also be gained from the environment by radiation and conduction. Depending on environmental conditions, these will increase the rate of heat storage, further driving the increase in core temperature and further increasing the amount of heat that must be lost in the form of sweat to minimize heat gain.

The eccrine glands secrete sweat onto the surface of the skin, which allows for evaporative cooling when the water is converted from a liquid to water vapor. The amount of heat loss is defined by the latent heat of evaporation for a given amount of water (the phase change from liquid to water vapor), requiring 2.45 J/kg. Therefore, the amount of evaporative cooling is determined by sweat rate and the environmental conditions that affect evaporation, such as temperature, relative humidity, and air movement. It is important to point out that in very humid conditions, sweat will accumulate on the skin, forming large droplets that will fall from the surface of the skin and not evaporate. This will not cool the skin and, therefore, will not cool the blood perfusing the skin and will not aid in minimizing the rate of heat gain.

During exercise, particularly in a hot environment, the increase in sweating that accompanies the rise in core temperature is the primary source of fluid and electrolyte loss in humans. The concentration of sodium in sweat is approximately 40 to 60 meq/l and chloride is approximately 30 to 45 meq/l. At a sweat rate of 1 l/hr, the sodium loss is approximately 2% of total body sodium per hour. Although this does not represent a significant loss of whole body sodium, many endurance events last over 3 to 4 hr, during which this rate of sodium loss can represent a significant threat to the maintenance of fluid and electrolyte homeostasis. The concentration of electrolytes in sweat varies widely among individuals, according to different rates of sweating and according to the level of heat acclimation and physical fitness.[36] Sodium concentration in sweat decreases during the process of heat acclimation.[37] This will greatly impact the total amount of sodium loss and therefore the movement of water from the fluid compartments as described above. For more information on the effects of electrolyte loss and the impact on homeostasis and performance, refer to Chapters 5 to 8.

The increase in thermoregulatory sweating closely parallels the increase in body temperature.[38–40] Therefore, for a given rise in core temperature, sweat rate will increase to minimize additional heat gain via evaporative cooling. However, other factors will also influence sweat rate. For instance, Nadel et al.[39] independently varied core temperature, mean skin temperature, and local skin temperature while measuring sweat rate during rest and after exercise. They concluded that (1) at a constant skin temperature, sweat rate was proportional to core temperature; (2) at a constant core temperature, sweat rate was proportional to mean skin temperature; and (3) local skin temperature acts as a multiplier to the central control signal to determine local sweat rate.

Sweat rate is a function of the combined internal (related to the exercise intensity) and external (ambient temperature and humidity) thermal loads.[41] This fluid loss from sweating can be quite significant. In fact, values in excess of 30 g/min (1.8 l/hr) have been reported during exercise in the heat.[42]

Although the relative concentrations of electrolytes in the sweat are dependent on numerous factors, including adaptation to heat, sweat is ordinarily hypotonic relative to plasma[43] due to active reabsorption within the sweat gland. Profuse sweating will therefore result in a decline in fluid volume but an increase in plasma osmolality. The resulting hypohydration will result in an increased core temperature during exercise in the heat. Because it has been shown that hypohydration does not influence the rate of aerobic or anaerobic metabolism during exercise,[44,45] this increased heat storage results from hypohydration-mediated or osmolality-mediated decreases in heat loss mechanisms.[46] However, the physiological mechanism responsible for the reduced sweating is still poorly understood. Attempting to independently manipulate volume and osmolality has been one approach to investigate these factors. Sawka et al.[32] have shown that plasma hyperosmolality is strongly related to reduced sweating rates during hypohydration. It has also been reported by Harrison and co-workers[28] that plasma hyperosmolality will elevate core temperature responses during exercise and heat stress, despite the maintenance of euhydration. Fortney et al.[47] showed that the esophageal temperature threshold for cutaneous vasodilation increased after isotonic hypovolemia induced by diuretics. Sweat gland sensitivity was also reduced, as evident by the attenuated increase in sweat rate for a given increase in core temperature. It appears that hypertonicity increases the core temperature threshold for sweating.[48] In short, hypohydration and hypertonicity have been shown to either reduce sweat rate and skin blood flow or to result in an elevation in core temperature at a given level of exercise and heat stress. In addition to the effects of hypovolemia on temperature regulation, hypovolemia will also alter the hemodynamic responses during exercise, as discussed below.

D. KIDNEY FLUID LOSS AND CONSERVATION

The role of the kidney in fluid balance during exercise and recovery has been expertly reviewed by Zambraski.[49,50] The kidney serves to filter large amounts of plasma and to produce urine for the excretion of the by-products of metabolism. Approximately 1 ml of urine per minute will be produced at rest, containing approximately 140 meq/l of sodium and 40 meq/l of potassium. During exercise, the renal response is to decrease the excretion of water and sodium. During moderate to heavy exercise in athletes, the urine production by the kidneys may be reduced up to 60%.[50] In addition, sodium excretion may decline with moderate exercise, most likely via increased tubular sodium absorption.[50]

However, Zambraski makes the point that in the context of whole-body water loss and sodium conservation during prolonged exercise, the potential conservation of fluid and sodium from the kidney is negligible. He states that the major role and significance, especially during exercise, transcend a simple reduction of water and sodium excretion or a redistribution of renal blood flow. The actual amount of water retained due to decreased urinary excretion is relatively small, ranging from 0.2 to 0.75 ml/min. At the high end of this range, only 135 ml of water would be conserved during exercise lasting 3 hr. Consequently, this water loss is almost negligible in light of the volumes of water loss from sweating. The amount of water that can be conserved due to a reduction in urinary flow rate is quite small.[49]

These calculations demonstrate the relatively minor role of the kidney in fluid and sodium regulation during exercise. The true importance of this organ with regard to fluid balance is observed during recovery from exercise and long-term fluid and pressure regulation.[50] This last point stems from the observation that the kidneys have the primary responsibility for controlling total body sodium. Therefore, for restoration of fluid in any one body fluid compartment to occur without a further decrease from another compartment, total body water and sodium must increase. These changes in fluid and sodium can only result from a change in the renal regulation of sodium balance.

As multiday endurance events become more popular, studies investigating the role of the kidneys in long-term regulation of electrolyte and fluid balance under extreme conditions will be necessary. Races such as the Raid Gauloises and the ECO-challenge require athletes to compete up to 20 hr a day for 4 to 5 days, often without adequate hydration. Little information is available regarding how the combined effects of severe dehydration, continuous exercise, and lack of adequate dietary sodium intake over an expanded period of time may be impacted by kidney function.

E. RESPIRATORY WATER LOSS

During ventilation in an exercising person, air is humidified as it enters the lungs. By the time the person exhales, the expired air is nearly 100% saturated with water vapor, thereby contributing to total body water loss. The amount of water loss with ventilation will vary depending on the level of exercise intensity (i.e., respiratory water loss rises with increasing metabolic rate, driving ventilation). Although small compared to sweating, significant water loss from breathing alone can occur during heavy, prolonged exercise. Mitchell et al.[51] estimated these respiratory water losses to be approximately 120 ml/hr. This water loss, however, is also dependent on the water vapor content of the *inspired* air. Because the amount of water in the air is dependent on temperature, cold air will contain relatively small amounts of water. When the cold air is inhaled, the air is warmed by the body and the relative humidity is very low. This requires significant amounts of water from the lungs to saturate the air, contributing to the amount of fluid loss.

V. CARDIOVASCULAR CONSEQUENCES OF HYPOHYDRATION

Hypohydration compromises the ability of the cardiovascular system to respond to both exercise and heat stress, and the effect of hypohydration is greater for exercise in a hot environment. During hypohydration, reduced blood volume leads to a diminished venous return of blood to the heart (i.e., reduced preload). Due to the Frank–Starling mechanism, stroke volume will be less for a given contractile state of the heart. Reduced venous return and stroke volume may not be manifest in a hypohydrated individual resting in the supine position, and due to the exquisite regulation by the arterial and cardiopulmonary baroreflexes, the *initial* blood pressure and heart rate responses to upright posture and exercise may even appear normal. However, with the addition of either exercise or heat stress, reductions in blood volume become readily apparent. Vasodilation in skeletal muscle vascular beds (exercise) or cutaneous vascular beds (heat stress) further decreases venous return to the heart and cardiac preload. Under these conditions, baroreflex-mediated increases in heart rate, contractility, and vasoconstriction are necessary to maintain arterial pressure at appropriate levels. Thus, in order to maintain adequate blood flow to critical regions (e.g., the brain and heart), blood flow to other regions may be compromised during exercise or heat stress.

Let us consider in more detail the cardiovascular responses to dynamic exercise such as running and cycling. During exercise in a cool environment, the normal response includes vasodilation of the exercising muscle and reflex vasoconstriction of the vascular beds in inactive skeletal muscle, the kidney, and the visceral organs. For moderate levels of exercise, this is adequate to prevent arterial pressure from falling with the drop in vascular resistance in the active muscle. The vasoconstriction also serves the purpose of shunting a high percentage of the cardiac output to the exercising muscle. However, during heavy exercise with large muscle mass (e.g., when both arm and leg exercise are performed simultaneously), some vasoconstriction may even occur in the active muscle vascular beds in order to maintain appropriate levels of arterial pressure.[52] Hypohydration adversely affects these reflex adjustments by reducing stroke volume. In an effort to compensate for reduced stroke volume and maintain cardiac output and muscle blood flow, the heart rate response becomes exaggerated.[44] For example, Saltin[53] studied exercise responses in ten individuals before and after dehydration that resulted in body weight loss of ~4%. While oxygen consumption during submaximal exercise (45% $\dot{V}O_2$peak) was unaffected by dehydration, heart rate was higher after dehydration by ~13 beats per minute. It is likely that this degree of dehydration also results in greater vasoconstriction and may lead to decreased blood flow to the active muscle.

Cardiovascular responses to heat stress parallel those to dynamic exercise. During heat stress, the normal response includes vasodilation of the skin in conjunction with sweating and reflex vasoconstriction of the renal and splanchnic circulations. The rise in skin blood serves to transfer heat from the core to the skin, where evaporative cooling can dissipate heat to the atmosphere. As with exercise, blood flow is shunted away from several vascular beds by vasoconstriction so that arterial pressure may be maintained despite the drop in cutaneous vascular resistance. In addition, splanchnic vasoconstriction will permit the translocation of blood from this compliant circulation to the skin.[23] Recent studies have demonstrated that during a challenge to arterial pressure similar to standing, the baroreflexes will decrease skin vasodilation and sweating in order to defend arterial pressure at an appropriate level.[25] Hypohydration adversely affects these adjustments during heating by reducing venous return and stroke volume. As a result, when hypohydration is superimposed on heat stress, reduced cutaneous vasodilation and sweating, exaggerated heart rate increases, and excessive increases in body core temperature are evident.[54,55]

The effect of hypohydration on the cardiovascular system is even more pronounced when exercise is performed in a hot environment. The combination of vasodilation in exercising muscle and skin rapidly surpasses the reduced capacity of the cardiovascular system during hypohydration. Data from a study by Nadel and co-workers[56] (Figure 5) illustrate this effect. Subjects cycled for 30 min at 55% $\dot{V}O_2$peak in a hot environment (35°C) under both euhydrated and hypohydrated conditions. When the subjects were euhydrated, the normal rise in core temperature during exercise led to a progressive decline in stroke volume (as cutaneous blood flow increased). Accordingly, heart rate increased in an attempt to maintain cardiac output. In contrast, when the subjects were hypohydrated, stroke volume was initially lower and fell to lower levels as exercise progressed. Despite the greater heart rate response, cardiac output remained lower than under euhydrated conditions throughout the exercise trial (~2 l/min less) and core temperature rose excessively.

VI. GUIDELINES FOR FLUID REPLACEMENT

In 1996, the American College of Sports Medicine (ACSM) released a position stand regarding exercise and fluid replacement,[57] as summarized in Table 1. The ACSM guidelines represent the logical conclusion of decades of scientific research on athletes and serve as a model for the recommendations listed below. Our intention in this review is to highlight some of the key studies and scientific rationale underlying these guidelines.

In general terms, fluid and electrolyte replacement for the athlete takes place in three stages. First, fluid and electrolyte replacement needs to occur during preparation for exercise. Initiating exercise with a fluid deficit dramatically impairs performance.[32,53,58-60] Second, critical fluid and electrolyte replacement should occur throughout exercise[61-64] in an attempt to match water losses from sweating. Third, fluid and electrolytes need to be replaced during recovery, or postexercise.[65-68] Because different factors influence hydration status and the ability to replace fluids and electrolytes during each of these three stages, each stage will be discussed separately here, and distinct recommendations for fluid and electrolyte replacement will be provided for each.

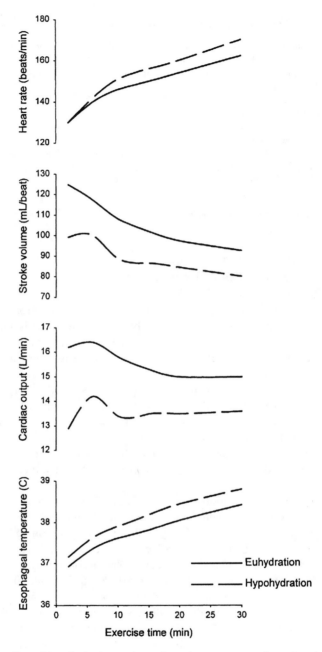

FIGURE 5 Effect of hypohydration on hemodynamic responses to dynamic submaximal exercise. (Data adapted from Nadel et al.[56])

TABLE 1   Guidelines for Fluid Replacement

1. Consume a balanced diet and drink adequate fluids during 24 hr preceding exercise.
2. Drink 500 ml of fluid 2 hr before exercise.
3. During exercise, drink fluids early and at regular intervals. The goal is to replace fluid at a rate equal to what is lost in sweating (up to what can be tolerated).
4. Fluid should be cooler than ambient temperature (15 to 22°C), flavored for palatability, and readily available.
5. Additionally, if exercise will be longer than 1 hr, proper amounts of carbohydrates and/or electrolytes should be included in fluids.
   A. The addition of carbohydrates should allow for 30 to 60 g/hr. This can be achieved by consuming 600 to 1200 ml/hr of a 4 to 8% carbohydrate solution.
   B. The addition of sodium at 0.5 to 0.7 g/l increases palatability, promotes fluid retention, and avoids hyponatremia.

Adapted from the American College of Sports Medicine position stand on exercise and fluid replacement.[57]

A. PRE-EXERCISE HYDRATION AND PREPARATION FOR EXERCISE

Well before exercise begins, steps should be taken to assure proper fluid and electrolyte balance for the upcoming exercise bout. When exercise is started from an inadequately hydrated state, temperature regulation is compromised. As discussed above, the result is an excessive rise in body core temperature and exaggerated cardiovascular responses for a given work load. Under these circumstances, endurance and performance are compromised. Hypohydration affects aerobically fit individuals to a greater degree than less fit individuals. When euhydrated, aerobically fit individuals tolerate heat stress well due largely to training-induced hypervolemia, which allows a fit individual to better maintain cardiac filling pressure during cutaneous vasodilation. However, studies have shown that this advantage is lost during hypohydration,[69,70] making pre-exercise hydration in athletes even more important.

The impact of hypohydration on endurance and performance is well documented.[53,58–60] Early work by Saltin[53] and Craig and Cummings[58] established that in well-controlled studies, physiologically induced hypohydration to a moderate degree (2 to 4% loss of body weight) effectively reduced work capacity. More recently, Armstrong et al.[59] studied the effect of pharmacologically induced dehydration on running performance on a track during 1500-, 5000-, and 10,000-m time trials. In these studies, athletes underwent dehydration until they had lost ~2% of body weight. While this mild dehydration did not reduce $\dot{V}O_2$max, it reduced time to exhaustion on a treadmill by 6.2%. Performance during the 1500-m run was not reduced; however, performance at 5000 and 10,000 m was reduced by 6.7 and 6.3%. Further analysis of the data suggested that dehydration equal to only 1% of body weight would have increased running time 10, 23, and 94 sec for the three distances. Similar work capacity decrements for dehydration of ~1% have been reported by Pichan and colleagues for cycling.[60]

Because proper levels of hydration are achievable at rest by consuming ample fluids with meals, one should consume a balanced diet and drink adequate fluids during the 24 hr preceding exercise. In a healthy individual following a meal, fluid absorption is facilitated by the abundant electrolytes in the diet. Thus, hydration with fluids during meals is convenient, because under these conditions almost any fluid will be readily absorbed. On a practical note, production of "clear and copious" urine is a crude but effective indicator of proper hydration status. In contrast, infrequent urination with small quantities of darkly colored urine is an indicator of hypohydration that is in need of amelioration. To "top off" the system prior to exercising, one should drink 500 ml of fluid 2 hr before the workout. This allows appropriate time for the water to be absorbed by the gastrointestinal tract and for the kidney to excrete any excess fluid.[45,57]

B. EXERCISE OF SHORT-DURATION (<1 HR)

Fluid and electrolyte replacement should occur throughout exercise in an attempt to match water losses from sweating. Without adequate fluid replacement during exercise, progressive fluid losses will undermine thermoregulation and result in increasing loss of performance. Body core temperature is best maintained and exercise performance is highest when body fluid levels are maintained at resting values, which can only be achieved by consuming an amount of fluid equal to what is lost during exercise. This is illustrated by a study from Walsh and colleagues,[63] who studied the effect of the low levels of dehydration that develop during moderate cycling for 60 min in the heat. Subjects underwent two identical bouts of cycling on different days with and without fluid replacement. With fluid replacement at the onset and throughout exercise, dehydration was reduced from 1.8% of body weight without fluid replacement to 0.2% of body weight with replacement. This resulted in a reduced perception of effort during the 60 min of moderate cycling. During subsequent high-intensity cycling to exhaustion, endurance increased 50% with fluid replacement compared to no fluid replacement. Similar results were found by Below and co-workers.[64] These studies demonstrate that even when exercise is initiated from a euhydrated state, sufficient hypohydration develops during exercise of 1 hr duration to warrant fluid replacement.

Montain and Coyle[71] studied the effect of early versus late fluid replacement during exercise. In this study, subjects who ingested ~1.2 l of fluid (which matched expected sweat losses) at the onset of exercise had a smaller rise in core temperature and heart rate over 1 hr of exercise than subjects drinking the same volume of fluid 40 min after the onset of exercise. This supports the concept that replacement is best achieved by early ingestion of fluids (i.e., rehydrate before a significant fluid deficit has occurred).

For practical reasons, the drinking schedule should be selected to maximize fluid absorption across the gastrointestinal tract. The gastric emptying rate is a rate-limiting step in this process,[72] and the factors which influence gastric emptying rate are well characterized.[73–75] The current consensus is that gastric volume is the primary factor controlling gastric emptying during running and cycling, with fluid content (i.e., caloric and osmotic content) being secondary. Thus, the goal becomes maintaining the highest gastric volume that is comfortable for the athlete, with the caveat that higher gastric volumes which are associated with gastric distress lead to a decrease in the rate of emptying. For the average individual who sweats 1 l/hr while exercising in the heat, a drinking schedule consisting of 250 ml of water every 15 min might satisfy these requirements. This schedule would provide adequate fluid to the system to match that lost by sweating (1 l/hr), would maintain a high gastric volume (i.e., enhance gastric emptying), and would be well tolerated by most individuals. Despite all the evidence in favor of matching fluid intake to sweat losses, many athletes consume insufficient fluids while exercising. In addition to using a planned drinking schedule, voluntary fluid consumption can be increased by cooling beverages (15 to 22°C), adding flavoring or sweeteners, and, perhaps more importantly, making fluids readily available.[57,76]

Beyond consumption and gastric emptying, rehydration is affected by the rate of intestinal absorption of fluid.[77] Because the colon can absorb ~90% of the fluid it receives, the colon is often viewed as the site of most fluid absorption along the gastrointestinal tract. However, the proximal small intestine absorbs up to 60% of the fluid it receives from the stomach before the ingestate reaches the colon. Thus, factors influencing absorption in the early sections of the small intestine weigh heavily upon the ability to rehydrate effectively during exercise.

Water is absorbed passively in the intestine. Hypotonic solutions are readily absorbed down the osmotic gradient. One might expect that hypertonic solutions are poorly absorbed. On the contrary, fluid can be absorbed across the small intestine against an osmotic gradient due to the active uptake of solutes, particularly carbohydrates and sodium. The movement of these solutes out of the intestinal lumen and into the bloodstream carries with it large quantities of water. The impact of carbohydrates and sodium on intestinal absorption has been extensively studied.[77-80] Intestinal absorption is good for hypertonic solutions up to ~400 mosmol/kg, with enhanced water and sodium absorption across the proximal intestine when compared to isotonic and hypotonic solutions. Furthermore, the presence of multiple carbohydrate forms (e.g., glucose, fructose, maltodextrins, sucrose) stimulates greater water absorption than fluids containing single carbohydrate forms.[81] This is most likely due to the independent active transport pathways available for each carbohydrate form.

C. EXERCISE OF LONGER DURATION (>1 HR)

As with exercise of short duration, replacement fluid should be readily available, cooler than ambient temperature, and flavored for palatability. Montain and Coyle[62] studied the effect of varying rates of fluid replacement during exercise in eight cyclists. On separate days, each cyclist rode for 2 hr in a warm environment while drinking a quantity of sports drink sufficient to replace approximately 0, 20, 48, or 81% of the fluids lost during exercise. They found that the physiologic strain was directly related to the degree of fluid deficit that developed during exercise. The rise in core temperature, heart rate, and the fall in stroke volume during extended exercise all correlate with the degree of dehydration. Thus, the goal for fluid replacement during exercise of longer duration continues to be matching fluid intake to fluid losses. Two additional goals must be considered for exercise that lasts more than an hour. First, carbohydrates should be added to increase fluid absorption in the intestine and to support maintenance of blood glucose levels. Second, sodium should be included to replace losses in sweat and to promote absorption of fluid.

Carbohydrate intake during aerobic exercise can postpone the development of fatigue by promoting the maintenance of blood glucose levels. This issue is covered in detail in Chapters 3 and 11 of this text. However, in the context of fluid replacement during exercise, several key issues regarding the benefits of carbohydrate solutions need to be emphasized here. First, sweetened fluids, when preferred by the athlete, will be consumed in greater volume than plain water during exercise.[76] Second, as mentioned above, fluids containing carbohydrates (and in particular multiple carbohydrate forms) stimulate water absorption in the small intestine.[81] Studies have shown that carbohydrate solutions of up to ~8% facilitate fluid uptake; however, solutions with >10% will impair fluid uptake and may even lead to gastrointestinal distress.[57,79] Finally, Hamilton and colleagues[61] studied the effect of fluid replacement and glucose infusions on cardiovascular responses to exercise. During 2 hr of moderate cycling exercise, fluid replacement with water sufficient to maintain body weight reduced cardiovascular drift (i.e., stroke volume and cardiac output were maintained, and the rise in core temperature was less) compared to no fluid replacement. However, cardiovascular drift was further reduced by the addition of a glucose infusion versus fluid replacement alone. More recent evidence suggests that for exercise <1 hr in duration, performance may be enhanced by including carbohydrates in the fluid replacement.[64]

During prolonged exercise, particularly events lasting >4 to 5 hr, including sodium in replacement fluids is advisable. In addition to increasing palatability, small amounts of sodium facilitate fluid uptake in the intestines as the sodium (along with carbohydrates) is actively transported from the lumen to the bloodstream. Furthermore, as noted above, a sodium debt develops during prolonged exercise, and this is exaggerated in hot environments. While the degree of sodium debt is generally minor when compared to the substantial dehydration that can occur, water replacement in the absence of supplemental sodium during extended exercise can lead to hyponatremia or decreased plasma sodium concentrations.[82] Classically, hyponatremia is associated with individuals who drink plain water in excess of their sweat losses or who are less physically conditioned and thus produce a more salty sweat (i.e., more sodium is lost). As plasma sodium falls below 130 meq/l, symptoms of hyponatremia may occur, including lethargy, confusion, seizures, or loss of consciousness. The problem of hyponatremia is not restricted to competitive athletic events; every year individuals suffer from exercise-induced hyponatremia while hiking in Grand Canyon National Park.[83]

D. REPLACEMENT AFTER EXERCISE

Sodium content of replacement fluid during recovery from exercise may be more important than that during exercise. Most research has shown that after prolonged exercise, particularly in the heat, restoration of total body water balance can only be achieved through the addition of sodium to the replacement fluid.[65,67]

As indicated above, during exercise in the heat, plasma volume and osmolality are maintained at the expense of tissue fluids. Thus, rehydration with plain water leads to early plasma volume expansion and a decrease in plasma osmolality. The drive to drink becomes diminished as the osmotic drive is removed. Also, the renin–angiotensin–aldosterone pathway is suppressed,[66] so that further water and sodium are lost by increased urine production. Addition of sodium to drinking water prevents the drop in osmotic drive and decreases the amount of fluid and sodium that is lost via the kidney during rehydration. Maughan and Leiper[67] studied the effect of varying sodium levels on rehydration following dehydration by exercise in the heat. Subjects exercised until they had lost 2% of their body weight. Over the next 30 min, the subjects consumed fluid equal to 1.5 times what had been lost, and then urine production was assessed for 5.5 hr. Each subject underwent this protocol on four occasions so that the sodium content of the replacement fluid could be varied. The results demonstrated that the fraction of water that is retained is related to the sodium concentration of the fluid ingested. Only 36% of the lowest sodium content fluid (2 mmol/l) was retained, whereas 74% of the highest sodium content fluid (100 mmol/l) was retained. In effect, excess fluid must be consumed (beyond that lost in sweat) to restore total body water balance;[68] without the inclusion of sodium, balance will not be restored due to excess urinary loss of water.

VII. SPECIAL CONSIDERATIONS

A. AGE

As the "baby-boomer" population ages and advances in health care and medicine continue, the number of people classified as "older" or "elderly" in the U.S. is rapidly increasing. This has led to broadened interest regarding factors that impact the health of the aged population. Germane to the topic of this chapter, epidemiological evidence indicates that mortality and morbidity rates are increased in the elderly during climactic heat waves.[84,85] Of 280 heat-related deaths reviewed by a coroner during a 5-day period in St. Louis, Missouri in 1966, 277 were over the age of 60 years. Based on epidemiological evidence, Jones et al.[86] determined that adults over the age of 65 have a 10- to 12-fold greater risk of developing heat stroke than do persons under 65 years. In his thorough review of body fluid regulation and age, Kenney[87] cautions against interpreting this to confer that aging results in decreased tolerance to heat stress. Variability in activity level, training status, methods, and subject screening for underlying diseases has led to confounding information.

Evidence suggests that hypohydration in older individuals may impact circulatory and thermoregulatory function to a greater extent than in the young, although this has not been adequately investigated. Skin blood flow is known to be lower in older individuals for a given rise in core temperature, as an effect of a reduced vasodilator sensitivity.[88] However, when the effects of chronic disease and a more sedentary lifestyle are minimized, heat tolerance does not appear to be compromised by age.[87]

Maximal and near-maximal cardiac output appear to be reduced in the elderly, independent of training status.[89,90] Of greater importance during hypohydration is that aging alters the determinants of cardiac output to a greater dependence on stroke volume to compensate for a reduced heart rate. A reduced venous return during hypohydration thereby could have a greater effect on cardiac output in older individuals. A reduced plasma volume in older individuals is a common observation,[91] which also may impact venous return, although as pointed out earlier this may only reflect the higher body fat and lower lean muscle mass with aging. Redistribution of blood flow from the splanchnic and renal regions is also reduced in older individuals during passive heating[92] and exercise in the heat.[93] This could also impact blood pressure regulation and fluid shifts between the compartments. The splanchnic region is highly compliant, and a relative inability to redistribute blood flow from this region during dehydration could exacerbate the impact of a reduced plasma volume. In addition, older individuals are not able to redistribute blood flow from the renal circulation to the same extent as the young. As pointed out by Zambraski[50] and discussed above, the small amount of fluid conserved by changes in renal blood flow may not have much importance during exercise or immediately following exercise. However, the long-term effects of altered renal function with aging during prolonged hypohydration are in need of further investigation.

How might the recommendation for fluid replacement during exercise differ in this population? As of yet, no comprehensive studies addressing this issue have been reported. Of importance is the observation that the thirst drive is reduced as a function of age.[94] This may indicate that older individuals need to be more conscientious about adequately hydrating prior to exercise and to begin drinking fluids well before they become thirsty.

B. ALTITUDE

Unacclimated individuals undergo a plasma volume contraction when acutely exposed to moderate high altitude. This is the result of many factors, including increased renal sodium and water excretion (natriuresis and diuresis) and decreased voluntary sodium and water intake.[95] Respiratory water losses are increased by high ventilatory rates and typically dry air. The result is an increase in hematocrit and hemoglobin that is thought to improve oxygen delivery to the tissues by increasing the oxygen-carrying capacity of the blood; however, this comes at the cost of a reduced blood volume, stroke volume, and cardiac output. With acclimation and its associated increase in red blood cell production, plasma and blood volume will return to prealtitude levels.

Hypoxic stimulation of the peripheral chemoreceptors appears to be the trigger for the changes in water and sodium metabolism associated with altitude.[96] Swenson and colleagues[97] studied natriuresis and diuresis in humans subjected to 6 hr of hypoxia (breathing 12% O_2 in an environmental chamber). In this study, the isocapnic hypoxic ventilatory response (HVR) was measured as a surrogate for peripheral chemoreceptor responsiveness. HVR correlated with the magnitude of natriuresis and diuresis, supporting the concept that chemoreceptors drive the water and sodium losses that occur with altitude. Likewise, administration of almitrine, a direct stimulant of the peripheral chemoreceptors, leads to natriuresis and diuresis.[98] Studies of humans at altitude or in hypobaric chambers have suggested that, in addition to decreased plasma volume, total body water and extracellular and intracellular fluids are reduced.[95]

Pugh[99] performed a classic series of studies at the extreme altitude of 5790 m (19,000 ft, The Silver Hut, on the Ming Bo glacier, Himalayas). During these studies, whole-body water turnover increased from sea-level values of 2.9 l/day to 3.9 l/day at altitude. Water turnover was further increased to 5.0 l/day during periods of high activity, such as climbing 5 to 7 hr/day. Thus, fluid replacement needs are significantly higher at altitude compared to sea level.

VIII. SUMMARY

Thermoregulation and the ability to prevent excessive increases in core temperature during exercise are dependent upon the ability to increase blood flow to the skin and to sweat. When exercise is performed in a hypohydrated state, the ability to increase skin blood flow and thus to transfer heat from the body core to the skin is markedly reduced. In addition to decreasing skin vasodilation, hypohydration and hyperosmolality limit the rate of sweating during exercise, reducing the ability to dissipate heat via evaporative cooling. These detrimental effects of dehydration on thermoregulation have been observed after fluid losses of as little as 1% of body weight. Therefore, replacement of fluid and electrolytes in preparation for, during, and after exercise is of paramount concern to the athlete. This chapter provides a scientific rationale and presents general guidelines to assist the athlete in preventing the development of exercise-induced dehydration and its associated effects on endurance and performance.

REFERENCES

1. Ganong, W.F., *Review of Medical Physiology,* 18th ed., Appleton & Lange, Stamford, CT, 1995.
2. Guyton, A.C. and Hall, J.E., *Textbook of Medical Physiology,* 9th ed., W.B. Saunders, Philadelphia, 1996.

3. Knochel, J.P., Clinical complications of body fluid and electrolyte balance, in *Body Fluid Balance,* Buskirk, E.R. and Puhl, S.M., Eds., CRC Press, Boca Raton, FL, 1996.
4. Greenleaf, J.E. and Harrison, M.H., Water and electrolytes, in *Nutrition and Aerobic Exercise. ACS Symposium No. 294,* Layman, D.K., Ed., American Chemical Society, Washington, D.C., 1986, 107.
5. Loeppky, J.A., Myhre, L.G., Venters, M.D., and Luft, U.C., Total body water and lean body mass estimated by ethanol dilution, *J. Appl. Physiol.,* 42, 803, 1977.
6. Sawka, M.N. and Pandolf, K.B., Effect of body water loss on physiological function and exercise performance, in *Fluid Homeostasis During Exercise,* Gisolfi, C.V. and Lamb, D.R., Eds., Cooper Publishing Group, Carmel, IN, 1990.
7. Olszewski, W., Engeset, A., Jaeger, P.M., Sodolowski, J., and Theodorsen, L., Flow and composition of leg lymph in normal men during venous stasis, muscular activity, and local hyperthermia, *Acta Physiol. Scand.,* 99, 149, 1977.
8. Mohsenin, V. and Gonzalez, R.R., Tissue pressure and plasma oncotic pressure during exercise, *J. Appl. Physiol.,* 56, 102, 1984.
9. Miles, D.S., Sawka, M.N., Glaser, R.M., and Petrofsky, J.S., Plasma volume shifts during progressive arm and leg exercise, *J. Appl. Physiol.,* 54, 491, 1983.
10. Bealer, S.L., Haddy, F.J., Diana, J.N., Grega, G.J., Manning, R.D., Jr., Rose, J.C., and Gann, D.S., Neuroendocrine mechanisms of plasma volume regulation, *Fed. Proc.,* 45, 2455, 1985.
11. Mubarak, S.J. and Hargens, A.R., Clinical use of the wick-catheter technique, in *Tissue Fluid Pressure and Composition,* Hargens, A.R., Ed., Williams and Wilkins, Baltimore, 1981, 261.
12. Roztocil, K., Prerovsky, I., Jandova, R., Widimsky, J., and Oliva, I., Transcapillary escape rate of albumin in juvenile hypertension, *Clin. Physiol.,* 3, 289, 1983.
13. Pivarnik, J.M., Kayrouz, T., and Senay, L.C., Jr., Plasma volume and protein content in progressive exercise: influence of cyclooxygenase inhibitors, *Med. Sci. Sports Exercise,* 17, 153, 1985.
14. Edwards, R.J. and Harrison, M.H., Intravascular volume and protein responses to running exercise, *Med. Sci. Sports Exercise,* 16, 247, 1984.
15. Aronson, P.S., Distribution of sodium chloride across cell membranes, in *The Regulation of Sodium and Chloride Balance,* Seldin, D.W. and Geibisch, G., Eds., Raven Press, New York, 1990, 3.
16. Adolf, E.F., Blood changes in dehydration, in *Physiology of Man in the Desert,* Adolf, E.F., Ed., Interscience, New York, 1947, 160.
17. Senay, L.C., Jr., Plasma volumes and constituent of heat exposed men before and after acclimatization, *J. Appl. Physiol.,* 38, 570, 1975.
18. Senay, L.C., Jr., Temperature regulation and hypohydration: a singular view., *J. Appl. Physiol.,* 47, 1, 1979.
19. Senay, L.C., Jr., Relationship of evaporative rates to serum [Na$^+$], [K$^+$] and osmolarity in acute heat stress, *J. Appl. Physiol.,* 25, 149, 1968.
20. Nose, H., Mack, G.W., Shi, X., and Nadel, E.R., Shift in body fluid compartments after dehydration in humans, *J. Appl. Physiol.,* 65, 318, 1988.
21. Kozlowski, S. and Saltin, B., Effect of sweat loss on body fluids, *J. Appl. Physiol.,* 19, 1119, 1964.
22. Harrison, M.H., Heat and exercise: effects on blood volume, *Sports Med.,* 3, 214, 1986.
23. Rowell, L.B., Human cardiovascular adjustments to exercise and thermal stress, *Physiol. Rev.,* 54, 75, 1974.
24. Johnson, J.M. and Park, M.K., Effect of heat stress on cutaneous vascular responses to the initiation of exercise, *J. Appl. Physiol.,* 53, 744, 1982.
25. Kellogg, D.L., Jr., Johnson, J.M., and Kosiba, W.A., Baroreflex control of the cutaneous active vasodilator system in humans, *Circ. Res.,* 66, 1420, 1990.
26. Hagan, R.D., Diaz, F.J., and Horvath, S.M., Plasma volume changes with movement to supine and standing positions, *J. Appl. Physiol.,* 45, 414, 1978.
27. Harrison, M.H., Effects of thermal stress and exercise on blood volume in humans, *Physiol. Rev.,* 65, 149, 1985.

28. Harrison, M.H., Edwards, R.J., and Fennessy, P.A., Intravascular volume and tonicity as factors in the regulation of body temperature, *J. Appl. Physiol.,* 44, 69, 1978.

29. Senay, L.C., Jr., Rogers, G., and Jooste, P., Changes in blood plasma during progressive treadmill and cycle exercise, *J. Appl. Physiol.,* 49, 59, 1980.

30. Pivarnik, J.M., Leeds, E.M., and Wilkerson, J.E., Effects of endurance exercise on metabolic water production and plasma volume, *J. Appl. Physiol.,* 56, 613, 1984.

31. Sawka, M.N., Francesconi, R.P., Pimental, N.A., and Pandolf, K.B., Hydration and vascular fluid shifts during exercise in the heat, *J. Appl. Physiol.,* 56, 91, 1984.

32. Sawka, M.N., Young, A.J., Francesconi, R.P., Muza, S.R., and Pandolf, K.B., Thermoregulatory and blood responses during exercise at graded hypohydration levels, *J. Appl. Physiol.,* 59, 1394, 1985.

33. Costill, D.L. and Fink, W.J., Plasma volume changes following exercise and thermal dehydration, *J. Appl. Physiol.,* 37, 521, 1974.

34. Smith, E.E., Guyton, A.C., Davis Manning, R., and White, R.J., Integrated mechanisms of cardiovascular response and control during exercise in the normal human, *Progr. Cardiovasc. Dis.,* 18, 421, 1976.

35. Diaz, F.J., Bransford, D.R., Kobayashi, K., Horvath, S.M., and McMurray, R.G., Plasma volume changes during rest and exercise in different postures in a hot humid environment, *J. Appl. Physiol.,* 47, 798, 1979.

36. Costill, D.L., Sweating: its composition and effects on body fluids, in *The Marathon: Physiological, Medical, Epidemiological and Psychological Studies,* Milvy, P., Ed., New York Academy of Science, New York, 1977, 160.

37. Costill, D.L. and Sparks, E., Rapid fluid replacement following thermal dehydration, *J. Appl. Physiol.,* 34, 299, 1973.

38. Saltin, B., Gagge, A.P., and Stolwijk, J.A.J., Body temperatures and sweating during thermal transients caused by exercise, *J. Appl. Physiol.,* 28, 318, 1970.

39. Nadel, E.R., Bullard, R.W., and Stolwijk, J.A.J., Importance of skin temperature in the regulation of sweating, *J. Appl. Physiol.,* 31, 80, 1971.

40. Nadel, E.R., Mitchell, J.W., Saltin, B., and Stolwijk, J.A.J., Peripheral modifications to the central drive for sweating, *J. Appl. Physiol.,* 31, 828, 1971.

41. Nadel, E.R., Cafarelli, E., Roberts, M.F., and Wenger, C.B., Circulatory regulation during exercise in different ambient temperatures, *J. Appl. Physiol.,* 46(3), 430, 1979.

42. Shapiro, Y., Pandolf, K.B., and Goldman, R.F., Predicting sweat loss responses to exercise, environment and clothing, *Eur. J. Appl. Physiol.,* 48, 83, 1982.

43. Pivarnik, J.M., Water and electrolytes during exercise, in *Nutrition and Exercise and Sport,* Hickson, J.F. and Wolinsky, I., Eds., CRC Press, Boca Raton, FL, 1989, 185.

44. Saltin, B., Circulatory response to submaximal and maximal exercise after thermal dehydration, *J. Appl. Physiol.,* 19, 1125, 1964.

45. Greenleaf, J.E. and Castle, B.L., Exercise temperature regulation in man during hypohydration and hyperhydration, *J. Appl. Physiol.,* 30, 847, 1971.

46. Sawka, M.N., Hubbard, R.W., Francesconi, R.P., and Horstman, D.H., Effects of acute plasma volume expansion on altering exercise–heat performance, *Eur. J. Appl. Physiol.,* 51, 303, 1983.

47. Fortney, S.M., Nadel, E.R., Wenger, C.B., and Bove, J.R., Effect of blood volume on sweating rate and body fluids in exercising humans, *J. Appl. Physiol.,* 51, 1594, 1981.

48. Fortney, S.M., Wenger, C.B., Bove, J.R., and Nadel, E.R., Effect of hyperosmolality on control of blood flow and sweating, *J. Appl. Physiol.,* 57, 1688, 1984.

49. Zambraski, E.J., Renal regulation of fluid homeostasis during exercise, in *Perspectives in Exercise Science and Sports Medicine,* Gisolfi, C.V. and Lamb, D.R., Eds., Cooper Publishing Group, Carmel, IN, 1990, 247.

50. Zambraski, E.J., The kidney and body fluid balance during exercise, in *Body Fluid Balance: Exercise and Sport,* Buskirk, E.R. and Puhl, S.M., Eds., CRC Press, Boca Raton, FL, 1996, 75.

51. Mitchell, J.W., Nadel, E.R., and Stolwijk, J.A., Respiratory water losses during exercise, *J. Appl. Physiol.,* 32, 474, 1972.

52. Rowell, L.B., *Human Cardiovascular Control,* Oxford University Press, New York, 1993.

77. Gisolfi, C.V., Exercise, intestinal absorption, and rehydration, *Sports Sci. Exchange,* 4, 1991.
78. Gisolfi, C.V., Summers, R.W., Schedl, H.P., Bleiler, T.L., and Oppliger, R.A., Human intestinal water absorption: direct vs indirect measurements, *Am. J. Physiol.,* 258, G216, 1990.
79. Gisolfi, C.V., Summers, R.W., Schedl, H.P., and Bleiler, T.L., Intestinal water absorption from select carbohydrate solutions in humans, *J. Appl. Physiol.,* 73, 2142, 1992.
80. Shi, X., Summers, R.W., Schedl, H.P., Chang, R.T., Lambert, G.P., and Gisolfi, C.V., Effects of solution osmolality on absorption of select fluid replacement solutions in human duodenojejunum, *J. Appl. Physiol.,* 77, 1178, 1994.
81. Shi, X., Summers, R.W., Schedl, H.P., Flanagan, S.W., Chang, R., and Gisolfi, C.V., Effects of carbohydrate type and concentration and solution osmolality on water absorption, *Med. Sci. Sports Exercise,* 27, 1607, 1995.
82. Noakes, T.D., Goodwin, N., Rayner, B.L., Branken, T., and Taylor, R.K.N., Water intoxication: a possible complication during endurance exercise, *Med. Sci. Sports Exercise,* 17, 370, 1985.
83. Shopes, E.M., Drowning in the desert: exercise-induced hyponatremia at the Grand Canyon, *J. Emer. Nurs.,* 23, 586, 1997.
84. Oechsli, F.W. and Buechley, R.W., Excess mortality associated with three Los Angeles September hot spells, *Environ. Res.,* 3, 277, 1970.
85. Ellis, F.P., Exton-Smith, A.N., Foster, K.G., and Weiner, J.S., Eccrine sweating and mortality during heat waves in very young and very old persons, *Isr. J. Med.,* 12, 815, 1976.
86. Jones, S.T., Liang, A.P., Kilbourne, E.M., Griffin, M.R., Patracia, P.A., Fite Wassilak, S.G., Mullan, R.J., Herrick, R.F., Donnell, H.D., Choi, K., and Thacker, S.B., Morbidity and mortality associated with the July 1980 heat wave in St. Louis and Kansas City, MO, *J. Am. Med. Assoc.,* 247, 3327, 1982.
87. Kenney, W.L., Body fluid and temperature regulation as a function of age, in *Exercise in Older Adults,* Lamb, D.R., Gisolfi, C.V., and Nadel, E., Eds., Cooper Publishing, Carmel, IN, 1995, 305.
88. Kenney, W.L., Morgan, A.L., Farquhar, W.B., Brooks, E.M., Pierzga, J.M., and Derr, J.A., Decreased active vasodilator sensitivity in aged skin, *Am. J. Physiol.,* 272, H1609, 1997.
89. Ogawa, T., Spina, R.J., Martin, W.H., Kohrt, W.M., Schechtman, K.B., Holloszy, J.O., and Ehsani, A.A., Effects of aging, sex, and physical training on cardiovascular responses to exercise, *Circulation,* 86, 494, 1992.
90. Minson, C.T. and Kenney, W.L., Age and cardiac output during cycle exercise in thermoneutral and warm environments, *Med. Sci. Sports Exercise,* 29, 75, 1997.
91. Davy, K.P. and Seals, D.R., Total blood volume in healthy young and older men, *J. Appl. Physiol.,* 76, 2059, 1994.
92. Minson, C.T., Wladkowski, S.L., Cardell, A.F., Pawelczyk, J.A., and Kenney, W.L., Age alters the cardiovascular response to direct passive heating, *J. Appl. Physiol.,* 84, 1323, 1998.
93. Ho, C.W., Beard, J.L., Farrell, P.A., Minson, C.T., and Kenney, W.L., Age, fitness, and regional blood flow during exercise in the heat, *J. Appl. Physiol.,* 82, 1126, 1997.
94. Mack, G.W., Weseman, C.A., Langhans, G.W., Scherzer, H., Gillen, C.M., and Nadel, E.R., Body fluid in dehydrated healthy older men: thirst and renal osmoregulation, *J. Appl. Physiol.,* 76, 1615, 1994.
95. Hoyt, R.W. and Honig, A., Body fluid and energy metabolism at high altitude, in *Handbook of Physiology, Section 4: Environmental Physiology,* Fregly, M.J. and Blatteis, C.M., Eds., American Physiological Society, Bethesda, MD, 1996, chap. 55.
96. Honig, A., Peripheral arterial chemoreceptors and reflex control of sodium and water homeostasis, *Am. J. Physiol.,* 257, R1282, 1989.
97. Swenson, E.R., Duncan, T.B., Goldberg, S.V., Ramirez, G., Ahmad, S., and Schoene, R.B., Diuretic effect of acute hypoxia in humans: relationship to hypoxic ventilatory responsiveness and renal hormones, *J. Appl. Physiol.,* 78, 377, 1995.
98. Koller, E.A., Schopen, M., Keller, M., Lang, R.E., and Vallotton, M.B., Ventilatory, circulatory, endocrine, and renal effects of almitrine infusion in man: a contribution to high altitude physiology, *Eur. J. Appl. Physiol.,* 58, 419, 1989.
99. Pugh, L.G.C.E., Physiological and medical aspects of the Himalayan scientific and mountaineering expedition, 1960–61, *Br. Med. J.,* 2, 621, 1962.

53. Saltin, B., Aerobic and anaerobic work capacity after dehydration, *J. Appl. Physiol.,* 1964.

54. Ekblom, B., Greenleaf, C.J., Greenleaf, J.E., and Hermansen, L., Temperature regulatic exercise dehydration in man, *Acta Physiol. Scand.,* 79, 475, 1970.

55. Senay, L.C., Jr., Temperature regulation and hypohydration: a singular view, *J. Appl.* 47, 1, 1979.

56. Nadel, E.R., Fortney, S.M., and Wenger, C.B., Effect of hydration state on circula thermal regulations, *J. Appl. Physiol.,* 49, 715, 1980.

57. Convertino, V.A., Armstrong, L.E., Coyle, E.F., Mack, G.W., Sawka, M.N., Senay, L.C Sherman, W.M., American College of Sports Medicine Position Stand: exercise and placement, *Med. Sci. Sports Exercise,* 28, i, 1996.

58. Craig, F.N. and Cummings, E.G., Dehydration and muscular work, *J. Appl. Physiol.,* 1966.

59. Armstrong, L.E., Costill, D.L., and Fink, W.J., Influence of diuretic-induced dehydr competitive running performance, *Med. Sci. Sports Exercise,* 17, 456, 1985.

60. Pichan, G., Gauttam, R.K., Tomar, O.S., and Bajaj, A.C., Effect of primary hypohyd physical work capacity, *Int. J. Biometeorol.,* 32, 176, 1988.

61. Hamilton, M.T., Gonzalez-Alonso, J., Montain, S.J., and Coyle, E.F., Fluid replacer glucose infusion during exercise prevent cardiovascular drift, *J. Appl. Physiol.,* 71, 8?

62. Montain, S.J. and Coyle, E.F., Influence of graded dehydration on hyperthermia and c: cular drift during exercise, *J. Appl. Physiol.,* 73, 1340, 1992.

63. Walsh, R.M., Noakes, T.D., Hawley, J.A., and Dennis, S.C., Impaired high-intensity performance time at low levels of dehydration, *Int. J. Sports Med.,* 15, 392, 1994.

64. Below, P.R., Mora-Rodrigues, R., Gonzalez-Alonso, J., and Coyle, E.F., Fluid and carb ingestion independently improve performance during 1 h of intense exercise, *Med. Sc Exercise,* 27, 200, 1995.

65. Nose, H., Mack, G.W., Shi, X., and Nadel, E.R., Role of osmolality and plasma volum rehydration in humans, *J. Appl. Physiol.,* 65, 325, 1988.

66. Nose, H., Mack, G.W., Shi, X., and Nadel, E.R., Involvement of sodium retention h during rehydration in humans, *J. Appl. Physiol.,* 65, 332, 1988.

67. Maughan, R.J. and Leiper, J.B., Sodium intake and post-exercise rehydration in man *Appl. Physiol.,* 71, 311, 1995.

68. Shirreffs, S.M., Taylor, A.J., Leiper, J.B., and Maughan, R.J., Post-exercise rehydration effects of volume consumed and drink sodium content, *Med. Sci. Sports Exercise,* 2 1996.

69. Buskirk, E.R., Iampietro, P.F., and Bass, D.E., Work performance after dehydration: e physical conditioning and heat acclimatization, *J. Appl. Physiol.,* 12, 189, 1958.

70. Cadarette, B.S., Sawka, M.N., Toner, M.M., and Pandolf, K.B., Aerobic fitness hypohydration response to exercise–heat stress, *Aviat. Space Environ. Med.,* 55, 507,

71. Montain, S.J. and Coyle, E.F., Influence of the timing of fluid ingestion on temperatur lation during exercise, *J. Appl. Physiol.,* 75, 688, 1993.

72. Duchman, S.M., Ryan, A.J., Schedl, H.P., Summers, R.W., Bleiler, T.L., and Gisolf Upper limit for intestinal absorption of a dilute glucose solution in men at rest, *Med. Sci Exercise,* 29, 482, 1997.

73. Houmard, J.A., Egan, P.C., Johns, R.A., Neufer, P.D., Chenier, T.C., and Israel, R.G., emptying during 1 h of cycling and running at 75% VO_2max, *Med. Sci. Sports Exercise,* 2 1991.

74. Mitchell, J.B. and Voss, K.W., The influence of volume on gastric emptying and fluid 1 during prolonged exercise, *Med. Sci. Sports Exercise,* 23, 314, 1991.

75. Noakes, T.D., Rehrer, N.J., and Maughan, R.J., The importance of volume in regulating emptying, *Med. Sci. Sports Exercise,* 23, 307, 1991.

76. Wilmore, J.H., Morton, A.R., Gilbey, H.J., and Wood, R.J., Role of taste preference o intake during and after 90 min of running at 60% of VO_{2max} in the heat, *Med. Sci. Exercise,* 30, 587, 1998.

SUPPLEMENTS CONTAINING MACROELEMENTS

Chapter 10

MAGNESIUM, PHOSPHATE, AND CALCIUM SUPPLEMENTATION AND HUMAN PHYSICAL PERFORMANCE*,**

Henry C. Lukaski

CONTENTS

---

* Mention of a trademark or proprietary product does not constitute a guarantee of warranty of the product by the U.S. Department of Agriculture and does not imply its approval to the exclusion of other products that may also be suitable.
** U.S. Department of Agriculture, Agricultural Research Service, Northern Plains Area is an equal opportunity/affirmative action employer and all agency services are available without discrimination.

I. INTRODUCTION

As athletes seek to improve and optimize performance, they explore various sources of information ranging from radical changes in diet to the use of nutritional supplements to advances in training and technique. Because advertisements claim that supplements promote remarkable and beneficial effects on performance, athletes are willing to indiscriminately use various nutritional supplements to boost their performance without regard to the credibility of the claims or the safety of the product. Supplement use among athletes, recreational and elite, is widespread; it ranges from 6 to 100%,[1] which surpasses the reported 40 to 60% rate of supplement consumption in the U.S. population.[2] Although the efficacy of nutritional supplements on performance has been discussed,[3,4] the effects of supplemental magnesium, phosphate, and calcium have received limited attention.

The role of macromineral, excluding the electrolytes, supplementation on exercise metabolism and physical performance has been the topic of occasional interest among sports scientists. In contrast to the numerous studies involving supplementation with vitamins and iron, there has been only sporadic consideration of the ergogenic potential of magnesium, phosphate, and calcium. Primary interest in magnesium and phosphate arises from their key roles in cellular energy metabolism. Calcium, in contrast, has been examined not as a potential facilitator of energy utilization but as a regulator of the maintenance of body structure, bone. This chapter summarizes the fundamental roles of these mineral elements in physiological functions relating to energy expenditure and critically reviews the findings that describe the effects of supplemental magnesium, phosphate, and calcium on physiological and biochemical aspects of human performance.

II. MAGNESIUM

Total body content of magnesium in an adult ranges from 20 to 30 g, of which the majority (55%) is stored in bone, at least 45% located within cells, and a minimal proportion found in the extracellular fluid. As an intracellular cation, magnesium plays a fundamental role in more than 300 enzymatic reactions in which the components of food are metabolized to provide chemical energy and the synthesis of new macromolecules.[5] Some of these activities include glycolysis, protein and fat metabolism, adenosine triphosphate (ATP) hydrolysis, and the second messenger system. Magnesium also acts as a physiological regulator of membrane stability and neuromuscular, cardiovascular, immune, and hormonal functions. Overall, magnesium may be considered as a central nutrient in the regulation of cellular energy metabolism, the integration of physiological systems, and thus a potentially limiting factor in physical performance.

A. MAGNESIUM SUPPLEMENTATION AND PERFORMANCE

Awareness of the importance of magnesium in virtually all aspects of cellular and biological systems stimulated interest in the effects of magnesium nutriture on physical performance.[6] Heightened interest in the importance of magnesium in physical performance paralleled the observation[7] that muscle spasms in a competitive tennis player with magnesium depletion, characterized by hypomagnesemia, were eliminated with daily magnesium supplementation (500 mg/day) for a few days.

1. Magnesium Supplementation and Physiological Function

Generalized magnesium supplementation may impact cellular function in physically active individuals (Table 1). Physical and mental stressors promote changes in secretion of glucocorticoid hormones, membrane stability, and glucose and lactate metabolism. Long-distance runners supplemented for 2 weeks with magnesium (360 mg/day) and placebo in a crossover designed experiment had significantly reduced plasma concentrations of cortisol (0.3 to 0.22 µmol/l) and aldosterone (0.48 to 0.25 nmol/l) during a standardized running test.[8] Similarly, a 3-week period of magnesium supplementation (360 mg/day), as compared to placebo treatment, improved cellular membrane stability as indicated by decreased plasma concentrations (10 to 30%) of myoglobin, urea, and some enzymes from liver and skeletal muscle after a marathon run.[9] Improvements in insulin sensitivity (i.e., reduced plasma glucose and insulin concentrations) occurred in trained swimmers and rowers supplemented with magnesium as compared to other athletes in the control groups.[10,11] Magnesium supplementation also promoted a concurrent elimination of lactic acid from the blood (15.5 versus 14.9 mmol/l) immediately following a strenuous and controlled rowing ergometer test.[11] These findings suggest that generalized magnesium supplementation may be beneficial to physical performance. Indeed, mean endurance running time increased from 17 to almost 19 min after 3 weeks of magnesium supplementation (360 mg/day) in trained runners.[12,13] The beneficial effects of magnesium supplementation in each of these studies, however, generally were small and probably of limited biological significance.

Magnesium supplementation is not consistently associated with favorable effects on function and performance (Table 1). Thirty-nine men participated in a double-blind, crossover experiment to examine the effects of magnesium supplementation (390 mg/day or placebo for 25 days with a 3-week washout period between treatments) on maximal and submaximal performance.[14] Magnesium supplementation impacted some metabolic responses during maximal work with small but nonsignificant increases in oxygen uptake [l/min, 7.6%; ml/(kg·min), 6.3%] and carbon dioxide production (6.5%) and a significant increase in total energy output

TABLE 1 Biochemical and Physiological Responses During Exercise to Magnesium Supplementation

	Response
Generalized Mg supplementation	
Golf et al.[8]	↓ stress response
Bertschat et al.[9]	↓ cell membrane permeability
Pohlmann[10]	↑ insulin sensitivity
Münch[11]	↓ lactate accumulation
Mands[12] and Kappes[13]	↑ endurance running time
Vecchiet et al.[14]	↑ total energy output
Terblanche et al.[15]	No improvement in marathon performance
Mg supplementation of Mg-depleted subjects	
Golf et al.[17]	↓ cell membrane permeability
Brilla and Haley[18]	↑ strength gain
Lukaski et al.[20]	↑ Mg retention, ↑ efficiency of energy use, ↓ HR during exercise

(15.5%). During submaximal work, supplemental magnesium exerted small and nonsignificant improvements in function, including reduced heart rate (6%) and decreased ventilatory rate, oxygen utilization, and carbon dioxide production (10.8, 16.4, and 9.9%, respectively), with no change in respiratory exchange ratio. Similarly, marathon runners supplemented with magnesium (365 mg/day for 6 weeks) showed no improvement in running performance, as well as no increase in resistance to muscle damage or muscle function.[15] These findings confirm that magnesium supplementation per se does not enhance physiological function or performance when magnesium status is normal.[16]

2. Magnesium Supplementation in Magnesium-Depleted Individuals

Supplementation of magnesium to magnesium-depleted individuals results in significant improvements in physiological function and some measures of performance (Table 1). Female competitive athletes with plasma magnesium concentrations at the low end of the range of normal values received a magnesium supplement (360 mg/day) for 3 weeks and responded with significant reductions in serum total creatine kinase and creatine kinase isoenzyme from skeletal muscle after training as compared to other athletes receiving a placebo.[17] Similarly, serum lactate concentration and oxygen consumption during an exhaustive rowing-ergometer test decreased significantly in male competitive rowers supplemented with magnesium (360 mg/day for 4 weeks) as compared to the rowers receiving a placebo.[11]

Supplemental magnesium may also influence strength gain and power.[18] Young men participating in a strength training program consumed their usual diets and received either a magnesium supplement or a placebo such that daily magnesium intakes were 507 or 250 mg/day, respectively. Although both groups gained strength, peak knee-extension torque increased significantly more in the men supplemented with magnesium. Thus, a magnesium intake of 250 mg/day, which is less than the recommendation of 420 mg/day,[19] permitted strength gain, but further increases in strength were attained with an intake exceeding 500 mg/day, which is about 20% greater than the current recommended dietary intake.[19]

Restricted dietary magnesium impacts physiological responses during exercise. Postmenopausal women who consumed diets containing adequate (320 mg/day for 35 days), low (180 mg/day for 91 days), then adequate (380 mg/day for 49 days) magnesium demonstrated decreased muscular efficiency during submaximal work.[20] Low magnesium intake resulted in a significant increase (12%) in oxygen consumption and heart rate (10 bpm) during progressive ergocycle work. Magnesium balance was negative, indicating a net loss of magnesium, and skeletal muscle magnesium concentration decreased significantly when dietary magnesium was 180 mg/day. These findings indicate that dietary magnesium deprivation induces magnesium loss from the body, depletes muscle magnesium stores, and adversely influences muscle energy efficiency.

III. PHOSPHATE

Phosphorus is an essential mineral element that is found in all cells; it is the sixth most abundant element in the body. The primary sites of phosphorus storage in the body include bone (85%) and skeletal muscle (14%). Phosphate serves a variety of biological functions including stabilization of proteins, polysaccharides, phospholipids, nucleic acids, and hydroxyapatite. Phosphate also performs key functions in energy metabolism, such as the maintenance of the high energy bonds of ATP and creatine phosphate (CP), and is required for the activities of phosphorylation and dephosphorylation enzymes, as well as phosphoenolpyruvate, a rate-limiting enzyme in glycolysis. Awareness of these key functions of phosphate in preservation of ATP and CP and the optimal activity of phosphoenolpyruvate has prompted studies of phosphate supplementation on physical performance.

A. PHOSPHATE LOADING AS AN ERGOGENIC AID

Reports of supplementation of phosphate salts to enhance physical performance began in the 1920s and concluded that phosphates decrease fatigue of athletes and workers.[21] Although these results were provocative, the original studies were hampered by poor experimental designs. Nevertheless, the early findings served as the stimulus for recent investigations that examined the effects of phosphate supplementation on performance.

1. Rationale for Use of Phosphate Salts

The theoretical basis for a beneficial effect of phosphate loading on physical performance includes its potential roles in acid–base balance, oxygen delivery to tissues, glycolysis, and recharging of high-energy phosphate compounds. For high-intensity activities, phosphate may act as buffer to reduce accumulation of H^+ and thus decrease the onset of fatigue and exhaustion.[22] Increased intracellular phosphate has been shown to stimulate red blood cell (RBC) glycolysis and increase RBC 2,3-diphosphoglycerate (2,3-DPG) concentration,[23,24] thereby reducing the affinity of oxyhemoglobin for oxygen[25] and improving peripheral oxygen delivery. Phosphate loading may also stimulate glycolysis or increase the concentration of inorganic phosphate, which hypothetically facilitates the resynthesis of CP in working muscle.[26] Any of these mechanisms, therefore, could enhance anaerobic and possibly aerobic performance.

2. Phosphate Supplementation Trials

The effects of phosphate loading on exercise performance are inconsistent (Table 2). Some studies report enhanced functional responses and improved exercise performance. During a 7-week experimental period, ten well-trained male runners participated in a double-blind crossover trial of acute phosphate supplementation (4 g/day for 3 days) with a sodium citrate placebo at weekly intervals.[27] Phosphate loading resulted in significantly increased serum phosphate and erythrocyte 2,3-DPG concentrations and peak oxygen consumption. Peak oxygen uptake was significantly correlated with the increase in 2,3-DPG concentration ($r = 0.81$). Also, lactate concentration during submaximal work was attenuated. Similarly, phosphate (4 g of tribasic sodium phosphate), as compared to placebo, supplementation of male runners for 6 days in a crossover design elicited a significant increase in peak aerobic power and a decrease in ventilatory anaerobic threshold.[28] Phosphate loading, however, affected neither serum phosphate nor RBC 2,3-DPG concentrations. Five-mile performance run times were not affected with phosphate supplementation. In a follow-up study, Kreider et al.[29] supplemented six male cyclists and triathletes with either phosphate (4 g tribasic sodium phosphate) or a glucose placebo for 3 days in a crossover design before testing. They confirmed that phosphate supplementation was associated with an increased anaerobic threshold and reported increased myocardial ejection fraction and fractional shortening assessed with two-dimensional echocardiography and an improved endurance performance during a simulated 40-km time trial, with a significant increase in serum phosphorus but no change in RBC 2,3-DPG. Bredle et al.[30] also found that phosphate loading improved cardiovascular function and reduced cardiac output during submaximal work. Among moderately trained cyclists, phosphate loading (3.6 g sodium phosphate) compared to placebo for 3 days before testing was associated with a significant increase in peak aerobic capacity without demonstrable change in either plasma phosphate or RBC 2,3-DPG concentrations.[31]

Other studies demonstrated no benefit of phosphate supplementation on exercise performance. Duffy and Conlee[32] examined the acute (1.24 g 1 hr before exercise) and chronic (3.73 g/day for 6 days preceding exercise) effects of phosphate supplementation on some measures of exercise performance and function among 11 untrained men and found no significant effect of phosphate treatment on

TABLE 2 Effects of Phosphate Supplementation on Performance

Source	Supplement	PO$_4$ Dose	Duration	Ergogenic Effect	Change in Phosphate (mmol/l)	
					Supplement[a]	Exercise[b]
Cade et al.[27]	NaH$_2$PO$_4$	3.2 g/day	3 days	6–12% ↑ V̇O$_2$peak ↓ submaximal lactate	0.05	0.19
Duffy and Conlee[32]	Stim-O-Stam[c]	1.24 g/day 3.37 g/day	1 hr[d] 6 days	No performance improvements No performance improvements	NR[e] NR[e]	NR[e] NR[e]
Bredle et al.[30]	CaHPO$_4$	22.2 g/day	4 days	No performance improvements	0.40	0.30
Mannix et al.[33]	CaHPO$_4$	15.5 g/day	3 hr[d]	No performance improvements	0.18	0.15
Stewart et al.[31]	NaH$_2$PO$_4$	2.9 g/day	3 days	10% ↑ V̇O$_2$peak 20% ↑ time to exhaustion	0.01	0.30
Kreider et al.[28]	Na$_3$PO$_4$	2.3 g/day	6 days	9% ↑ V̇O$_2$ peak 12% ↑ V̇O$_2$ at anaerobic threshold	0.16	0.70
Kreider et al.[29]	Na$_3$PO$_4$	2.3 g/day	3 and 4 days	9% ↑ V̇O$_2$ peak 10% ↑ V̇O$_2$ at anaerobic threshold 8% ↓ in 40K performance time	0.06	0.18
Galloway et al.[35]	Na$_2$HPO$_4$	15.5 g	90 min[d]	No performance improvements	0.07	0.06

[a] Change in plasma phosphate concentration after phosphate supplementation.
[b] Change in plasma phosphate concentration after exercise.
[c] Stim-O-Stam: each tablet contained 200 mg Na$_2$HPO$_4$, 186.8 mg NaH$_2$PO$_4$, 27.5 mg K$_3$PO$_4$, and 30 mg ascorbic acid; each subject consumed three tablets.
[d] Immediately before the exercise test.
[e] Not reported.

treadmill endurance, leg muscular power, or peak oxygen uptake. Similarly, Mannix et al.[33] found no benefit of acute phosphate loading (22.2 g ingested 3 hr before testing) on oxygen delivery and cardiovascular function during exercise.

Differences in experimental designs and treatments may contribute to the heterogeneity of these findings.[34] Small sample sizes (six to ten subjects) and differences in aerobic fitness levels (untrained and trained subjects) limit application of the findings to the population of healthy young men. Similarly, the use of different types of exercise (endurance and peak aerobic power tests) is another confounding variable. Phosphate loading yields performance-enhancing[27–29,31] and no effects during peak intensity exercise, as well as positive[28,29] and null[32,33,35] functional effects during submaximal work.

The lack of use of a consistent dose of supplemental phosphate, both the amount and the chemical form (Table 2), and a failure to assess dietary phosphate intake further contribute to the inconsistent experimental findings. Studies have used both sodium and calcium phosphate supplements. The use of sodium, as compared to calcium, phosphate has some practical limitations.[34] Sodium phosphate tends to produce smaller increases in plasma phosphate concentration than calcium phosphate. Also, it requires about four times more sodium phosphate than calcium phosphate to deliver the same total dose of elemental phosphorus. Sodium phosphate also has been reported to cause gastrointestinal disturbances,[27] which may adversely influence performance results.

In addition, not all studies have demonstrated the efficacy of phosphate supplementation with measurements of increased plasma phosphate or RBC 2,3-DPG concentrations. This limitation is significant because failure to document increases in erythrocyte 2,3-DPG suggests that the theoretical basis for phosphate loading, to increase oxygen delivery to tissues, is untenable. Thus, if phosphate loading has a beneficial effect on performance (Table 2), it is small and of questionable physiological significance, because the studies that produced the largest difference in plasma phosphate concentration as a result of supplementation[30,33] failed to demonstrate an ergogenic effect. Furthermore, the magnitude of change in plasma phosphate concentration following exercise generally exceeds the size of the change achieved through supplementation (Table 2).

A recent study, however, that overcame these limitations demonstrated that phosphate loading did not benefit performance. Galloway et al.[35] supplemented trained and untrained men with either a phosphate supplement (22.2 g/day) or a placebo 90 min before exercise testing in a crossover design. Dietary intakes of phosphate were similar among the trained (2335 and 2279 mg/day) and untrained (2033 and 1866 mg/day) men during the placebo and supplementation trials, respectively. There were no differences in plasma phosphate, 2,3-DPG, endurance time, peak oxygen consumption, or postexercise lactate accumulation in blood in response to phosphate loading. They concluded that acute phosphate loading is not effective as an ergogenic aid and that aerobic fitness level does not affect the response to phosphate supplementation.

IV. CALCIUM

Calcium is another mineral element with multiple biological roles. Although calcium is best known for its structural role in bones and teeth, it is acknowledged that calcium is required by all cells for their specialized functions. Intracellular calcium acts as a second messenger and enables cells to respond to stimuli such as neural input and hormonal signals. Movement of calcium from intracellular compartments to the cytosol triggers cell division, secretion of chemicals, contraction, and movement. A number of calcium-dependent enzymes also facilitate blood-clotting mechanisms.

The skeleton is the principal site of calcium storage in the body. With more than 99% of body calcium in bone, this reservoir acts dynamically to maintain the calcium concentration in the extracellular fluid. Short-term insufficiency of dietary calcium results in transient loss of calcium from bone. However, chronic and long-term inadequate calcium intake can adversely affect bone quality and strength.

A. CALCIUM SUPPLEMENTATION, PHYSICAL ACTIVITY, AND INJURY

The theoretical basis to support the use of supplemental calcium to positively impact metabolic responses during exercise is very limited. Some preliminary data[36] suggest that consumption of a hypertonic calcium solution (1 to 1.5 l of a 1.5% calcium gluconate) may maintain plasma volume and attenuate increases in body temperature during exercise in the heat (39.4°C). A more plausible hypothesis for the use of supplemental calcium is the maintenance of bone quality and the prevention of injuries to bone and connective and soft tissue.

Calcium supplements[37] and the adoption of a program of weight-bearing activity[38] have been used to prevent and to treat age-related bone loss in nonosteoporotic women. However, when both treatment interventions have been applied, no additive effects were found in elderly women.[39]

Calcium supplementation apparently does not influence the risk of developing bone stress injuries. Supplementation of healthy male military recruits with 500 mg of calcium (0.3 g calcium carbonate and 2.94 g calcium lactate-gluconate), as compared to placebo, had no effect on the frequency of overuse injuries during 9 weeks of physical training.[40] Importantly, mean daily calcium intakes were 872 and 976 mg/day, which represents 70 to 80% of the Recommended Dietary Allowance (RDA),[19] respectively, for the supplemented and placebo-treated recruits. This finding suggests that a calcium intake of at least 800 mg/day is protective against overuse bone injuries and that additional calcium provides no further benefit.

An etiological factor in the development of muscle cramps during exercise may be intracellular, specifically sarcoplasmic reticulum, calcium depletion.[41] Although it has been proposed that small amounts of supplemental calcium (100 to 150 mg/day) might be beneficial in ameliorating muscle cramping,[41] there are no experimental data to support this hypothesis.

V. NUTRITIONAL CONSIDERATIONS

Calcium, phosphate, and magnesium are mineral elements that are stored principally in bone. When dietary intake is less than body losses of these minerals, the maintenance of the physiological functions in nonosseous tissues that require calcium, phosphate, and magnesium is supported by a mobilization of the mineral elements from bone. In addition, homeostatic adaptations are implemented that increase absorption and decrease mineral losses. These dynamic responses serve to preserve the content of these essential nutrients and thus to maintain biological function. These adaptations, which maintain the extracellular concentration of these mineral elements, complicate the routine assessment of magnesium, phosphorus, and calcium nutritional status because of the general lack of availability of a sensitive and specific blood biochemical marker of mild and moderate mineral deficiency.

A. ADVERSE EFFECTS OF SUPPLEMENTATION

Generalized use of mineral supplements can have adverse effects on function and health. There is no evidence that large doses of supplemental magnesium are harmful to individuals with normal renal function. Early symptoms of magnesium toxicity include nausea, vomiting, and hypotension. Increased serum magnesium can occur when individuals with impaired renal function chronically consume magnesium-containing drugs, such as antacids or cathartics,[42] because more than 20% of magnesium from various salts can be absorbed. Ingestion of magnesium supplements in amounts exceeding 500 mg/day often causes gastrointestinal disturbances, particularly diarrhea, in some individuals and may exert a negative effect on phosphate balance.[43]

Dietary phosphorus or supplemental phosphate may influence calcium metabolism. There was no change in the calcium balance of men when phosphorus intake increased from 800 mg/day (i.e., RDA is 700 mg/day for men[19]) to up to 2000 mg/d with a calcium intake of 200 to 2000 mg/day.[44] Similarly, varying phosphorus intake had no effect on the calcium balance of perimenopausal women.[45] Urinary calcium excretion varied inversely with dietary phosphorus and calcium balance did not change, which implies that fecal calcium losses varied directly with phosphorus intake.[44,45] Thus, dietary phosphorus and supplemental phosphate apparently exert important effects on calcium metabolism (i.e., decreased intestinal absorption and decreased renal excretion of calcium), but these effects probably negate each other so that overall calcium balance is not affected. The mechanism by which phosphorus intake might decrease intestinal calcium absorption is related to calcitriol production. Serum calcitriol concentration decreased in men fed increasing amounts of dietary phosphorus from less than 500 mg/day to 3000 mg/day.[46] Thus, the ability of calcium metabolism to adapt to changes in phosphorus intake, from diet or supplement use, apparently depends on the ability of the kidney to respond with changes in calcitriol production.

Although no adverse effects have been observed in many healthy adults consuming large doses of supplemental calcium, high intakes may induce constipation and may increase the risk of urinary stone formation in some men. A high calcium intake may inhibit the intestinal absorption of iron, zinc, and other essential minerals.[47]

Recent evidence indicates important differences between acute and chronic use of calcium supplements in iron metabolism. Among healthy adults with adequate iron nutritional status and consuming 15 mg iron and less than 320 mg calcium daily, short-term calcium supplementation (1200 mg/day provided as 400 mg calcium in each of three meals) significantly decreased nonheme iron absorption from 15.8 to 4.7%.[48] However, no significant effects on blood biochemical measures of iron nutriture were found in healthy adults after 6 months of calcium supplementation (1200 mg/day).[48] Thus, any short-term changes in nonheme iron absorption associated with calcium supplementation apparently are normalized over time by homeostatic controls.

VI. SUMMARY AND CONCLUSIONS

Because magnesium, phosphate, and calcium play fundamental roles in the regulation of energy metabolism and body structure, there has been interest in the effect of supplementation of these minerals on physical performance and injury prevention. The majority of the experimental evidence indicates that the generalized use of supplemental magnesium, phosphate, and calcium does not provide an ergogenic benefit to physically active individuals.

Magnesium supplementation of magnesium-adequate athletes can result in some minor improvements in metabolic function, including membrane stability, reduction in stress hormone response, insulin sensitivity, and lactate disposal during exercise. There is a conspicuous lack of evidence supporting performance improvements in magnesium-adequate individuals supplemented with magnesium. In contrast, magnesium-depleted individuals supplemented with magnesium have responded with significant and beneficial functional responses, including enhancement of strength gain, improvement of efficiency of energy utilization, and a decrease in heart rate during submaximal work.

The use of phosphate loading to gain performance benefits has yielded inconsistent results. Differences in experimental designs (i.e., amount and chemical form of phosphate compounds, duration of supplementation regimen, training status of subjects, type of exercise protocol, etc.) have complicated the interpretation of the experimental results. It is clear, however, that the observed changes in plasma phosphate were not consistent with the dose of the phosphate supplement. Furthermore, the measured changes in erythrocyte 2,3-DPG did not support the fundamental hypothesis that phosphate loading promotes oxygen delivery to tissues by increasing RBC 2,3-DPG.

The role of calcium supplementation in performance has not examined metabolic function but alternatively has addressed the hypothesis that supplemental calcium prevents exercise-induced injuries. Limited evidence suggests that a daily threshold of 800 mg of calcium is adequate to prevent overuse injuries because supplementation with additional calcium (500 mg/day) did not significantly impact the incidence of stress-related injuries.

The findings summarized in this review confirm the results of large-scale surveys[49–51] of athletes who received vitamin and mineral supplements. The generalized use of supplemental magnesium, phosphate, and calcium does not support performance improvements if individual athletes have adequate nutritional status.

The generalized use of nutritional supplements is not recommended unless under the supervision of a physician or a registered dietitian. This guideline is presented because indiscriminate use of some nutritional supplements may lead to adverse nutritional and health consequences that are dependent on the amount of the supplement and duration of its use.

Two professional organizations provide advice to individuals who seek to use nutritional supplements to enhance performance. Both the American Dietetics Association[52] and the American College of Sports Medicine[53] state that the proper nutritional strategy to promote health and optimal performance is to obtain adequate nutrients from a wide variety of foods. Use of nutritional supplements is appropriate when scientific evidence supports safety and effectiveness. Because some groups of physically active individuals (i.e., young athletes, participants in sporting activities that require weight standards for competition, overweight individuals beginning an exercise program, and older active people) may be at increased risk of nutrient depletion, the use of a balanced nutritional supplement, not exceeding the recommended or safe and adequate daily intake, may be consumed as a short-term preventive measure.

REFERENCES

1. Burke, L.M. and Read, R.S.D., Dietary supplements in sport, *Sports Med.,* 15, 43–65, 1993.
2. Stewart, M.L., McDonald, J.T., Levy, A.S., Schucker, R.E., and Henderson, D.P., Vitamin/mineral supplement use: a telephone survey of adults in the United States, *J. Am. Diet. Assoc.,* 85, 1585–1590, 1985.
3. Bucci, L., *Nutrients as Ergogenic Aids for Sports and Exercise,* CRC Press, Boca Raton, FL, 1993.
4. Lukaski, H.C., Vitamin and mineral metabolism and exercise performance, in *Perspectives in Exercise Science and Sports Medicine,* Vol. 12, Spriet, L., Hargreaves, M., and Lamb, D.B., Eds., Cooper Publishing Group, Carmel, IN, 1999, 261–313.
5. Shils, M.E., Magnesium, in *Modern Nutrition in Health and Disease,* 8th ed., Shils, M.E., Olson, J.A., and Shike, M., Eds., Lea & Febiger, Philadelphia, 1994, 164–184.
6. Brilla, L.R. and Lombardi, V.P., Magnesium in sports physiology and performance, in *Sports Nutrition: Minerals and Electrolytes,* Kies, C.V. and Driskell, J.A., Eds., CRC Press, Boca Raton, FL, 1995, 139–177.
7. Liu, L., Borowski, G., and Rose, L.I., Hypomagnesemia in a tennis player, *Physician Sportsmed.,* 11, 79–80, 1983.
8. Golf, S., Happel, O., and Graef, V., Plasma aldosterone, cortisol, and electrolyte concentrations in physical exercise after magnesium supplementation, *J. Clin. Chem. Biochem.,* 22, 717–721, 1984.

9. Bertschat, F., Golf, S.W., Riediger, H., Graef, V., and Ising, H., Protective effects of magnesium on release of proteins from muscle cells during a marathon run, *Magnesium Bull.,* 8, 310–313, 1986.

10. Pohlmann, U., Magnesiumstoffwechsel bei Schwimmern, dissertation, Giessen, Germany, 1991.

11. Münch, J., Einfluß einer Langzemagnesiumsupplemenierung auf physiologische und Biochemische Parameter unter Wettkampfspezifischen Belastungen bei Ruderern, dissertation, Giessen, Germany, 1992.

12. Mands, C., Magnesiumsubstitution bei Langstreckenläufern und ihr Einfluß auf das Körperliche, Kardiorespiratorische und Metabolische Leitsungsvermögen, dissertation, Giessen, Germany, 1987.

13. Kappes, P., Einfluß von Magnesiumsubstitution auf das Kardiorespiratorische, Metabolische und Körperliche Leitsungsvermögen von Ausdauertrainierten Frauen, dissertation, Giessen, Germany, 1994.

14. Vecchiet, L., Pieralisi, G., D'Ovidio, M., Dragani, L., Felzani, G., Mincarini, A., Giamberardino, M.A., Borella, P., Bargellini, A., and Piovanelli, P., Effects of magnesium supplementation on maximal and submaximal effort, in *Magnesium and Physical Activity,* Vecchiet, L., Ed., Parthenon Publishing Group, London, 1995, 227–237.

15. Terblanche, S., Noakes, T.D., Dennis, S.C., Marais, D.W., and Eckert, M., Failure of magnesium supplementation to influence marathon running performance or recovery in magnesium-replete subjects, *Int. J. Sport Nutr.,* 2, 154–164, 1992.

16. Borella, P., Bargellini, A., and Ambrosini, G., Magnesium supplementation in adults with marginal deficiency: response in blood indices, urine and saliva, *Magnesium Bull.,* 16, 1–4, 1994.

17. Golf, S., Graef, V., Gerlach, H.-J., and Seim, K.E., Changes in serum creatine kinase and serum creatine kinase MB activities during training and magnesium supplementation in elite female athletes, *Magnesium Bull.,* 2, 43–46, 1983.

18. Brilla, L.R. and Haley, T.F., Effect of magnesium supplementation on strength training in humans, *J. Am. Coll. Nutr.,* 11, 326–329, 1992.

19. Institute of Medicine, Food and Nutrition Board, *Dietary Reference Intakes for Calcium, Phosphorus, Magnesium, Vitamin D, and Fluoride,* National Academy Press, Washington, D.C., 1997.

20. Lukaski, H.C., Milne, D.B., and Nielsen, F.H., Decreased efficiency during exercise among postmenopausal women fed a low magnesium diet, *FASEB J.,* 11, A147, 1997.

21. Bucci, L.R., Micronutrient supplementation and ergogenesis — minerals, in *Nutrients as Ergogenic Aids for Sports and Exercise,* CRC Press, Boca Raton, FL, 1993, 65–67.

22. Horswill, C.A., Effects of bicarbonate, citrate, and phosphate loading on performance, *Int. J. Sport Nutr.,* 5, S111–S119, 1995.

23. Lichtman, M.A., Miller, D.R., Cohen, J., and Waterhouse, C., Reduced red cell glycolysis, 2,3-diphosphoglycerate and adenosine triphosphate concentration, and increased hemoglobin–oxygen affinity caused by hypophosphatemia, *Ann. Intern. Med.,* 74, 562–58, 1971.

24. Tsuboi, K.K. and Fukunaga, K., Inorganic phosphate and enhance glucose degradation by intact erythrocytes, *J. Biol. Chem.,* 240, 2806–2810, 1965.

25. Benesch R. and Benesch, R.E., Intracellular organic phosphates as regulators of oxygen release by hemoglobin, *Nature,* 221, 618–622, 1969.

26. Chastiotis, D., The regulation of glycogen phosphorylase and glycogen breakdown in human skeletal muscle, *Acta Physiol. Scand. Suppl.,* 518, 1–68, 1983.

27. Cade, R., Conte, M., Zauner, C., Mars, D., Peterson, J., Lunne, D., Hommen, N., and Packer, D., Effects of phosphate loading on 2,3-diphosphoglycerate and maximal oxygen uptake. *Med. Sci. Sports Exercise,* 16, 263–268, 1984.

28. Kreider, R.B., Miller, G.W., Williams, M.H., Somma, C.T., and Nasser, T., Effects of phosphate loading on oxygen uptake, ventilatory anaerobic threshold, and run performance, *Med. Sci. Sports Exercise,* 22, 250–256, 1990.

29. Kreider, R.B., Miller, G.W., Schenck, D., Cortes, C.W., Miriel, V., Somma, C.T., Rowland, P., Turner, C., and Hill, D., Effects of phosphate loading on metabolic and metabolic responses to maximal and endurance exercise, *Int. J . Sport Nutr.,* 2, 20–47, 1992.

30. Bredle, D., Stager, J., Brechue, W., and Farber, M., Phosphate supplementation, cardiovascular function, and exercise performance in humans, *J. Appl. Physiol.*, 65, 1821–1826, 1988.

31. Stewart, I., McNaughton, L., Davies, P., and Tristram, S., Phosphate loading and the effects on VO_2max in trained cyclists, *Res. Q. Exercise Sport*, 61, 80–84, 1990.

32. Duffy, D.J. and Conlee, R.K., Effects of phosphate loading on leg power and high intensity treadmill exercise, *Med. Sci. Sports Exercise*, 18, 674–677, 1986.

33. Mannix, E.T., Stager, J.M., Harris, A., and Farber, M.O., Oxygen delivery and cardiac output during exercise following oral phosphate–glucose, *Med. Sci. Sports Exercise*, 22, 341–347, 1990.

34. Tremblay, M.S., Galloway, S.D., and Sexsmith, J.R., Ergogenic effects of phosphate loading: physiological fact or methodological fiction? *Can. J. Appl. Physiol.*, 19, 1–11, 1994.

35. Galloway, S.D.R., Tremblay, M.S., Sexsmith, J.R., and Roberts, C.J., The effects of acute phosphate supplementation in subjects with different aerobic fitness levels, *Eur. J. Appl. Physiol.*, 72, 224–230, 1996.

36. Greenleaf, J.E. and Brock, P.J., Na^+ and Ca^{+2} ingestion: plasma volume–electrolyte distribution at rest and exercise, *J. Appl. Physiol.*, 48, 838–847, 1980.

37. Reid, I.R., Ames, R.W., Evans, M.C., Gamble, G.D., and Sharpe, S.J., Long-term effects of calcium supplementation on bone loss and fractures in postmenopausal women: a randomized controlled study, *Am. J. Med.*, 98, 331–335, 1995.

38. Berard, A., Bravo, G., and Gauthier, P., Meta-analysis of the effectiveness of physical activity for the prevention of bone loss in postmenopausal women, *Osteoporos. Int.*, 7, 331–337, 1997.

39. Smith, E.L., Reddan, W., and Smith, P.E., Physical activity and calcium modalities for bone mineral increase in aged women, *Med. Sci. Sports Exercise*, 13, 60–64, 1981.

40. Schwellnus, M.P. and Jordaan, G., Does calcium supplementation prevent bone stress injuries? A clinical trial, *Int. J. Sport Nutr.*, 2, 165–174, 1992.

41. Williams, M.H., The role of minerals in physical activity, in *Nutritional Aspects of Human Physical Performance*, 2nd ed., Charles C Thomas, Springfield, IL, 1985, 186–195.

42. Mordes, J.P. and Wacker, E.C., Excess magnesium, *Pharmacol. Rev.*, 29, 274–300, 1977.

43. Spencer, H., Minerals and mineral interactions in human beings, *J. Am. Diet. Assoc.*, 86, 864–867, 1986.

44. Spencer, H., Kramer, L., Osis, D., and Norris, C., Effect of phosphorous on the absorption of calcium and on the calcium balance in man, *J. Nutr.*, 108, 447–457, 1978.

45. Heaney, R.P. and Recker, R.R., Effects of nitrogen, phosphorous and caffeine on calcium balance in women, *J. Lab. Clin. Med.*, 99, 46–55, 1982.

46. Portale, A.A., Halloran, B.P., Murphy, M.M., and Morris, R.C., Oral intake of phosphorous can determine the serum concentration of 1,25-dihydroxyvitamin D by determining its production rate in humans, *J. Clin. Invest.*, 77, 7–12, 1986.

47. Greger, J.L., Effect of variations in dietary protein, phosphorous, electrolytes, and vitamin D on calcium and zinc metabolism, in *Nutrient Interactions*, Bodwell, C.E. and Erdman, J.W., Eds., Marcel Dekker, New York, 1988, 205–227.

48. Minihane, A.M. and Fairweather-Tait, S.J., Effect of calcium supplementation on daily non-heme iron absorption and long-term iron status, *Am. J. Clin. Nutr.*, 68, 96–102, 1998.

49. Weight, L.M., Myburgh, K.H., and Noakes, T.D., Vitamin and mineral supplementation: effects on the running performance of trained athletes, *Am. J. Clin. Nutr.*, 47, 192–195, 1988.

50. Tellford, S., Catchpole, E.A., Deakin, V., Hahn, A.G., and Plank, A.W., The effect of 7 to 8 months of vitamin/mineral supplementation on athletic performance, *Int. J. Sport Nutr.*, 2, 135–153, 1992.

51. Singh, A., Moses, F.M., and Deuster, P.A., Chronic multivitamin–mineral supplementation does not enhance physical performance, *Med. Sci. Sports Exercise*, 24, 726–732, 1992.

52. American Dietetics Association, Position of the American Dietetics Association: vitamin and mineral supplementation, *J. Am. Diet. Assoc.*, 96, 73–77, 1996.

53. American College of Sports Medicine, *Current Comment: Vitamin and Mineral Supplements and Exercise*, American College of Sports Medicine, Indianapolis, 1998.

Chapter 11

SPORTS BEVERAGES

Julie H. Burns
Jacqueline R. Berning

CONTENTS

0-8493-8196-7/99/$0.00+$.50
© 1999 by CRC Press LLC

I. INTRODUCTION

The physiological and performance effects of macronutrients, electrolytes, fluids, and macroelements on exercise and sport have been reviewed in detail in other chapters of this book. The focus of this chapter is the use of sports beverages during sport and activity. The rationale and use of many commonly consumed beverages and the various ingredients they contain as they relate to the maintenance of hydration and performance enhancement are provided. Guidelines and practical considerations for the use of sports beverages before, during, and after physical activity are also presented.

The development of the very first sports beverage, Gatorade® Thirst Quencher, was based on Scandinavian research conducted in the 1930s and continuing into the 1960s that demonstrated a performance-enhancing role for carbohydrates during endurance exercise.[1,2] Researchers at the University of Florida, Gainesville, developed Gatorade®, a scientifically formulated beverage comprised, at that time, of glucose and electrolytes, with the goal of enhancing the performance of the school's football team — the Florida Gators. The success of the Gator football team in the mid to late 1960s was attributed in large part to the players' use of Gatorade®. As a result, a multimillion-dollar sports beverage industry was born. Annual sales for sports drinks now total more than $2 billion.[3]

There are at least 25 different sports drinks available in the U.S. today, and many other beverages, such as fruit juice, soda, coffee, and bottled, tap, and caffeinated water, are marketed as "sports" drinks. Because of the wide variability in the components of beverages used by athletes during exercise (e.g., a fluid replacement beverage like Gatorade®, Powerade®, or Allsport® versus diluted fruit juice), determining whether a particular beverage is suitable will depend on when and why it is being consumed. Energy and hydration requirements during physical activity are vastly different from requirements before activity (e.g., during the precompetition meal or immediately prior to exercise) and after exercise. The ideal beverage for sport should taste good and meet all of the nutrient, electrolyte, and fluid requirements for the particular phase of activity so that performance is enhanced and all physiological benefits of hydration can be realized.

II. RATIONALE FOR COMPONENTS ADDED TO SPORTS BEVERAGES

A. FUNDAMENTAL CONCEPTS

The types of fluids that athletes classify as "sports" drinks vary widely and may include any kind of fluid consumed before, during, or after activity. In this chapter, sports drinks will refer to those formulated for quick replacement of fluids and electrolytes lost during exercise and that provide carbohydrate fuel to working muscles (usually called fluid replacement beverages or isotonic beverages). Sports drinks generally contain a carbohydrate source, various electrolytes, and water. Some sports drinks also supply supplemental vitamins, minerals, and other ingredients, such as glycerol, choline, and carbonation.

B. FLUID BALANCE AND REGULATION

Regular fluid intake is essential for maintaining a body temperature that maximizes human performance. Adequate fluid balance maintains blood volume, which in turn supplies blood to the skin for body temperature regulation. Exercise produces heat, which must be eliminated from the body to maintain appropriate body temperature. The human body is not efficient at converting potential energy from oxygen and nutrients into mechanical energy. During exercise, only about one-fourth of this potential energy is converted into mechanical energy, leaving approximately 75% of the total energy produced as heat. Most of the heat generated by exercising muscles is transferred to the blood, where it circulates through the body and raises core temperature. The amount of heat produced during exercise, even in physically fit individuals, is enough to raise core body temperatures by 18°C every 5 to 8 min. Without effective means to dissipate this heat, moderate to high-intensity exercise could raise body temperatures to lethal levels within 15 to 30 min.

The body maintains appropriate temperatures by a system referred to as thermoregulation. As heat is generated in the muscles during exercise, it is transferred via the blood to the body's core. Increased core temperature results in increased blood flow to the skin, where, in cool to moderate ambient temperatures, heat is transferred to the environment by convection, radiation, and evaporation. Environmental conditions have a large impact on thermoregulation. When ambient temperatures are warm to hot, the body must dissipate both the heat produced during exercise and the heat absorbed from the environment. When this occurs, the body relies solely on the evaporation of sweat to maintain appropriate body temperature. Thus, maintaining hydration becomes crucial when ambient temperatures reach or exceed 36°C.

Humidity affects the body's ability to dissipate heat to even a greater extent than air temperatures. As humidity increases, the rate at which sweat evaporates decreases, which means more sweat drips off the body instead of being transferred from the body to the environment. The combined effects of a hot, humid environment and the large metabolic heat load of exercise leave the thermoregulatory system unable to cope adequately. Ensuring proper and adequate fluid intake is one of the ways to prevent an overtaxing of the thermoregulatory system and subsequent heat injury or illness.

Body fluid balance of healthy individuals is maintained on a daily basis by factors that control the intake and output of both water and electrolytes. Antidiuretic hormone (vasopressin) and the renin–angiotensin–aldosterone system are hormonal mechanisms that control the osmolality, sodium content, and volume of extracellular fluids and play a major role in the regulation of fluid balance. There is a continuous loss of water from the skin and respiratory tract plus intermittent losses from the kidneys and gastrointestinal tract. When fluid is lost from the body in the form of sweat, plasma volume decreases and plasma osmolality increases. The kidneys, under hormonal control, regulate water and solute excretion in excess of the obligatory urine loss. When the body is subjected to hot environments, whether the heat load is imposed internally by exercise or externally by environment, certain hormonal adjustments occur to maintain bodily function. The body maintains balance by conserving both water and sodium. To this end, the pituitary gland releases antidiuretic hormone to increase water absorption from the kidneys, which causes the urine to become more concentrated, thus conserving fluid and making the urine a dark gold color. This feedback process helps the body to hold on to much needed body water and preserve blood volume. At the same time, aldosterone is released from the adrenal cortex and acts upon the renal tubules to increase the reabsorption of sodium, which helps maintain the correct osmotic pressure. These reactions also increase the thirst mechanism in the body. However, in situations where water losses are increased acutely, such as during intense athletic workouts or competition, thirst response can be delayed, making it difficult for athletes to ingest enough fluid to offset the volume of fluid that is lost.

The replacement of electrolytes, particularly sodium, in combination with water, is essential for effective rehydration. When sufficient amounts of sodium and water are ingested, plasma osmolality and sodium concentration do not decline. When both water and sodium are consumed, circulating levels of vasopressin and aldosterone are maintained, and excess urine output that would otherwise occur is prevented. Several researchers[4–6] have found that rehydration with water alone dilutes the blood rapidly, increases its volume, and stimulates urine output. Blood dilution lowers both the sodium- and volume-dependent part of the thirst drive, thus removing much of the drive to drink and slowing fluid replacement efforts (see also Section II.F).

Another electrolyte that is involved with maintaining body fluids is potassium. Potassium is the major ion of the intracellular fluid. As the major electrolyte inside body cells, potassium works in close association with sodium and chloride to maintain body fluids and generate electrical impulses in nerves and muscles, including the heart. Potassium balance, like sodium balance, is also regulated by aldosterone. Potassium regulation in the body is quite precise, and deficiencies are rare, except in cases of fasting, diarrhea, and some diuretic therapies.

C. FLUID ABSORPTION

Most athletes believe that as soon as they ingest a fluid, it is available immediately for absorption. However, the speed at which fluid is absorbed depends upon a number of different factors. These variables include the amount of fluid consumed, the type of fluid ingested, the osmolality of the fluid consumed, and the gastric emptying rate.

The proximal small intestines (duodenum and jejunum) are the primary site of fluid absorption; approximately 50 to 60% of any given fluid load is absorbed here. The colon, on the other hand, absorbs a greater percentage (approximately 80 to 90%) of the fluid it receives, but the colon receives very little fluid and accounts for only about 15% of the total fluid load. Intestinal fluid absorption is a passive process and can occur against an osmotic gradient. The intestinal mucosa is a semipermeable membrane with relatively large aqueous channels. Thus, in the presence of an osmotic gradient, there is a large and rapid movement of water across the duodenojejunum, compared with only a modest water flux across the colon.[7] Water-soluble electrolytes, such as sodium, move rapidly across the proximal intestines. Water movement occurs passively and is generally dependent upon solute absorption. However, Leiper and Maughan[8] found that infusion of a hypotonic solution through the jejunum increased water absorption with increasing solute absorption. These results suggest that the greater osmotic gradient promoted greater water movement from the intestinal lumen to the blood. It is also true that although water movement is usually passive, water can be absorbed against a concentration gradient.

1. Glucose and Sodium

Because glucose is actively absorbed in the intestines, it can markedly increase both sodium and water absorption. It has been known for over 70 years that the small intestines absorb certain hexoses faster than others.[9,10] Cori[11] first suggested selectivity of the intestinal membrane for simple sugars. Cori found that sugars disappeared from the intestine at strikingly different rates: galactose > glucose > fructose > mannose > xylose > arabinose. It was established that galactose and glucose were actively absorbed against a concentration gradient and that fructose, mannose, xylose, and arabinose were not. According to Crane,[12] glucose and sodium associate with a carrier in the microvilli of the intestinal cell. The complex travels to the inner side of the membrane where it disassociates, releasing the glucose and sodium. The sodium is then actively transported out of the cell, while the glucose is emptied into the bloodstream. The sodium ion attaches to the carrier and changes the configuration of the carrier, which allows the glucose molecule to attach for transfer across the membrane. The carrier then assumes another shape when the site brings potassium out of the cell. Early studies indicated that water absorption was maximized when luminal glucose concentrations ranged from 1 to 3% (55 to 140 mM);[13] however, most sports drinks contain two to three times this quantity without causing adverse gastrointestinal symptoms. If, on the other hand, the concentration of glucose in the lumen reaches 10% (550% mosmol), it can cause fluid secretions and gastrointestinal distress.[14]

Clinical trials have shown that sucrose, when used in equimolar concentrations as glucose, is as effective as glucose in the treatment of dehydration secondary to diarrhea caused by cholera, rotavirus, and other noncholera pathogens.[15] Glucose polymers offer the potential advantage of reducing osmolality and increasing the quantity of glucose. In the treatment of diarrheal diseases, increasing the carbohydrate concentration beyond certain limits can lead to hypernatremia.[16] In another study,[17] no differences were found in fluid absorption from the intestinal perfusion of plain water or from a hypotonic carbohydrate–electrolyte solution formulated with glucose polymers.

2. Osmolality

Sports drinks are either hypertonic, isotonic, or hypotonic. Some evidence indicates that hypotonic solutions are more efficacious than isotonic solutions in maximizing water absorption;[18] others, however, have not found this to always be the case.[19–21] A recent study by Ryan and colleagues[21] examined the effect of hypohydration (–2.7% body weight) on gastric emptying and intestinal water flux using three carbohydrate–electrolyte solutions of varying concentrations (6, 8, and 9%). The researchers found that gastric emptying and water flux were not impaired when subjects were hypohydrated to approximately 3% during moderate exercise when either water or a 6% carbohydrate–electrolyte solution was ingested. Hyperosmolality (>400 mosmol), as in the 8 and 9% carbohydrate–electrolyte solutions (and some commercially available sports drinks; see Table 1), reduces water flux in the proximal intestine.

D. PERFORMANCE EFFECTS

1. Fundamental Concepts

The two nutrients most likely to affect performance are fluids and carbohydrate, both components of sports drinks. An inadequate supply of carbohydrate fuel

TABLE 1 Select Commercial Sports Drink Comparison

Beverage (8-oz/240-ml Serving)	Calories	Carbs (g)	% Carbs	Sodium (mg)	Potassium (mg)	Carbohydrate Ingredients
Gatorade® (Quaker Oats, Chicago, IL)	50	14	6	110	30	Sucrose, fructose, glucose
Powerade® (The Coca-Cola Company, Atlanta, GA)	70	19	8	55	30	High-fructose corn syrup, glucose polymers (maltodextrins)
Allsport® (Pepsico, Purchase, NY)	70	19	8	55	55	High-fructose corn syrup, also contains 10% daily value for thiamin, niacin, B_6, pantothenic acid, and B_{12} and is carbonated
10-K® (Suntory Water Group, Inc. Marietta, GA)	60	15	6	55	30	Sucrose, fructose
Exceed® (Weider Health & Fitness, Woodland Hills, CA)	70	17	7	50	45	Glucose polymers, fructose
Cytomax® (Champion Nutrition, Concord, CA)	66	13	5	53	100	Corn starch, fructose, glucose
Hydra Fuel® (Twinlabs, Hauppauge, NY)	66	16	7	25	50	Glucose polymers, glucose, fructose
Quickick® (Quickick, Baton Rouge, LA)	67	16	7	100	23	High-fructose corn syrup
1st Ade® (American Beverages, Verona, PA)	60	16	7	55	25	High-fructose corn syrup, glucose, sucrose, fructose
Endura® (Meta Genics, Inc., San Clemente, CA)	60	15	6	46	80	Glucose polymers, fructose
Hy-5® (Grey Eagle Enterprises, Maryland Heights, MO)	50	13	6	40	70	Maltodextrins
Race Day® (Internnutria Sports, Framingham, MA)	70	17	6	100	222	Maltodextrins, sucrose, fructose; also contains choline

leads to early fatigue, while suboptimal fluid intake before and during exercise causes physiological consequences that may affect performance. When athletes consume fluids voluntarily during exercise, they usually replace less than one-half of their body fluid loss,[22] which not only compromises cardiovascular function and performance but places the athlete at risk for heat-related injury.

Carbohydrate feedings prior to exercise have been shown to improve performance.[23] Greater gains in performance are seen when both pre-exercise and during-exercise carbohydrate feedings are used together.[24] Pre-exercise carbohydrate meals should include between 200 and 350 g of carbohydrate in the 3 to 6 hr leading up to exercise and can be consumed in either liquid or solid form.[25]

The timing and frequency of food and fluid intake before, during, and after exercise may affect exercise capacity and performance because these variables determine the amount and availability of fuel.[26] Behavioral strategies such as the adoption of frequent carbohydrate-rich meals with adequate fluids (like high-carbohydrate supplements, fruit juices, sports drinks, and water) allow athletes to meet their high energy, fluid, and carbohydrate needs.[26] A recent study[27] looked at whether combining a pre-exercise carbohydrate meal with the ingestion of a carbohydrate–electrolyte solution (sports drink) was more effective in improving endurance than a carbohydrate–electrolyte solution alone. As expected, the carbohydrate–electrolyte solution consumed during exercise improved endurance running capacity. Further improvements in performance were seen with the combination of the carbohydrate–electrolyte solution and the pre-exercise carbohydrate meal that provided 2.5 g carbohydrate per kilogram body weight. These findings can be used by practicing sports nutritionists and others as they plan and make recommendations for fluid intake and precompetition meals.

2. Short-Duration Events

Athletes who participate in short-duration events may believe that they are not exposed to the same heat stress as endurance athletes and need not be concerned about fluid consumption or hydration. Contrary to these beliefs, athletes who participate in short-duration activities, such as sprint running in track and field, or stop-and-go sports like basketball, volleyball, or baseball may be just as likely to develop dehydration as are distance runners or ultramarathoners. While many athletes, such as sprinters, participate in short-duration events, they may have to run several heats before reaching a championship heat, which exposes them to both environmental and internal heat stresses. All individuals who participate in physical activity or sports should be educated on the guidelines for dehydration prevention and fluid replacement.

The benefit of carbohydrate intake during high-intensity intermittent efforts or short-duration events has not been routinely investigated. One of the first studies to examine the influence of carbohydrate in a sports drink on endurance capacity during intermittent high-intensity shuttle running was performed by Nicholas and colleagues.[28] Researchers devised a running protocol to simulate the efforts of stop-and-go sports, such as those required in football, soccer, and rugby. During the breaks and between the efforts, the subjects consumed fluids that either contained carbohydrate (sports drink) or did not (water placebo). When consuming the sports drink, subjects ran 2 min longer (8 min total) at the end of 75 minutes of "play" compared to running on the water placebo. Thus, sports drink helped to maintain high-intensity efforts during high-intensity activities that consisted of intermittent sprinting, running, and jogging. This research prompted more interest in the efficacy of carbohydrate feedings during more intense exercise lasting less than 60 min or for intermittent high-intensity exercise. Davis et al.[29] demonstrated that a sports drink consumed before and during stop-and-go sports, like basketball, helps delay fatigue and maintains hydration. Sixteen physically active but untrained subjects (seven women, nine men) ingested an 18% carbohydrate beverage just prior to repeated 1-min cycling bouts on a bicycle ergometer at 120 to 130% $\dot{V}O_2max$ that were separated by 3 min of rest. A 6% carbohydrate–electrolyte beverage was ingested every 20 min until subjects fatigued. Plasma glucose and insulin levels were higher, ratings for perceived exertion for the legs were lower, and time to fatigue was delayed when subjects consumed the carbohydrate–electrolyte beverage versus an artificially flavored placebo (see also Section III.C).

3. Endurance Events

Marathoners talk of "hitting the wall." Cyclists speak of "bonking." Both groups attribute their fatigue in long events to drained fuel stores. Along with replacing fluids in the body, athletes who participate in activities that last longer than an hour, or in endurance events, also need to be concerned about providing the brain and muscles with a continuous supply of carbohydrate energy. When exercise lasts longer than an hour, blood glucose levels start to dwindle. After 1 to 3 hr of continuous cycling, running, or swimming at 65 to 80% of maximum effort, or after repeated bouts of intense sprinting at 85% plus of maximum effort, muscle glycogen stores may become depleted. In addition, if only water is being consumed, blood glucose levels may be very low (hypoglycemia) and will result in a higher use of muscle glycogen. When muscle glycogen levels are low and blood glucose levels have dropped, no matter how fast athletes will their bodies to go, they cannot physically respond, and they "hit the wall." The liver generally supplies glucose to maintain blood sugar for proper functioning of the central nervous system. As the muscles run out of glycogen, they will begin to take up glucose that is available in the blood, placing a drain on the liver glycogen stores. The longer the exercise bout, the greater the utilization of blood glucose by the muscles for energy (Figure 1). It has been suggested that carbohydrate feedings improve performance by maintaining blood glucose levels at a time when muscle glycogen stores are diminished. This allows carbohydrate utilization and energy production to continue at high rates.[30]

Athletes can help maintain their bodies' supply of energy by consuming about 15 to 30 g of carbohydrate every half hour during exercise.[31] Most 8- to 12-oz (240- to 355-ml) servings of commercial sports drinks provide about 15 to 20 g of carbohydrate; therefore drinking 8 to 12 oz (240 to 355 ml) of a commercial sports

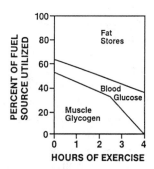

FIGURE 1   Energy sources during prolonged exercise at 70% of aerobic capacity. Blood glucose needs to be maintained after 2 to 3 hr of exercise because it becomes the primary source of fuel. (From Burke, E.R. and Berning, J.R., *Training Nutrition: The Diet and Nutrition Guide for Peak Performance*, Cooper Publishing Group, Carmel, IN, 1996, 39. With permission.)

drink every 30 min should help to delay the fatigue that occurs when muscle and liver glycogen are depleted, while also helping replace fluid losses.

E. CARBOHYDRATES

Carbohydrates are an important ingredient in sports drinks because they supply energy for working muscles. Sports drinks consumed during exercise help maintain blood glucose concentration, enhance carbohydrate oxidation,[32] and blunt the increase in stress hormones (renin angiotestin-I, adrenocorticotropic hormone, and cortisol).[33] While there is agreement about the inclusion of carbohydrate as the energy source for performance enhancement, the type(s) and blend of carbohydrate for optimal fluid and energy delivery based on gastric emptying and absorption rates continue to be researched.

1. Type and Mix of Carbohydrate

Research has shown that sports drinks that contain multiple carbohydrate sources, such as sucrose, glucose, and fructose, help stimulate fluid absorption and are effective in speeding energy to muscles.[34] Most commercially available sports drinks contain a blend of one or more of the following carbohydrates: glucose, sucrose, fructose, glucose polymers (2 glucose units), and maltodextrins (at least 5 glucose units). Fructose should not be the sole or predominant source of carbohydrate (not to exceed a 1:1 molar ratio with glucose).[35] Fructose alone or in high amounts is passively absorbed. Because of passive, slow absorption, fructose tends to sit in the gut and draw fluid in the wrong direction, causing gastrointestinal distress in some individuals.[36–38] Glucose and fructose (as fructose or as sucrose), when present together, facilitate the absorption of fluids during exercise. There does not appear to be an advantage to using glucose polymers over free glucose when the percentage of carbohydrate remains the same.[39]

2. Concentration of Carbohydrate

Much of the initial work done with sports beverages focused on identifying an optimal concentration of carbohydrate that would enhance performance, while still promoting gastric emptying. Davis et al. determined that a 6% carbohydrate solution entered the bloodstream as quickly as water and showed an improvement in endurance capacity with the carbohydrate solution.[40] Researchers then studied the rates of absorption of a sports beverage (a 6% carbohydrate–electrolyte solution), distilled water, and a 10% glucose solution.[14] The solutions were infused directly into the small intestine. The sports beverage was absorbed more rapidly from the intestine than either the water or 10% glucose solution. Thus, the addition of carbohydrate to the sports beverage enhanced the intestinal absorption of water. For optimal absorption and performance, the American College of Sports Medicine (ACSM) recommends that a sports drink contain 4 to 8% carbohydrate (about 38 to 77 cal or 9.5 to 19 g carbohydrate per 8 oz/240 ml);[38] there is no additional performance advantage, however, to consuming an 8 or 10% solution,[41] and concentrations of 8% and higher can actually lead to a saturation of intestinal wall solute transporters, so that carbohydrate remains in the intestinal lumen and counteracts absorption.[20,35]

F. ELECTROLYTES

Electrolytes (sodium, chloride, and potassium) are necessary for the maintenance of fluid balance and for muscle contraction and relaxation (see other chapters in this volume for a detailed discussion). The presence of sodium in a sports drink is of primary importance in that it both imparts physiological benefits and improves palatability.

1. Sodium

Sodium is a macroelement found in large concentrations in extracellular fluid. The sodium in sports drinks assists in maintaining body fluid balance in plasma volume and total body fluid balance. Sodium in sports drinks enhances beverage taste and replaces sodium lost in sweat. Sodium enhances intestinal absorption of fluids and stimulates thirst by maintaining or increasing plasma osmolality, which encourages the consumption of fluid during exercise.[42] Most sports beverages contain from 10 to 25 meq Na per liter or 55 to 110 mg per 8-oz (240-ml) serving. Gatorade® has 20 meq Na per liter or 110 mg per 8 oz (240 ml), and Powerade® and Allsport® each have about 12.5 meq/l or 55 mg per 8-oz (240-ml) serving (see Table 1). The sweat of a well-trained athlete may contain about 40 to 50 meq/l,[43] although sweat sodium concentrations are highly variable and total sodium loss may be quite high due to the large volume of sweat produced by athletes. Because sports drinks contain less sodium than sweat does, consuming them is not likely to lead to an electrolyte overload.[44]

a. Palatability

Sodium, in conjunction with carbohydrate and flavoring, enhances the palatability of sports drinks and promotes increased fluid consumption. The improvement in palatability and subsequent increased fluid intake is one reason for including sodium in a sports beverage.

b. Thirst Stimulator

Sodium consumed during exercise also serves to drive the thirst mechanism. Wilk and Bar-Or[45] demonstrated that the hydration effect of sodium was not solely due to enhanced taste. Twelve boys (ages 9 to 12) exercised under hot conditions and were provided unlimited access to either water, grape-flavored water, or a grape-flavored sports beverage containing 6% carbohydrate and 18 mmol sodium. When water only was offered, the boys became dehydrated. When the sports drink was offered, they drank almost twice as much fluid and stayed well-hydrated throughout the exercise. The grape-flavored water was not as beneficial as the sports drink from a hydration standpoint. The authors concluded that the addition of a 6% carbohydrate–electrolyte solution (containing 18 mmol/l of Na), along with the flavoring, stimulated adequate drinking that prevented dehydration. The cumulative effects of drinking a palatable beverage early and throughout the periods of exercise also helped to maintain a positive hydration status in children.

To test whether additional sodium added to a sports beverage would aid in rehydration, Wemple et al. compared a standard 6% carbohydrate solution with 25 meq Na per liter to a 6% carbohydrate solution with extra sodium (50 meq Na per liter) and a placebo (no Na).[46] During a 3-hr recovery following exercise, subjects drank voluntarily from one of the three beverages. The results showed that the beverage with 25 meq/l stimulated the greatest fluid intake, while smaller volumes of the placebo and the higher sodium solution (50 meq/l) were consumed. The researchers[46] suggested that the higher sodium solution may have suppressed physiologic thirst by rapidly restoring and maintaining plasma volume or that the saltiness reduced the palatability of the beverage so that subjects consumed less. Based on this study, additional sodium added to a standard sports drink (at least at a level of 50 meq/l or about 275 mg/8 oz) does not appear to assist in the rehydration phase and may actually hinder the process.

c. Absorption

Transportation of sodium occurs in the intestine via glucose–sodium co-transporters.[47] To study the effects of fluid absorption in the human small intestine, researchers used carbohydrate–electrolyte solutions containing three different sodium concentrations (1, 25, and 50 meq of Na) utilizing a segmental perfusion technique at rest in a neutral environment.[48] The data suggest that the level of carbohydrate in the solution is a more important factor in determining intestinal water absorption than the sodium concentration. The authors[48] suggest that the addition of sodium to fluid replacement beverages may not be a factor in fluid absorption when the amount and blend of carbohydrate (e.g., glucose and fructose) optimize the recruitment of solute transporters in the intestinal wall.

2. Potassium

As discussed previously, sodium is the electrolyte of primary importance in a sports drink. Other electrolytes, including potassium and chloride, are also lost in sweat and are included in some commercially available drinks. Potassium is the major ion of the intracellular fluid. As the major electrolyte inside body cells, potassium works in close association with sodium and chloride to maintain body fluids and generate electrical impulses in nerves and muscles. A pound (0.5 kg) of sweat contains about 80 to 100 mg potassium, and estimated losses during 2 to 3 hr of hard exercise may total close to 300 to 800 mg.[49] Even though the amount of potassium lost in sweat is not likely to create a potassium deficiency,[50] Nadel et al.[51] suggested that the inclusion of potassium in beverages consumed after sweat loss may aid in the rehydration of water in the intracellular space.[51] Cunningham[52] suggested that additional potassium may be needed during and after exercise sessions or activities when sweat losses are very high and that more studies are needed to assess the potential relationship between plasma potassium and performance. While additional potassium would help replace losses incurred during exercise, potassium does not play a key functional role in the way that sodium does (i.e., potassium is not needed for fluid absorption; it does not help maintain plasma volume, which is probably the key fluid compartment and most limited compartment needed to be maintained during exercise; and it does not drive fluid intake via taste or physiologic thirst).[42]

While many commercial sports drinks provide from 30 to 55 mg potassium per 8-oz (240-ml) serving, losses that range from 80 to 100 mg/lb (0.5 kg) of sweat lost may be more appropriately replaced by high-potassium foods and drinks. Potassium is found in a wide range of foods. Good sources include fruits, many vegetables, and fresh meat, poultry, and fish.[53] Athletes should be advised not to take potassium supplements because they can cause a dangerously high potassium level, resulting in an abnormal heartbeat.[44]

3. Other Electrolytes

Unlike sodium, potassium, and chloride, other electrolytes, such as magnesium and calcium, are not lost in substantial amounts in sweat and are not needed in a fluid replacement beverage used during exercise.[54]

G. OTHER COMPONENTS
1. Vitamins

Currently, no data exist demonstrating a beneficial performance effect for vitamins added to sports drinks.[55] A study was performed to determine the effect of nicotinic acid (vitamin B_3) on performance. Nicotinic acid was added to water or a carbohydrate–electrolyte sports beverage during a time trial following prolonged cycling.[56] The beverage did not improve the capacity to perform high-intensity exercise and may have even impaired performance, through its effect of inhibiting fatty acids. Niacin appeared to inhibit the release and/or utilization of free fatty acids, which may have caused the body to rely on muscle glycogen as the only source of fuel. The authors speculate that the supply of muscle glycogen may have been prematurely depleted.

Overall vitamin loss in sweat, even for water-soluble vitamins, is miniscule.[55] Nevertheless, one commercially available sports drink, Allsport®, adds 10% of the daily value for thiamin, niacin, vitamin B_6, pantothenic acid, and vitamin B_{12}. These vitamins, while important in energy metabolism and in the maintenance of healthy circulation, are more appropriately obtained from the diet. To illustrate, chicken, fish, pork, liver, and kidney provide excellent sources of vitamin B_6 and B_{12}, while many whole grains, nuts, legumes, and fortified cereals supply reasonable amounts of vitamin B_1 (thiamin), B_3 (niacin), and some B_6 and B_{12} (fortified cereals).[53] Athletes who consume the recommended amount of carbohydrate (at least 60% of calories from carbohydrate) should consume several servings of breads, cereals, and grains daily; these foods are not only excellent sources of many of the B vitamins but are excellent sources of the key fuel for physical activity, carbohydrate.

2. Choline

Choline is a form of fat that has been implicated in endurance performance. Specifically, choline is an amine precursor for the neurotransmitter acetylcholine and for lecithin, a component of lipoproteins involved in lipid transport. While one study showed that choline levels decreased from the start to finish of a marathon,[57] performance, as measured by time to fatigue and total work done, was not different compared to a control trial.[58] Even though research is still accumulating on the possible role of choline during exercise, one commercial sports drink that contains choline has already been developed and marketed to endurance athletes (see Table 1).

3. Glycerol

Another lipid compound, glycerol, has been used by some athletes in an attempt to hyperhydrate or increase total body water. Glycerol retains body fluids because it increases plasma osmolality, causing a reduction in urine output. Several studies have been published investigating the effect of glycerol loading on core temperature, sweat rate, or heart rate during exercise,[59–63] and data are equivocal. One study showed an endurance performance benefit with glycerol loading alone, or pre-exercise loading plus the use of fluids with carbohydrate, during cycling.[61] Another report, however, found that glycerol loading alone was no more efficacious than the ingestion of a carbohydrate–electrolyte drink during exercise.[59] Latzka et al.[60] suggest that if adequate hydration is maintained before and during exercise, then pre-exercise hyperhydration with glycerol confers no additional benefits in maintaining physiological functions. Inder and colleagues[63] recently studied the effect of glycerol and the arginine vasopressin analog despressin (DDAVP) on hydration and exercise performance in triathletes ingesting usual volumes of prerace fluids. No changes in sweat volume, plasma sodium, renin, or hemoglobin were seen with either glycerol or DDAVP. The authors concluded that neither glycerol nor DDAVP administered prior to training or competition in a thermoneutral environment provides any advantage over conventional fluid replacement.

Products that contain glycerol are available on the market. These glycerol products are marketed as "hyperhydraters," and instructions for preparing the product according to individual body weight are generally provided. Some athletes purchase glycerol at a health food store and take it as directed. More research is needed on the performance effects and potential side effects of consuming sports drinks that contain glycerol during exercise before a recommendation for the use of glycerol can be made.

4. Carbonation

There are many characteristics that impact the volume of fluid that will be voluntarily consumed during exercise. The palatability of a beverage includes flavor, taste, mouthfeel, and temperature.[42] Mouthfeel, including "throatburn," has been implicated as a factor in determining the amount of fluid consumed during activity. Recent research demonstrated that carbonation added to a sports drink reduced fluid intake.[64] When subjects were allowed limited time to consume fluids during a break from exercise, they ingested significantly less of a carbonated fluid (when carbonation was above 2.3 vol CO_2) compared to a noncarbonated fluid. Complaints of throatburn and a "bloated stomach" feeling were recorded on a survey whenever a carbonated beverage was consumed. Another study cited higher rates of heartburn sensation after subjects running on a treadmill consumed a 6% carbonated beverage compared to a 6 and 10% noncarbonated drink.[65]

Allsport®, a commercially available sports drink, is carbonated to a level of 1.2 vol CO_2. An unpublished study[66] conducted and discussed by Passe et al.[64] directly compared Allsport® to a noncarbonated control drink following 90 min of exercise. Significantly less of the carbonated beverage was consumed ($p < 0.001$) compared to the control noncarbonated beverage. The researchers noted that additional research is needed to study the relationship between carbonation and other constituents in the drink, such as carbohydrate level, electrolytes, and flavor intensity, and drinking behavior.

5. Amino Acids

The rationale for adding amino acids to an oral rehydration beverage is based on the observation that amino acids have multiple transport pathways, stimulate sodium and water absorption independently of glucose, and provide added nutritional value in cases of diarrheal diseases.[67,68] In a clinical trial, headed by Naline,[69] an oral rehydration solution containing both glucose and glycine provided more effective fluid absorption than a solution containing either glucose or glycine alone. A later study by Shi et al.,[70] however, indicated that glycine had no beneficial effect over and above a sucrose/glucose solution. Further testing in humans, especially in those who are dehydrated from physical activity, needs to be performed before adding amino acids to sports drinks can be justified.

III. TYPES OF BEVERAGES CONSUMED DURING PHYSICAL ACTIVITY

The ACSM 1996 position stand on exercise and fluid replacement[38] emphasizes that athletes will perform at their best when fluid intake closely matches fluid loss from sweating. The main reason that athletes do not adequately match fluid losses during exercise is that enough fluids are not consumed before or during exercise bouts.[22] Obviously, drinking most any type of fluid will help maintain fluid balance. However, beverages that contain carbohydrate and electrolytes, like sodium and potassium, may be beneficial under many circumstances in sport. Beverages that are commonly consumed during exercise are discussed and compared in this section.

A. COMMERCIALLY AVAILABLE SPORTS DRINKS

Commercially available sports drinks are designed to be palatable to encourage intake during exercise. At the 1998 ACSM meeting in Orlando, a poster presented by Passe et al.[71] highlighted the importance of palatability in a sports beverage. Forty-nine athletes were studied to determine whether the perception of a 6% carbohydrate beverage changed with exercise. The researchers first measured how much the athletes liked ten different flavors of a 6% carbohydrate–electrolyte beverage and plain water while at rest. Palatability was measured using a sensory scale. At a later date, when the athletes returned for exercise, they received their most preferred flavor, least preferred flavor, or water. The researchers found that the least preferred flavors at rest were consumed in significantly greater quantities than water when offered during exercise. This occurred even though these beverages were liked less than water at rest. The "liking scores" for the least preferred flavors increased dramatically from sedentary to exercise conditions, surpassing plain water. The flavors that were liked the most at rest continued to be favored and consumed in the largest quantities during exercise. The authors concluded that the taste of a beverage is extremely important in promoting intake and that palatability can change substantially during exercise, a practical tip to pass on to athletes.

Athletes often ask which fluid replacement beverage they should use. This is really a matter of personal preference when absorption, palatability, and performance effects are similar. Athletes should experiment with several different drinks during training to identify which drink or drinks perform the best for them. For competitions, such as in races, athletes should train with the sports drink that will be served on race day or arrange to have a bottle of their preferred sports drink available at each fluid station.

Sports drinks that fall between the range of 4 and 8% (see Table 1) should not be diluted, as this will cause the carbohydrate content of the drink to fall below the 30 to 60 g/hr cited in the ACSM fluid position stand as necessary to maintain the oxidation of carbohydrates and delay fatigue.[38]

B. FRUIT JUICES

Some athletes use fruit juice as their sports drink during exercise. Fruit juice tends not to be an ideal fluid replacement beverage during exercise because of its high carbohydrate (10% for orange juice) and low sodium content (see Table 2). As discussed in Section II, the concentration of carbohydrate should be less than 8% to maximize absorption and reduce stomach discomfort. Fruit juice also contains a high level of fructose, along with sucrose and glucose. Even when fruit juices are diluted by 50% to bring the carbohydrate concentration within range (from 10% to 5% for orange juice), the sodium content (6 mg per 8 oz/240 ml) is still not high enough to stimulate voluntary drinking or assist in the maintenance of fluid balance.

Postexercise training, fruit juice may be used to replace glycogen and fluids, but because of its low sodium content, lightly salted foods should also be eaten to help restore water balance. Research is needed to determine how diluted fruit juice compares to a commercial sports drinks in terms of palatability and volume of fluid consumed voluntarily during exercise.

C. WATER

Water is one of the most essential nutrients for life and for sports performance. Drinking too little water or losing too much through sweating impairs performance. Water in the body provides many key functions. Water in blood transports glucose, oxygen, and fats to working muscles and carries away metabolic by-products such as carbon dioxide and lactic acid. During exercise, water absorbs heat from the muscle, dissipates it through sweat, and regulates body temperature. The water in saliva and gastric secretions helps digest foods and in urine eliminates metabolic waste products. Throughout the body, water lubricates the joints and provides a cushion for organs and tissues.[44]

One of the most widely debated topics is the issue of whether water or a sports drink should be consumed during activity lasting less than 60 min. The 1996 ACSM fluid guidelines discussed in Section IV provide specific recommendations for fluid consumption before and during exercise.[38] The position paper stated that while preliminary data existed to support a performance enhancement for exercise lasting less than 60 min with proper carbohydrate intake (from the diet or consumed during exercise), plain water was as effective for exercise lasting less than

TABLE 2 Select Beverage Comparison

Beverage (8 oz/240 ml Prepared)	Calories	Carbs (g)	% Carbs	Sodium (mg)	Potassium (mg)	Carbohydrate Ingredients
Pedialyte® (Abbott Laboratories, Abbott Park, IL)	24	6	2.5	248	187	Glucose
Coca-Cola® (The Coca-Cola Company, Atlanta, GA)	103	27	11	6	0	High-fructose corn syrup, sucrose
Diet soft drinks	1	0	0	2–8	18–100	None
Orange juice	104	25	10	6	436	Fructose, sucrose, glucose
Water	0	0	0	Low	Low	None

1 hr. Since the ACSM guidelines have been released, research supporting the performance effects of drinking a carbohydrate–electrolyte beverage during shorter duration and intermittent exercise has continued to accumulate.[29,72–76] While the mechanism by which carbohydrate improves performance during moderate to high-intensity protocols is not clear, the results from several studies are encouraging. Some sports nutritionists working with athletes who perform moderate to high-intensity exercise lasting less than 60 min may wish to consider suggesting that their athletes experiment with using a carbohydrate–electrolyte beverage during activity for possible performance improvements.

Water as a sports drink does not provide energy to enhance performance or electrolytes to maintain fluid balance and stimulate thirst (see Table 2). Water does, however, replace fluids lost from sweat and is readily available and inexpensive, if taken from the tap. Many athletes choose to alternate their intake of water with a sports drink during exercise.

D. HOMEMADE SPORTS DRINKS

Homemade sports drinks are sometimes recommended by sports nutritionists as a low-cost way to replace fluids during exercise. The composition of a home-made sports drink, in terms of carbohydrate and electrolyte levels, may come close to matching a commercially prepared drink, but often lacks the flavor, appeal, mouthfeel, and shelf life of a commercially made sports drinks. Product stability is no small consideration as athletes attempt to avoid bacterial exposure to reduce risk of illness during heavy training. Research is needed to determine whether an athlete will like and therefore drink enough of a homemade sports drink to prevent dehydration during exercise.

For the recreational athlete, the homemade drink may be an option and is less costly than commercial products. The homemade sports drink found in Nancy Clark's *The New York City Marathon Cookbook* is as follows:[77,*]

Nancy Clark's Homemade Sports Drink
Ingredients
    1 tablespoon (15 g) sugar
    1 pinch (1/16th teaspoon/.5 g) salt
    1 tablespoon orange juice (7.5 ml) or 2 tablespoons (15 ml) lemon juice
    7.5 ounces (225 ml) ice water
Directions
    1. Dissolve the sugar and salt in a small amount of hot water in a glass.
    2. Add the juice and remaining ice water.
Yield: 1 serving
Calories: 50
Sodium (mg) 119
Potassium (mg) 30

---

* Used with permission from the author.

E. SOFT DRINKS

Soft drinks are not acceptable sports drinks during exercise for several reasons. They contain too much carbohydrate (about 10 to 11% for Coke®* and Pepsi®**), the wrong mix of carbohydrate (mostly high-fructose corn syrup and sucrose), little sodium (about 6 mg/8 oz), no potassium, and are carbonated (see Table 2). Carbonation in soft drinks turns into carbon dioxide gas in the stomach and can cause abdominal cramps, nausea, bloating, and diarrhea. The caffeine found in many soft drinks increases fluid loss by stimulating urine production. In practice, most athletes have trouble "chugging" carbonated soft drinks and are not able to consume enough fluids to prevent dehydration.

Some athletes drink soft drinks with their pregame meal that is usually eaten about 4 hr prior to exercise. Caffeine-free, nondiet soft drinks are a better choice from a hydration and carbohydrate standpoint. For athletes who like to drink carbonated beverages, some sports nutritionists recommend that players make their own "soft drink" by mixing at least 12 oz (355 ml) of fruit juice with some carbonated water (like seltzer) to improve the nutritional content of the beverage.

F. ORAL REHYDRATION SOLUTIONS

Oral rehydration solutions (ORS), recommended by the World Health Organization for the treatment of acute diarrhea, have a sodium content of 60 to 90 mmol/l.[78] In contrast, the sodium content of most sports drinks is in the range of 10 to 25 mmol/l or 55 to 110 mg per 8 oz (240 ml) and in some cases even lower (see Tables 1 and 2). As discussed in Section II.F, when higher levels of sodium are added to sports drinks, less volume is consumed, due to either suppressed physiologic thirst or reduced palatability. Thus the extra sodium found in ORS does not appear to be warranted or ideal for use as a fluid replacement beverage during exercise.

ORS also differ from sports drinks in that their carbohydrate concentration is formulated to be low (~2.5%) to promote rapid absorption (about 2.5%). Glucose is the sole carbohydrate source in ORS. Research has shown a lack of performance enhancement when low-dose carbohydrate beverages (~2.5%), similar to an ORS, are consumed during exercise.[40,79]

G. CAFFEINATED BEVERAGES

Caffeine is banned by the International Olympic Committee because of its ability to enhance performance in some individuals. The level at which caffeine is banned is much greater than the amount necessary for performance enhancement.[80] An energy-enhancing effect is seen with only 1.5 to 3.0 mg (3.3 to 6.6 mg/kg) of

---

*Registered Trademark of Coca-Cola Company, Atlanta, Georgia.
**Registered Trademark of Pepsico Company, Somers, New York.

caffeine per pound.[81] For a 150-lb man, that amounts to only one 10-oz (295-ml) cup of coffee.[80]

Because caffeine has a diuretic effect[5,82] and thus promotes urine formation, athletes who use caffeine usually need to urinate within an hour after consumption of a caffeinated beverage. Two studies, however, looked at the hydration effects of caffeine during exercise when caffeine was taken prior to exercise; no effects were seen. Graham and Spriet[81] speculate that the extra adrenaline that circulates during exercise may block the diuretic effect of caffeine on the kidneys. An athlete who decides to use caffeine as an ergogenic aid should experiment with it during training to determine how it affects him or her individually.

Caffeine-containing beverages such as iced tea, hot tea, coffee, colas, caffeinated waters, and some new "energy drinks" that contain caffeine are poor choices as sports drinks because of their diuretic effect and variable carbohydrate content (see Table 2). Athletes should be encouraged to choose high-carbohydrate, noncaffeinated fluids immediately following exercise and to enjoy a caffeinated beverage in moderation later, if they desire.

H. ALCOHOL

Alcohol is a central nervous system depressant. Pure alcohol (200 proof) supplies 7 cal/g and is a source of energy that is metabolized more like a fat. Alcohol does not provide a significant amount of energy during exercise and must first be metabolized by the liver before it can be used by the muscle.[44] Drinking alcohol immediately prior to, or during, exercise will impair performance, because of its adverse effects on gross motor skills, such as balance and coordination. Alcohol may reduce glucose secretion from the liver, which may lead to hypoglycemia and early fatigue during endurance exercise. Alcohol may also be a contributing factor in hypothermia (medically urgent low body temperature) if consumed during exercise in cold weather.[44,83]

Alcohol should not be used to replace fluids immediately after exercise because of its diuretic effect (promotes urine production) and adverse effects on blood glucose and glycogen levels. The best drinks to consume following exercise contain carbohydrate, water, and electrolytes to replace glycogen and restore fluid balance. After competition and training, athletes may be dehydrated and have an empty stomach, both of which magnify the intoxicating effects of alcohol.[42] To maximize performance using nutrition, specifics on how to adequately replace fluids and glycogen immediately following exercise, including actual amounts and types of fluids and foods that are appropriate for each athlete, should be provided based on body weight and usual losses incurred. Fluids containing alcohol are discouraged immediately following exercise, and moderation should be practiced at subsequent times. Chronic alcohol use causes the loss of many nutrients from the body that are important for performance and health, including thiamin, vitamin B_6, and calcium.[84]

IV. FLUID GUIDELINES AND PRACTICAL TIPS FOR THE USE OF SPORTS DRINKS DURING PHYSICAL ACTIVITY

A. ACSM FLUID GUIDELINES

It is now well established and documented that dehydration affects physiologic performance. In recognition of these research findings, the ACSM published a position stand on exercise and fluid replacement.[38] The position stand was developed by a panel of experts in fluid hemostasis and related fields and provides clear and practical guidelines regarding fluid, carbohydrate, and electrolyte replenishment for athletes. Included in the paper are a number of practical recommendations for promoting optimal fluid intake before and during activity. The importance of an aggressive fluid replacement plan is emphasized throughout the position stand for the prevention of even slight dehydration during training and competition.[85]

1. Fluid Ingestion Before Exercise: ACSM Position Stand

It is recommended that individuals consume a nutritionally balanced diet and drink adequate fluids during the 24-hour period before an event, especially during the period that includes the meal prior to exercise, to promote proper hydration before exercise or competition.

The strategies listed in the position paper will increase body fluid as well as liver and muscle glycogen, delaying dehydration and fatigue. The most difficult part of this recommendation in practice is getting athletes to actually modify their eating and drinking habits. As noted by Murray in a *Sports Science Exchange*,[86] members of the 1996 British Olympic team were knowledgeable about the dangers of dehydration and low carbohydrate stores but were unaccustomed to eating in buffet lines when training for the Atlanta Olympics. They politely took just one beverage each as they passed through the line while their counterparts loaded up on three or four beverages. The British athletes lost an opportunity to hydrate and prepare themselves for their Olympic performance.

The position stand also states, "It is recommended that individuals drink about 500 ml (about 17 ounces) of fluid about 2 hours before exercise to promote adequate hydration and allow time for excretion of excess ingested water." Research has shown that athletes consuming fluid 1 hr before exercise have lower core temperatures and heart rates during exercise when compared with those who consumed no fluid.[87]

2. Fluid Ingestion During Exercise: ACSM Position Stand

During exercise, athletes should start drinking early and at regular intervals in an attempt to consume fluids at a rate sufficient to replace all the water lost through sweating, or consume the maximal amount that can be tolerated.

Performance and health are jeopardized when adequate amounts of fluids are not consumed during exercise. If inadequate replacement fluids are ingested, dehydration, glycogen depletion, and low blood glucose levels may occur, ultimately leading to reduced endurance, strength, and performance.

It is recommended that ingested fluids be cooler than ambient temperature (between 15–22 degrees C) and flavored to enhance palatability and promote fluid replacement. Fluids should be readily available and served in containers that allow adequate volumes to be ingested with ease and with minimal interruption of exercise.

Using drinks that are pleasing, appealing, and easily accessible will encourage athletes to drink more. Any step that increases the chances of athletes consuming more fluid while exercising will help decrease the extent of dehydration and reduce the risk of heat illness. Cooler fluids not only cool core body temperature but also leave the stomach more rapidly than warmer fluids, thus enhancing fluid absorption.

During intense exercise lasting longer than 1 hour, it is recommended that carbohydrates be ingested at a rate of 30–60 grams per hour to maintain oxidation of carbohydrates and delay fatigue. This rate of carbohydrate intake can be achieved without compromising fluid delivery by drinking 600–1200 ml per hour of solutions containing 4%–8% carbohydrates (gram per 100 ml). The carbohydrates can be sugars (glucose or sucrose) or starch (i.e. maltodextrins).

Much of the research investigating the ergogenic effects of carbohydrate feedings during exercise has found that ingestion of carbohydrate solutions containing various sugars results in improved exercise performance, provided at least 45 g of carbohydrate is ingested per hour.[88]

While the ACSM position stand recommends sports drinks for exercise lasting longer than 1 hr, it states that water consumption is equally effective for exercise lasting under 1 hr. The position stand states: "During exercise lasting less than 1 hour there is little evidence of physical performance differences between consuming a carbohydrate–electrolyte drink and plain water."

It has only been in recent years that scientists have looked at the nutrient needs of short-term exercise. As discussed in Section III.C, while more research needs to be done in this area, there appears to be a trend that indicates that carbohydrate ingestion may indeed benefit performance during shorter duration exercise.[72–76,89,90]

B. FLUIDS FOR RECOVERY

The ACSM position paper did not address the issue of recovery from exercise because the authors felt that the guidelines provided for fluid intake before and during exercise would prevent dehydration from occurring. While this is the ideal scenario, in practice, athletes generally do not consume enough fluids before and during activity to keep up with losses; on average, only about 50% of sweat losses are replaced with ad libitum intake.[22] For athletes who compete every day or train every day, it is extremely important that a rapid and complete rehydration strategy is followed. Rapid and complete rehydration can be ensured only by the ingestion of adequate amounts of water and sodium chloride.[51,91] Drinking plain water causes a decrease in plasma osmolality and partial restoration of plasma volume, resulting in a decrease in the drive to drink. Most sports science professionals recommend that athletes replace 100% of fluid lost by drinking a pint per pound of weight lost during exercise (or 1 l lost per kilogram). While this advice is good and well intended, it fails to account for the obligatory urine losses that occur during rehydration.[80] Gonzalez-Alonso and colleagues[5] have reported that obligatory urine losses during rehydration can represent 25 to 50% of the ingested fluid. Research by Shirreffs and colleagues[92] demonstrated that replenishment with 150% (1.5 pints or 24 oz/lb of weight lost) and 200% of losses fully restores hydration levels to normal. Based on this research, practitioners working with athletes should continue to encourage athletes to prehydrate, adopt the ACSM fluid guidelines, and consume at least 20 oz of fluid for every pound of weight lost during exercise for optimal recovery. The goal for the athlete is to replace at least 80% of the fluid lost before the next exercise or training session. Additionally, strategies for incorporating this higher fluid intake into the athlete's postexercise routine need to be devised. This updated postexercise rehydration recommendation is particularly important for the ultraendurance athlete or anyone who exercises in the heat and humidity, sweats profusely, trains more than once daily, or competes on back-to-back days. A recent paper by Horswill describes the main drivers of fluid replacement, including behavioral strategies for effective fluid replacement before, during, and after exercise.[42]

Lastly, when considering rehydration and the type of beverages that should be consumed, alcohol and beverages containing caffeine are contraindicated due to their diuretic effects at rest (see Section III).

C. PRACTICAL FLUID TIPS FOR YOUTH IN SPORT

Young children are more likely than adults to participate in physical activities that are less than 60 min in duration. Many youth soccer, t-ball, and basketball games are less than 60 min in duration. Children, like adults, do not tend to drink enough when fluids are offered ad libitum during exercise in hot and humid climates.[93,94] Children are different from adults in that for any given level of hypohydration, a child's core temperature rises faster than that of an adult, putting children at far greater risk for heat stress.[93] Children who participate in sports activities must be taught how to prevent dehydration by instructing them to drink "above and beyond thirst" and to drink at frequent intervals (i.e., every 20 min).[74,93,94] A rule of thumb based on the experience of Bar-Or et al.[93] is that a child 10 years of age or younger should drink until he or she does not feel thirsty and then should drink an additional half a glass of fluid (an extra one-third to one-half cup [80 to 100 ml]). Older children and adolescents should follow the same guidelines; they should, however, consume an additional one cup of fluid (8 oz/240 ml) after first drinking until they are not thirsty. When feasible, regulations for competition should be modified to allow children to leave the playing field periodically in order to drink and promote a positive hydration status.

Other concerns often encountered with keeping children well hydrated in sport are the palatability of the drink and the ability of the drink to stimulate further thirst. Prepubertal and early pubertal girls and boys prefer grape flavor to apple and orange flavors of sports drinks.[95] Meyer et al.[95] found this preference was apparent at rest, following a maximal exercise bout, and during a rehydration stage after prolonged exercise in hot, dry conditions. One of the hurdles in getting children to consume fluids can be overcome by providing fluids they like and will therefore drink. Using a sports drink that can maintain the drive to drink may help prevent active children from becoming dehydrated.

Research studies indicating that sports drinks may be beneficial for exercise lasting less than 1 hr may be particularly relevant for young active children who participate in age-group sports. Young swimmers, whose exercise time is less than an hour, participate in meets that usually last 1 to 2 days. Many child athletes may have to swim back-to-back heats, while others may have an hour or less between events and heats. Still others may swim early in the morning and then late in the day. While no research exists on carbohydrate supplementation and young age-group swimmers, a practical approach would be to encourage young swimmers who participate in all-day swimming events to consume sports drinks to assist in the maintenance of fluid balance and blood glucose levels. This approach may be applicable for other childhood sports as well. For example, a young soccer player may have only a 45-min practice, yet it may be scheduled immediately after school, when blood glucose and fluid levels are low. Providing a sports drink instead of water in this case may be more beneficial, as blood glucose, glycogen, and bodily fluids will be replenished with the sports drink.

Other practical suggestions for maintaining hydration include encouraging children to follow a drinking schedule; prehydration; using cool, flavored beverages; avoiding drinks with carbonation, caffeine, and alcohol; and practicing the guidelines for fluid consumption before, during, and after exercise during training.

V. SUMMARY

This chapter has identified the various components of sports drinks and their relationship to the maintenance of hydration and performance enhancement. In general, the components that are most critical include carbohydrate, water, and electrolytes — in particular, sodium. The adoption of behavioral strategies will help to maximize fluid intake and effectively replace fluid losses. The ideal sports performance diet incorporates the ACSM fluid guidelines, as well as fluid guidelines postexercise (with both type and amounts of fluid specified based on individual preferences), to minimize dehydration and ensure the complete restoration of fluids and glycogen stores.

Sport drinks and other beverages that athletes drink during exercise vary considerably in key attributes, including palatability and acceptance during exercise, absorption rates, retention of fluid, and performance enhancement. Athletes may wish to consider the different characteristics of each beverage when determining which type of fluid to consume during exercise and sport.

ACKNOWLEDGMENTS

The authors wish to graciously acknowledge the technical assistance of interns Katie Fitzgerald, Kim Henderson, and Alex Hoffman.

REFERENCES

1. Ahlborg, B., Bergstrom, J., Ekelund, L.G., and Hultman, E., Muscle glycogen and muscle electrolytes during prolonged physical exercise, *Acta Physiol. Scand.*, 70, 129, 1967.
2. Bergstrom, J., Hermansen, L., Hultman, E., and Saltin, B., Diet, muscle glycogen and physical performance, *Acta Physiol. Scand.*, 71, 140, 1967.
3. *Beverage Aisle Magazine*, 6, 32, 1997.
4. Costill, D.L. and Sparks, K.E., Rapid fluid replacement following thermal dehydration, *J. Appl. Physiol.*, 34, 299, 1973.
5. Gonzalez-Alonso, J., Heaps, C.L., and Coyle, E.F., Rehydration after exercise with common beverages and water, *Int. J. Sports Med.*, 13, 399, 1992.
6. Nose, H., Mack, G.W., Shi, X., and Nadel, E.R., Role of osmolality and plasma volume during rehydration in humans, *J. Appl. Physiol.*, 65, 325, 1998.
7. Gisolfi, C.V., Exercise, intestinal absorption and rehydration, *Sports Sci. Exchange (Gatorade Sports Sci. Inst.)*, 4, 32, 1991.
8. Leiper, J.B. and Maughan, R.J., Absorption of water and electrolytes from hypotonic, isotonic, and hypertonic solutions, *J. Physiol.*, 373, 95P, 1986.
9. Csaky, T.Z., Significance of sodium ions in active intestinal transport of non-electrolytes, *Am. J. Physiol.*, 201, 999, 1961.
10. Csaky, T.Z., A possible link between active and passive transport of electrolytes and non-electrolytes, *Fed. Proc.*, 22, 3, 1963.
11. Cori, C.F., The fate of sugar on the animal body. The rate of absorption of hexoses and pentoses from the intestinal tract, *J. Biol. Chem.*, 66, 7691, 1925.
12. Crane, R.K., Na-dependent transport in the intestine and other animal tissues, *Fed. Proc.*, 24, 1000, 1965.
13. Malawer, S.J., Interrelationship between jejunal absorption of sodium, glucose, and water in man, *Am. Soc. Clin. Invest.*, 44, 1072, 1965.
14. Gisolfi, C.V., Summers, R.W., Shedl, H.P., Bleiler, T.L., and Oppliger, R.A., Human intestinal water absorption: direct vs. indirect measurements, *Am. J. Physiol.*, 258, G216, 1990.
15. Ferreria, R.M.C. and Walker-Smith, J.A., Controversies in oral rehydration therapy: a way forward, *Gastroenterol. J. Club.*, 1, 2, 1989.
16. Sandu, B.K., Jones, B.J.M., Brooks, D.G.D., and Silk, D.B.A., Oral rehydration in acute infantile diarrhea with a glucose polymer electrolyte solution, *Arch. Dis. Child.*, 57, 152, 1982.

17. Wheeler, K.B. and Banwell, J.G., Intestinal water and electrolytes flux of glucose–polymer electrolyte solutions, *Med. Sci. Sports Exercise,* 18, 436, 1986.
18. Leiper, J.B. and Maughan, R.J., The effect of luminal tonicity on water absorption from a segment of the intact human jejunum, *J. Physiol.,* 378, 95, 1986.
19. Fortran, J.S., Levitan, R., Bikerman, V., Burrows, B.A., and Ingelfinger, F.J., The kinetics of water absorption in the human intestine, *Trans. Assoc. Am. Physicians,* 74, 195, 1961.
20. Gisolfi, C.V., Summers, R.W., Schedl, H.P., and Bleiler, T.L., Intestinal water absorption from select carbohydrate solutions in humans, *J. Appl. Physiol.,* 73(5), 21, 1992.
21. Ryan, A.J., Lambert, G.P., Shi, X., Chang, R.T., Summers, R.W., and Gisolfi, C.V., Effect of hypohydration on gastric emptying and intestinal absorption during exercise, *J. Appl. Physiol.,* 84, 1581, 1998.
22. Noakes, T.D., Adams, B.A., Myburgh, K.H., Greeff, C., Lotz, T., and Nathan, M., The danger of an inadequate water intake during prolonged exercise, *Eur. J. Appl. Physiol.,* 7, 210, 1988.
23. Sherman, W.M., Metabolism of sugars and physical performance, *Am. J. Clin. Nutr.,* 62, 2285, 1995.
24. Wright, D., Sherman, W.M., and Dernbach, A.R., Carbohydrate feedings before, during, or in combination improve cycling endurance performance, *J. Appl. Physiol.,* 71, 1982, 1991.
25. Coggan, A.R. and Swanson, S.C., Nutritional manipulations before and during endurance exercise: effects on performance, *Med. Sci. Sports Exercise,* 24, S331, 1992.
26. Hawley, J.A. and Burke, L.M., Effects of meal frequency and timing on physical performance, *Br. J. Nutr.,* 77, S91, 1997.
27. Chryssanthopoulos, C. and Williams, C., Pre-exercise carbohydrate meal and endurance running capacity when carbohydrates are ingested during exercise, *Int. J. Sports Med.,* 18, 543, 1997.
28. Nicholas, C.W., Williams, C., Lakomy, H.K.A., Phillips, G., and Nowitz, A., Influence of ingesting a carbohydrate–electrolyte solution on endurance capacity during intermittent, high-intensity shuttle running, *J. Sports Sci.,* 13, 283, 1995.
29. Davis, J.M., Jackson, D.A., Broadwell, M.S., Query, J.L., and Lambert, C.L., Carbohydrate drinks delay fatigue during intermittent, high-intensity cycling in active men and women, *Int. J. Sport Nutr.,* 7, 261, 1997.
30. Coggan, A.R. and Coyle, E.F., Reversal of fatigue during prolonged exercise by carbohydrate infusion or ingestion, *J. Appl. Physiol.,* 63, 2388, 1998.
31. Coyle, E.F. and Montain, S.J., Benefits of fluid replacement with carbohydrate during exercise, *Med. Sci. Sports Exercise,* 24, 5324, 1992.
32. Coyle, E.F., Coggan, A.R., Hemmert, M.K., and Ivy, J.L., Muscle glycogen utilization during prolonged strenuous exercise when fed carbohydrate, *J. Appl. Physiol.,* 61, 165, 1986.
33. Davis, J.M., Cokkinides, V.E., Burgess, W.A., and Bartoli, W.P., Effects of a carbohydrate–electrolyte drink or water on the stress hormone response to prolonged intense cycling: renin, angiotestin-I, aldosterone, ACTH, and cortisol, in *Hormones and Sport,* Vol. 55, Laron, Z. and Rogo, A.D., Eds., Serono Symposia Publication, Raven Press, New York, 1989, 193.
34. Shi, X., Summers, R.J., Schedl, H.P., Flanagan, S.W., Chang, R., and Gisolfi, C.V., Effects of carbohydrate type and concentration of solution osmolality on water absorption, *Med. Sci. Sports Exercise,* 27, 1607, 1995.
35. Schedl, H.P., Maughan, R.J., and Gisolfi, C.V., Intestinal absorption during rest and exercise: implications for formulating an oral rehydration solution (ORS), *Med. Sci. Sports Exercise,* 26, 267, 1994.
36. Massicotte, D., Peronnet, F., Brisson, G.R., and Hillaire-Marcel, C., Oxidation of a glucose polymer during exercise; comparison with glucose and fructose, *J. Appl. Physiol.,* 66, 179, 1989.
37. Murray, R., Paul, G.L., Seifert, J.G., Eddy, D.E., and Halaby, G.A., The effects of glucose, fructose, and sucrose ingestion during exercise, *Med. Sci. Sports Exercise,* 21, 275, 1989.
38. American College of Sports Medicine position stand on exercise and fluid replacement, *Med. Sci. Sports Exercise,* 28, i, 1996.
39. Koulmann, N., Melin, B., Jimenez, C., Charpenet, A., Savourney, G., and Bittel, J., Effects of different carbohydrate–electrolyte beverages on the appearance of ingested deuterium in body fluids during moderate exercise by humans in heat, *Eur. J. Appl. Physiol.,* 75, 525, 1997.

40. Davis, J.M., Lamb, D.R., Pate, R.R., Slentz, C.A., Burgess, W.A., and Bartoli, W.P., Carbohydrate–electrolyte drinks: effects on endurance cycling in the heat, *Am. J. Clin. Nutr.*, 48, 1023, 1988.

41. Murray, R., Seifert, J.G., Eddy, D.E., Paul, G.L., and Halaby, G.A., Carbohydrate feeding and exercise: effect of beverage carbohydrate content, *Eur. J. Appl. Physiol.*, 59, 152, 1989.

42. Horswill, C.A., Effective fluid replacement, *Int. J. Sport Nutr.*, 8(2), 175, 1998.

43. Costill, D., Water and electrolyte requirements during exercise, *Clin. Sports Med.*, 3, 369, 1984.

44. Coleman, E. *Diet, Exercise & Fitness,* 3rd ed., Nutrition Dimension, San Marcos, CA, 1996, chap. 7.

45. Wilk B. and Bar-Or, O., Effect of drink flavor and NaCl on voluntary drinking and hydration in boys exercising in heat, *J. Appl. Physiol.*, 80, 1112, 1996.

46. Wemple, R.D., Morocco, T.S., and Mack, G.S., Influence of sodium replacement on fluid ingestion following exercise-induced dehydration, *Int. J. Sports Med.*, 7, 104, 1997.

47. Sladen, G.E. and Dawson, A.M., Interrelationships between the absorption of glucose, sodium and water by the normal human jejunum, *J. Clin. Sci.*, 36, 119, 1969.

48. Gisolfi, C.V., Summers, R.H., Schedl, H.P., and Bleiler, T.L., Effect of sodium concentration in a carbohydrate–electrolyte solution on intestinal absorption, *Med. Sci. Sports Exercise,* 27, 1414, 1995.

49. Clark, N., *Nancy Clark's Sports Nutrition Guidebook,* 2nd ed., Human Kinetics, Champaign, IL, 1996, 197.

50. Costill, D.L., Cote, R., and Fink, W.J., Dietary potassium and heavy exercise: effects on muscle water and electrolytes, *Am. J. Clin. Nutr.*, 36, 266, 1982.

51. Nadel, E.R., Mack, G.W., and Nose, H., Influence of fluid replacement beverages on body fluid homeostasis during exercise and recovery, in *Perspectives in Exercise Science and Sports Medicine,* Vol. 3, Gisolfi, C.V. and Lamb, D., Eds., Benchmark Press, Indianapolis, 1988, 195.

52. Cunningham, J.J., Is potassium needed in sports drinks for fluid replacement during exercise? *Int. J. Sport Nutr.*, 7, 154, 1997.

53. Duyuff, R.L., *The American Dietetic Association's Complete Food and Nutrition Guide,* Chronimed Publishing, Minneapolis, 1996, chap. 4.

54. Costill, D., Water and electrolyte requirements during exercise, *Clin. Sports Med.*, 3, 639, 1984.

55. Murray, R. and Horswill, C.A., Nutrient requirements for competitive sports, in *Nutrition in Exercise and Sport,* 3rd ed., Wolinsky, I., Ed., CRC Press, Boca Raton, FL, 1997, 547.

56. Murray, R., Bartoli, W., Eddy, D., and Horn, M., Physiological and performance responses to nicotinic-acid ingestion during exercise, *Med. Sci. Sports Exercise,* 27, 1057, 1995.

57. Conlay, L.A., Wurtman, R.J., Blusztajn, K., Lopez, G., Coviella, I., Maher, T.J., and Evoniuk, G.E., Decreased plasma choline concentrations in marathon runners, *N. Engl. J. Med.,* 315, 892, 1986.

58. Spector, S.A., Jackman, M.R., Sabounjian, L.A., Sakkas, C., Landers, D.M., and Willis, W.T., Effect of choline supplementation on fatigue in trained cyclists, *Med. Sci. Sports Exercise,* 27, 668, 1995.

59. Lamb, D.R., Lightfoot, W.S., and Myhal, M., Prehydration with glycerol does not improve cycling performance vs. 6% CHO–electrolyte drink, *Med. Sci. Sports Exercise.* 29, S249 (Abstr.), 1997.

60. Latzka, W.A., Sawka, M.N., Montain, S.J., Skrinar, G.S., Fielding, R.A., Matott, R.P., and Pandolf, K.B., Hyperhydration: thermoregulatory effects during compensable exercise–heat stress, *J. Appl. Physiol,,* 83, 860, 1997.

61. Montner, P., Stark, D.M., Riedesel, M.L., Murata, G., Robergs, R., Timms, M., and Chick, T.L., Pre-exercise glycerol hydration improves cycling endurance time, *Int. J. Sports Med.,* 17, 27, 1996.

62. Murray, R., Eddy, D.E., Paul, G.L., Seifert, J.G., and Halaby, G.A., Physiological responses to glycerol ingestion during exercise, *J. Appl. Physiol.,* 71, 144, 1991.

63. Inder, W.J., Swanney, M.P., Donald, R.A., Prickett, C.R., and Hellmans, J., The effect of glycerol and desmopressin in exercise performance and hydration in triathletes, *Med. Sci. Sports Exercise,* 30, 1263, 1998.

64. Passe, D., Horn, M., and Murray, R., The effects of beverage carbonation on sensory responses and voluntary fluid intake following exercise, *Int. J. Sport Nutr.,* 7, 286, 1997.

65. Ryan, A.J., Navarre, A.E., and Gisolfi, C.V., Consumption of carbonated and non-carbonated sport drinks prolonged treadmill exercise in the heat, *Int. J. Sport Nutr.,* 1, 225, 1991.

66. Passe, D., Horn, M., and Murray, R., unpublished data, 1998.

67. Hellier, W.D.B., Thirumalai, C., and Holdsworth, C.D., The effect of amino acids and dipeptides on sodium and water absorption in man, *Gut,* 14, 41, 1973.

68. Stevens, B.R., Ross, H.J., and Wright, E.M., Multiple transport pathways for neutral amino acids in rabbit jejunal brush border vesicles, *J. Membr. Biol.,* 66, 213, 1982.

69. Naline, D.R., Cash, R.A., Rahman, M., and Yunus, M.D., Effect of glycine and glucose on sodium and water absorption from a segment of the intact human jejunum, *J. Physiol.,* 378, 95, 1986.

70. Shi, X., Summers, R.W., Schedl, H.P., Flanagan, S.W., Chang, R., and Gisolfi, C.V., Effects of carbohydrate type and concentration and solution osmolality on water absorption, *Med. Sci. Sports Exercise,* 27, 1607, 1995.

71. Passe, D., Horn, M., and Murray, R., Effect of beverage palatability on voluntary fluid intake during exercise, *Med. Sci. Sports Exercise,* 30, S156, 1998.

72. Ball, T.C., Headly, S.A., Vanderburgh, P.M., and Smith, J.C., Periodic carbohydrate replacement during 50 minutes of high intensity cycling improves subsequent sprint performance, *Int. J. Sport Nutr.,* 5, 151, 1995.

73. Nicholas, C.W., Williams, C., Phillips, G., and Nowitz, A., Influence of ingesting a carbohydrate–electrolyte solution on endurance capacity during intermittent, high intensity shuttle running, *J. Sports Sci.,* 13, 283, 1995.

74. Smith, K., Smith, N., Wishart, C., and Green, S., Effect of a carbohydrate–electrolyte beverage on fatigue during a soccer-related running test, *J. Sports Sci.,* 16, 502, 1998.

75. Vergauwen, L., Brouns, F., and Hespel, P., Carbohydrate supplementation improves stroke performance in tennis, *Med. Sci. Sports Exercise,* 30, 1289, 1998.

76. Wagenmakers, A.J M., Jeukendrup, A.E., Brouns, F., and Saris, W.H.M., Carbohydrate feedings improve 1 hour time trial cycling performance, *Med. Sci. Sports Exercise,* 28, S37, 1996.

77. Clark, N., *The New York City Marathon Cookbook,* Rutledge Hill Press, Nashville, 1994, 219.

78. Farthing, M.J.G., Oral rehydration therapy, *Pharm. Ther.,* 64, 477, 1963.

79. Burgess, W.A., Davis, J.M., Bartoli, W.P., and Woods, J.A., Failure of low dose carbohydrate feedings to attenuate glucoregulatory hormone responses and improve endurance performance, *Int. J. Sport Nutr.,* 1, 338, 1991.

80. Clark, N., Caffeine: a user's guide, *Physician Sports Med.,* 25(11), 1997.

81. Graham, T.E. and Spriet, L.L., Caffeine and exercise performance, *Sports Sci. Exchange (Gatorade Sports Sci. Inst.),* 9, 1, 1996.

82. Wemple, R.D., Lamb, D.R., and McKeever, K.H., Caffeine vs. caffeine-free sports drinks: effects on urine production at rest and during prolonged exercise, *Int. J. Sports Med.,* 18, 40, 1997.

83. Williams, M.H., Alcohol and sports performance, *Sports Sci. Exchange (Gatorade Sports Sci. Inst.),* 5, 5, 1992.

84. Dimeff, R.J., Steroids and other performance enhancers, in *Clinical Preventive Medicine,* Matzen, R.N. and Lang, R.S., Eds., C.V. Mosby, St. Louis, 1993, 367.

85. Murray, R., Fluid needs of athletes, in *Nutrition for Sport and Exercise,* Berning, J. and Steen, S., Eds., Aspen Publishing, Gaithersburg, MD, 1998.

86. Murray, R., Fluid replacement: The American College of Sports Medicine position stand, *Sports Sci. Exchange (Gatorade Sports Sci. Inst.),* 9, 4, 1996.

87. Greenleaf, J.E. and Castle, B.L., Exercise temperature regulation in man during hypohydration and hypothermia, *J. Appl. Physiol.,* 30, 847, 1971.

88. Coggan, A.R. and Coyle, E.F., Carbohydrate ingestion during prolonged exercise: effects on performance, in *Exercise and Sports Science Reviews,* Vol. 19, Holloszy, J.O., Ed., Williams and Wilkins, Baltimore, 1991, 1.

89. Below, P.R., Mora-Rodriquez, R., Gonzalez-Alonso, J., and Coyle, E.F., Fluid and carbohydrate ingestion independently improve performance during 1 hour of intense exercise, *Med. Sci. Sports Exercise,* 27, 200, 1994.

90. Walsh, R.M., Noakes, T.D., Hawley, J.A., and Dennis, S.C., Impaired intensity cycling performance time at low levels of dehydration, *Int. J. Sports Med.,* 15, 392, 1994.

91. Maughan, R., Leiper, J.B., and Shirreffs, S.M., Rehydration and recovery after exercise, *Sports Sci. Exchange (Gatorade Sports Sci. Inst.),* 9, 1, 1996.

92. Shirreffs, S.M., Taylor, A.J., Leiper, K.B., and Maughan, R.J., Post-exercise rehydration in man: effects of volume consumed and drink sodium content, *Med. Sci Sports Exercise,* 28, 1260, 1996.

93. Bar-Or, O., Dotan, R., Inbar, O., Rotshtein, A., and Zonder, H., Voluntary hypohydration in 10–12 year old boys, *J. Appl. Physiol. Respir. Environ. Exercise Physiol.,* 48, 104, 1980.

94. Bar-Or, O., Blimkie, C.J.R., Hay, J.A., MacDougall, J.C., Ward, D.S., and Wilson, W.M., Voluntary dehydration and heat intolerance in patients with cystic fibrosis, *Lancet,* 339, 696, 1992.

95. Meyer, F.O., Bar-Or, O., Salsberg, A., and Passe, D., Hypohydration during exercise in children: effect on thirst, drink preferences, and rehydration, *Int. J. Sport Nutr.,* 1, 22, 1994.

SUMMARY

Chapter 12

SUMMARY: MACROELEMENTS, WATER, AND ELECTROLYTES IN SPORTS NUTRITION

Judy A. Driskell
Ira Wolinsky

CONTENTS

I. INTRODUCTION

Numerous research papers on macroelements, water, and electrolytes in sports nutrition have been published in the last decade. The needs of athletes for some of these nutrients are higher than in the general population.

Currently, a committee of the National Academy of Sciences is updating the dietary recommendations. The new recommendations, known as Dietary Reference Intakes (DRIs), have been published for the macroelements calcium, phosphorus, and magnesium.[1] The DRIs include Adequate Intakes (AIs) for calcium and Recommended Dietary Allowances (RDAs) for phosphorus and magnesium. The committee of the National Academy of Sciences that set the DRIs believed that insufficient data were available to establish Estimated Average Requirements (EARs), and the EARs form the basis for setting the RDAs, so AIs were established for calcium. The committee believed that sufficient data were available to establish

EARs for phosphorus and magnesium; hence, RDAs were set for phosphorus and magnesium. Both the RDAs and the AIs are to be utilized in the evaluation of diets for nutrient adequacy. DRIs will be available for the other essential minerals in the next few years.

Many athletes reportedly consume less than adequate quantities of several of the macroelements and electrolytes. Athletes, like other Americans 2+ years of age, should follow the dietary recommendations of the Food Guide Pyramid[2] and the Dietary Guidelines for Americans.[3] Female varsity athletes were found to frequently snack on energy-dense foods that were low in micronutrients. Most surveys indicate that vitamin/mineral supplementation is more prevalent in athletes than in the general population.

II. MACROELEMENTS

The macroelements include calcium, phosphorus, and magnesium as well as the electrolytes. Reports indicate that athletes frequently have insufficient intakes of calcium, magnesium, and potassium and more than adequate intakes of phosphorus.

About 99% of the calcium in the body is found in the bones and teeth. Parathyroid hormone, calcitonin, and 1,25-dihydroxyvitamin D_3 are involved in the regulation of plasma calcium concentrations. Calcium phosphate in the skeleton gives vertebrates the support needed so they can be erect and support the weight of the body. Muscle mass and muscle strength are related to bone density. The gonadal hormones also influence bone density. Athletes, particularly females, often do not consume adequate amounts of calcium. Athletes should consume adequate amounts of calcium and vitamin D for proper functioning of the musculoskeletal system.

Phosphorus is involved in many reactions in the body, particularly those involved in energy metabolism. Parathyroid hormone and 1,25-dihydroxyvitamin D_3 influence blood phosphate levels; these levels are also influenced by estrogen and cortisol. Most individuals in the U.S. consume sufficient phosphorus. Phosphorus as phosphate is a component of the high-energy compounds adenosine triphosphate (ATP) and phosphocreatine (also called creatine phosphate). Several studies indicate that phosphate supplements, particularly sodium phosphate, have ergogenic value with regard to exercise performance, while no effect has been observed in other studies. Differences in study design, including the forms and amounts of phosphates ingested, likely influenced the findings. More well-designed studies are needed to evaluate the effects of phosphate loading in athletes involved in a variety of sports.

Magnesium is involved in many reactions in the body as an activator of many enzymes, including those producing ATP and the ATP–phosphocreatine cycle. Athletes frequently consume less than recommended quantities of magnesium, and marginal deficiency may be common in the general U.S. population. Low plasma magnesium concentrations have been associated with muscle spasms and cramps. The optimal level of magnesium for the athlete has not been established. Athletes should consume adequate dietary or supplemental magnesium or physical performance may be hampered.

III. WATER AND ELECTROLYTES

Water needs are generally considered along with electrolyte needs in the normal population as well as athletes. The 1989 *Recommended Dietary Allowances*[4] lists Minimum Daily Requirements for sodium, chloride, and potassium. Sodium, chloride, and potassium are electrolytes that function along with water with respect to fluid balance in the body. Fluid replacement (i.e., water plus electrolytes and sometimes sugars) is of paramount importance to the athlete.

Water is the most important nutrient for the human body. About 10% of the body's need for water comes from that formed in oxidative phosphorylation. Water serves a thermoregulatory function in that it helps cool the body, which is of importance to athletes. Hypohydration frequently occurs in physically active people, particularly if they are exercising in a hot environment. It is vital that an athlete stay hydrated at all times in order to attain and maintain peak physical performance. Thirst should not be relied upon as a signal that the body needs water. The recommended water intake for athletes is 1.5 ml/kcal expended.

Sodium is a cation found primarily in the body's extracellular fluid. Sodium movement is controlled by the Na^+K^+-activated adenosine triphosphatase (Na^+K^+–ATPase). The 1989 *Diet and Health* publication[5] recommends that individuals limit their daily sodium intake to ≤ 2400 mg. Sodium excretion in normal healthy individuals is under precise physiological control. Hyponatremia results in water intoxication. Hypernatremia results in hypohydration and hypovolemia. Exercise and heat adaptation produce a decline in the sodium concentration of sweat.

Chloride, a component of table salt ($NaCl$), is the major anion in extracellular fluid. Chloride, along with sodium, helps the body maintain acid–base balance. Deficiency of chloride due to dietary insufficiency is rare, but hypochloremia has been observed in individuals experiencing chronic vomiting, severe diarrhea, and excessive use of diuretics. Evidence exists that high dietary intakes of chloride (resulting in hyperchloremia) may induce hypertension. Chloride as part of fluid replacement appears to be beneficial in the treatment of muscle cramps, but large amounts may lead to hypertension.

Potassium is a cation found primarily intracellularly. Skeletal muscles contract after electrical changes occur on the cell membranes, causing sodium to enter the muscle cells and potassium to leave as a result of Na^+K^+–ATPase activity. Na^+K^+–ATPase activity is influenced by insulin and catecholamines. Neither the hyperkalemia or hypokalemia of exercise has been shown to be physiologically harmful. Any potassium lost in sweat is readily replaced by dietary potassium.

The composition of the body's fluids should be relatively constant. There is continuous exchange of fluid components in the body's internal compartments. Derangement of fluid balance is probably the most common physiological or medical disturbance in athletes. Dehydration at the level of 1% of body weight affects cardiovascular function. Water is the predominant component of plasma and is essential to the maintenance of blood volume. Thermoregulation is another important function of water. Some evidence indicates that hypohydration in older adults may influence circulatory and thermoregulatory functions more than in younger adults. Replacement of fluid and electrolytes before, during, and after exercise is of vital concern to the athlete.

IV. SUPPLEMENTS CONTAINING MACROELEMENTS

As athletes seek to improve their performance and reduce the severity of injuries, they may seek new dietary means toward this end. Athletes frequently take over-the-counter supplements containing macroelements. Supplements containing macroelements commonly taken by athletes include magnesium, phosphate, calcium, and electrolytes. Sports beverages containing water and electrolytes as well as sugar are consumed universally by athletes and by many nonathletes.

Magnesium supplementation of individuals inadequate in magnesium does result in improved efficiency of energy utilization, enhanced strength gain, and decreased heart rate during submaximal work. Magnesium supplementation of individuals having adequate magnesium status does not seem to enhance physical performance. Inconsistent results have been observed in phosphate loading studies, with differences in experimental designs likely complicating interpretation of research findings. Many individuals, particularly women, do not consume adequate amounts of calcium. Daily consumption of adequate amounts of calcium seems to be protective against overuse bone injuries. Calcium supplementation of individuals with adequate calcium status has not been observed to be beneficial. Supplemental magnesium, phosphate, and calcium given to individuals with adequate nutritional status do not support improvements in physical performance, although the findings with regard to phosphates remain controversial.

The composition of most commercial sports beverages with regard to calories, carbohydrate (both type and concentration), sodium, and potassium is given in Chapter 11. As expected, many athletes have a favorite sports beverage, generally influenced by the sensory characteristics of their choice. The American College of Sports Medicine[6] has published guidelines that are intended to minimize dehydration and ensure the complete restoration of fluids and glycogen stores. Fluid replacement before, during, and after an athletic event, especially those lasting over 1 hr, is of importance to all athletes. Sports beverages are an essential for the athlete.

V. IMPLICATIONS

More research is needed on macroelements, water, and electrolytes in relation to exercise and sport performance. Technically, electrolytes are macroelements, although electrolytes are generally thought of in terms of fluid replacement. Few double-blind, crossover, placebo-controlled studies involving macroelements and exercise have been conducted on humans. The initial macronutrient status of the subjects should be ascertained, and only subjects with adequate status should be used in supplementation studies. Exercise may affect the distribution of the macroelements in the various body tissues. Macroelements may be effective at some dosage levels but not others. Studies should be of sufficient duration for effects, if any, to be observed. Some gender differences may exist. The efficacy of supplementation with the various macroelements may vary with regard to different forms of physical activity and different performance measurements. Does supplementation affect the variables on a short-term or long-term basis? How well do subjects adapt to supplementation and training? What interactions exist among the various macroelements and with water that might influence exercise performance?

Macroelements, water, and electrolytes are of importance in sports nutrition. These nutrients are needed in adequate amounts for optimal physical performance. At the present time, data are insufficient for the establishment, with any degree of certainty, of macroelement, including electrolyte, requirements for sport or exercise.

REFERENCES

1. Institute of Medicine, *Dietary Reference Intakes: Calcium, Phosphorus, Magnesium, Vitamin D, and Fluoride* (prepublication copy), National Academy Press, Washington, D.C., 1997.
2. The Food Guide Pyramid, U.S. Department of Agriculture, Hyattsville, MD, 1992.
3. U.S. Departments of Agriculture and of Health and Human Services, Dietary Guidelines for Americans, U.S. Government Printing Office, Washington, D.C., 1995.
4. National Research Council, *Recommended Dietary Allowances*, 10th ed., National Academy Press, Washington, D.C., 1989.
5. National Research Council, *Diet and Health: Implications for Reducing Chronic Disease Risk*, National Academy Press, Washington, D.C., 1989.
6. American College of Sports Medicine, Position stand: exercise and fluid replacement, *Med. Sci. Sports Exercise*, 28, i, 1996.